Development of Specific Dosage Form: Wound Dressing

Development of Specific Dosage Form: Wound Dressing

Guest Editors

Mihaela Violeta Ghica
Madalina Georgiana Albu Kaya
Lacramioara Popa
Cristina Elena Dinu-Pirvu

MDPI

Basel • Beijing • Wuhan • Barcelona • Belgrade • Novi Sad • Cluj • Manchester

Guest Editors
Mihaela Violeta Ghica
Physical and Colloidal Chemistry Department
University of Medicine and Pharmacy Carol Davila
Bucharest
Romania

Madalina Georgiana Albu Kaya
Collagen Department
National Research and Development Institute for Textile and Leather
Bucharest
Romania

Lacramioara Popa
Physical and Colloidal Chemistry Department
University of Medicine and Pharmacy Carol Davila
Bucharest
Romania

Cristina Elena Dinu-Pirvu
Physical and Colloidal Chemistry Department
University of Medicine and Pharmacy Carol Davila
Bucharest
Romania

Editorial Office
MDPI AG
Grosspeteranlage 5
4052 Basel, Switzerland

This is a reprint of the Special Issue, published open access by the journal *Pharmaceuticals* (ISSN 1424-8247), freely accessible at: https://www.mdpi.com/journal/pharmaceuticals/special_issues/T0I75G7562.

For citation purposes, cite each article independently as indicated on the article page online and as indicated below:

Lastname, A.A.; Lastname, B.B. Article Title. *Journal Name* **Year**, *Volume Number*, Page Range.

ISBN 978-3-7258-6660-1 (Hbk)
ISBN 978-3-7258-6661-8 (PDF)
https://doi.org/10.3390/books978-3-7258-6661-8

Contents

About the Editors

Mihaela Violeta Ghica

Mihaela Violeta Ghica is a Professor, PhD, and Dr. Habil. in Pharmacy in the Department of Physical and Colloidal Chemistry, Faculty of Pharmacy, at Carol Davila University of Medicine and Pharmacy, Bucharest, Romania. She is also a Researcher at the Innovative Therapeutic Structures R&D Center at the same university. She holds a master's degree in Physical Chemistry and Applied Radiochemistry from the Faculty of Chemistry, University of Bucharest. She has 24 years of expertise in developing and characterising innovative biomaterials for precision treatment, advanced topical formulations, modern statistical experimental design strategies for drug delivery systems, and (bio)technological processes optimization. She has authored over 110 ISI articles and has an H-index of 25.

Madalina Georgiana Albu Kaya

Madalina Georgiana Albu Kaya is Vice President of the Scientific Council of INCDTP and a First-Degree Senior Researcher with a PhD in Chemistry from the Department of Collagen, Division Leather and Footwear Research Institute within the National Research and Development Institute for Textile and Leather, Bucharest, Romania. She has a master's in Physics and Applied Radiochemistry from the Faculty of Chemistry, University of Bucharest. She has 24 years of experience in the obtaining and characterization of collagen-based bioproducts. Her research experience includes collagen processing in different forms (gel, hydrogels, membranes, matrices (porous forms), tubular forms, powders, etc.) and the development of biomaterials from laboratory scale to market, as well as the characterization of collagen using modern equipment. She has published over 150 ISI articles and has an H-index of 30.

Lacramioara Popa

Lacramioara Popa is a Professor, PhD, and Dr. Habil. in Pharmacy in the Department of Physical and Colloidal Chemistry, Faculty of Pharmacy, at Carol Davila University of Medicine and Pharmacy, Bucharest, Romania. She is also a Researcher at the Innovative Therapeutic Structures R&D Center and President of the Ethics and Quality Assurance Commission, Faculty of Pharmacy, at the same university. She has 33 years of expertise in the integration of Quality by Design strategies in the development of drug delivery systems, the surface characterization of raw materials and pharmaceutical systems, and the medical applications of biopolymer chitosan. She has published over 75 ISI articles and has an H-index of 22.

Cristina Elena Dinu-Pirvu

Cristina Elena Dinu-Pirvu is a Professor, PhD, and Dr. Habil. in Pharmacy in the Department of Physical and Colloidal Chemistry, Faculty of Pharmacy, at Carol Davila University of Medicine and Pharmacy, Bucharest, Romania. She is also Coordinator of the Innovative Therapeutic Structures R&D Center, and Director of the Doctoral School at the same university. She has 33 years of expertise in the design and development of bioactive compound delivery systems for personalized medicine, functionalized nanoparticulate systems for theragnostic purposes, and valorization of the biopharmacological potential of medicinal and aromatic plants. She has published more than 120 ISI articles and has an H-index of 28.

Preface

Wound dressings have undergone substantial evolution in recent decades, progressing from simple protective coverings to advanced therapeutic systems designed to actively support and regulate the wound healing process. Because of the increasing prevalence of acute and chronic wounds and their significant clinical and economic burden, the development of innovative dosage forms for wound management remains a priority in pharmaceutical and biomedical research.

This Reprint integrates contributions from the Special Issue titled "Development of Specific Dosage Forms: Wound Dressing", published in *Pharmaceuticals*. The collected articles reflect current research efforts aimed at improving wound healing outcomes through the rational design of polymer-based materials, bioactive formulations, and multifunctional dressing systems.

The Reprint addresses a broad range of topics, including the formulation and characterization of polymeric dressings such as hydrogels, foams, films, nanofibrous scaffolds, and smart responsive materials; the incorporation of plant-derived bioactive compounds and active pharmaceutical ingredients to enhance antimicrobial activity, anti-inflammatory response, and tissue regeneration; and investigations into material structure, physicochemical properties, and biological interactions that influence healing performance. In addition, review articles provide critical overviews of electrospinning technologies and polymeric biomaterials, while a case report highlights the clinical relevance of biomaterial–cell interactions.

We sincerely thank all authors and reviewers whose contributions made this Special Issue possible. This Reprint is intended as a valuable resource for researchers, clinicians, and pharmaceutical scientists seeking to advance the development of effective and innovative wound dressing technologies.

Mihaela Violeta Ghica, Madalina Georgiana Albu Kaya, Lacramioara Popa, and Cristina Elena Dinu-Pirvu
Guest Editors

pharmaceuticals

MDPI

Editorial

Development of Specific Dosage Form: Wound Dressing—Current Progress and Novel Approaches

Mihaela Violeta Ghica [1,2], Mădălina Georgiana Albu Kaya [3,*], Lăcrămioara Popa [1,2,*] and Cristina Elena Dinu-Pîrvu [1,2]

1 Department of Physical and Colloidal Chemistry, Faculty of Pharmacy, Carol Davila University of Medicine and Pharmacy, 6 Traian Vuia Str., 020956 Bucharest, Romania; mihaela.ghica@umfcd.ro (M.V.G.); cristina.dinu@umfcd.ro (C.E.D.-P.)

2 Innovative Therapeutic Structures Research and Development Center (InnoTher), Carol Davila University of Medicine and Pharmacy, 6 Traian Vuia Str., 020956 Bucharest, Romania

3 National Research and Development Institute for Textiles and Leather, Division of Leather and Footwear Research Institute, Department of Collagen, 93 Ion Minulescu Str., 031215 Bucharest, Romania

* Correspondence: albu_mada@yahoo.com (M.G.A.K.); lacramioara.popa@umfcd.ro (L.P.)

This Special Issue, 'Development of Specific Dosage Form: Wound Dressing', highlights the current progress in the development of modern wound dressings, indicating how dynamic and challenging this field remains. Wound healing is a multifactorial controlled process in which complications such as inflammation, pain, infection, delayed repair, and chronic injuries continue to represent meaningful obstacles for both patients and healthcare systems [1,2].

Globally, the burden of cutaneous skin lesions has received continuous interest in medical management, despite modern therapeutic progress. Skin wounds caused by trauma, surgery, burns, or underlying diseases (diabetes mellitus, chronic venous insufficiency, cancer) not only cause physical and psychological challenges to patients, but also significant socioeconomic costs [3,4]. Worldwide, current estimates suggest that more than 40 million individuals suffer from skin lesions (acute and chronic), and the financial impact of wound care is considerable, ranging from USD 28 billion to nearly USD 97 billion annually [5,6].

Wound repair is far from a linear process because it implicates a cascade of overlapping and interdependent phases requiring the coordinated action of numerous cellular and molecular entities [7]. This complexity explains why complications are common and why conventional dressings that just protect the surface of the wound are often insufficient. To address these limitations, research has been oriented toward advanced wound dressings that can actively accelerate the healing process [8]. Materials science, nanotechnology, and pharmaceutical science have contributed to the development of various systems, including hydrogels, sponges, hydrocolloids, films, foams, alginates, and textile-based platforms, loaded with different bioactive agents or nanoparticles [9,10]. These innovations not only aim to provide biocompatibility, but also antimicrobial protection, controlled drug release, and stimulation of tissue regeneration [11].

Therefore, the design of active wound dressings needs to address multiple requirements simultaneously: maintain a moist environment at the lesion site, protect against microbial contamination, promote angiogenesis and reepithelialization, enable the controlled release of bioactive agents, and ensure patient compliance and comfort [12–16].

Recent advances have expanded the use of various materials and the applications of different strategies to promote the healing process. Natural, semisynthetic, and synthetic biopolymers, nanostructured carriers, and hybrid composites are being explored in various pharmaceutical formulations [17–20]. Many of them are loaded with plant-derived compounds, anti-inflammatory, analgesic, and antimicrobial agents, growth factors, or nanoparticles, offering multifunctional behavior ranging from the protective role of the traditional dressings to the therapeutic role of promoting skin repair [21–24]. Additionally, the development of smart modern dressings sensitive to pH, temperature, and enzymatic activity is a promising objective with significant clinical applicability [25]. Despite this innovative reassuring progress, many challenges remain, including increasing the scale of the manufacturing process, regulatory authorization, costs, and the requirement for clinical approval [26].

In this Special Issue, eleven works (eight original research articles, two review articles, and one case report) are published, illustrating the comprehensive nature of the current strategies for developing modern wound dressings. These studies highlight how biomaterials and multifunctional and drug delivery systems influence wound management, providing both therapeutic effects and long-term perspectives for clinical applications.

Before considering the development of bioactive wound dressings, it is important to mention that one article in this Special Issue investigated the key role of polymers in designing wound dressings that can accelerate wound healing. Wong et al. developed a new crystalline glucose/mannose film as a modern polymeric wound dressing that combines non-adhesive behavior with moisture regulation, biocompatibility, and biodegradability (Contribution 1). This new formulation demonstrated a cellulose II-like crystalline model, with a smooth surface, suitable vapor permeability, and high water absorption, which are properties required for tissue healing. In vivo analysis on rats revealed that the glucose/mannose film substantially accelerated wound healing through collagen maturation and inflammation decline, promoting rapid epithelialization compared to the commercial alginate and hydrocolloid controls.

Four contributions included in this Special Issue investigated the integration of plant extracts as multifunctional bioactive agents, highlighting the therapeutic effects of natural products in wound healing management, along with polymeric supports.

In this regard, Alzahrani et al. investigated the protective effects of *Amaranthus graecizans* L. (AG), rich in polyphenols, vitamins, and minerals, against nonalcoholic fatty liver disease, induced by hyperlipidemia in rats (Contribution 2). Male Wistar rats received a high-fat diet and were treated with graded doses of AG solution (100, 200, or 500 mg/kg body weight) for two months. Phytochemical analysis indicated abundant phenolic compounds (especially chlorogenic and gallic acids) alongside a high content of fibers, potassium, calcium, and vitamins. AG supplementation significantly improved lipid profiles, reduced liver enzyme levels, and repaired the histological structure of liver tissues in a dose-dependent manner. Higher doses (500 mg/kg of AG) led to notable decreases in hepatic fatty accumulation and improved hepatocyte integrity.

Asiri et Venkatesan analyzed the therapeutic role of *Myristica fragrans* essential oil (MEO) in the wound healing process using a full-thickness excision wound model on Wistar rats (Contribution 3). GC-MS analysis indicated that MEO is a bioactive substance rich in many constituents (nitrobenzoate esters, cineole derivatives, and sesquiterpenoids) known for their antioxidant and anti-inflammatory properties. Topical application of 10% MEO significantly accelerated wound reduction, promoting complete epithelialization due to a decrease in pro-inflammatory cytokines and macrophage marker CD68 expression, as well as an improved antioxidant balance. Moreover, MEO modulated the apoptotic pathways by decreasing the activity of Caspase-3, supporting the durability of fibroblasts and the deposition of the extracellular matrix. Histological analysis also confirmed the enhanced deposition of collagen, reepithelialization, and reduced inflammatory infiltration.

Hasatsri et al. developed a new foam dressing based on gelatin and *Eclipta prostrata* leaf extract, with antibacterial and anti-inflammatory effects, aiming to combine traditional herbal activity with an advanced biomaterial design (Contribution 4). This new formulation exhibited a uniform porous structure, which was optimal to promote cell migration and proliferation. The foam dressing maintained a slightly acidic pH (~5), appropriate for antibacterial activity and skin tissue regeneration. Physicochemical tests indicated good absorption, dehydration, and flexibility properties, which are required for the treatment of injuries with low exudate levels.

Furthermore, another contribution investigated the combined therapeutic effects of different natural components (curcumin, resveratrol, and baicalin) on in vitro wound healing (Contribution 5). Jagiełło et al. investigated the wound healing potential of these three natural bioflavonoids by using fibroblast cell lines (Balb3t3 and L929) to evaluate their cytotoxicity (MTT assay) and migration (scratch test). None of the analyzed bioactive substances demonstrated cytotoxic effects, but they exhibited stimulatory effects on fibroblast proliferation and migration. By applying the Brian and Cousens mathematical model, the optimal concentration intervals to maximize cell viability and wound obstruction rate were established, providing quantitative support for optimizing dosage in designing new bioactive dressings.

Another study included in this Special Issue presents a combination of a plant-derived essential oil with a nonsteroidal anti-inflammatory drug, demonstrating their therapeutic effects in wound care. In line with this aspect, Plugariu et al. developed an innovative thermosensitive hydrogel based on polyurethane, proposed for the controlled transdermal release of meloxicam in order to solve the low solubility of this drug and its systemic side effects (Contribution 6). The novel formulation showed a temperature-responsive sol–gel transition with a self-healing ability and nanomicellar structure, which facilitates the sustained release of meloxicam. Moreover, the incorporation of *Origanum compactum* essential oil enhanced the antimicrobial activity and permeability of the drug.

Apart from the chemical compounds derived from different plants, some works included in this Special Issue focused on the development of wound dressings by incorporating various active pharmaceutical ingredients. These new formulations demonstrate how different bioactive agents can be effectively loaded into polymeric matrices to promote antimicrobial protection, reduce inflammation, and accelerate tissue regeneration.

Tudoroiu et al. developed smart-film dressings based on collagen and hydroxyethylcellulose, incorporating naproxen and phenol red for the dual purpose of therapy and real-time wound monitoring (Contribution 7). By combining natural and semisynthetic polymers with a nonsteroidal anti-inflammatory drug and a pH indicator, these new formulations are pH-responsive drug delivery systems, representing a clinically meaningful platform for real-time post-burn wound evaluation and localized treatment, combining diagnostic and therapeutic functions for modern wound healing management.

Albu Kaya et al. presented the design of biocomposite sponges based on collagen and hyaluronic acid and loaded with metronidazole, intended for localized treatment of periodontitis (Contribution 8). Structural characterization revealed the maintenance of collagen triple helix integrity and a porous structure, which enhances moisture uptake and the diffusion of the incorporated drug. This research represents a promising localized drug delivery system that manages infections in oral injuries, highlighting the significant potential of these bioactive polymeric biocomposites for wound and tissue regeneration.

Alongside the eight original research contributions included in this Special Issue, two comprehensive review papers are included that present recent advances and future directions and strategies in wound management.

The first review article, authored by Aldahish et al., presents the advancing potential of electrospun nanofibers based on silk fibroin nanofibers in developing bioactive dressings for diabetic wound healing (Contribution 9). The review illustrates an overview of the pathophysiological barriers associated with chronic diabetic wounds (oxidative stress, prolonged inflammation, and damaged angiogenesis) and discusses how silk fibroin-based nanofibers can surmount these limitations. This work describes the particular characteristics of silk fibroin—such as its biocompatibility, architectural resemblance to the extracellular matrix, and mechanical flexibility—which favor cellular proliferation, angiogenesis, and tissue remodeling. Moreover, the review also presents recent electrospinning technology that offers meaningful information about fiber morphology, porosity, or drug-loading ability, allowing for the development of bioactive wound dressings that induce the sustained release of therapeutic agents.

The second review paper, authored by Sharma et al., investigates the application of biodegradable electrospun scaffolds as modern materials intended for the regeneration of cutaneous lesions (Contribution 10). This paper describes how many types of biopolymers (natural and synthetic, including collagen, hyaluronic acid, chitosan, cellulose, polylactides, and polyhydroxyalkanoates) can be transformed into nanofibrous structures that can mimic the extracellular matrix, enhancing cell adhesion, proliferation, and skin tissue remodeling. The paper examines key electrospinning parameters, such as polymer concentration, viscosity, voltage, flow rate, and collector distance, as well as their influence on fiber structure, mechanical efficiency, and biological reactions. Moreover, it also highlights the potential of multifunctional nanofibers that can incorporate different therapeutic agents such as antimicrobial, anti-inflammatory, or growth-promoting compounds to accelerate wound healing.

The last contribution included in this Special Issue is a case report authored by Saberianpour et al. that presents the biological interactions between the components of wound exudate and dressing biomaterials, discussing how they influence healing outcomes and establishing the potential biomarkers of wound progression (Contribution 11). Six patients with acute surgical wounds were treated using two general dressings: Atrauman (a hydrophobic polyester-based tulle dressing) and Melolin (a hydrophilic hydrocolloid dressing). Cellular and biochemical analyses indicated that efficient healing correlated with the retention of progenitor ($CD105^+$) and M2 macrophage cells on the Atrauman interface, while the absorption of these cells into Melolin was linked to the slower or impaired recovery. Moreover, Melolin adsorbed a broader range of inflammatory proteins, whereas Atrauman primarily bound albumin, limiting inflammatory activation.

Together, the original articles, reviews, and the case report collected in this Special Issue collectively form an overview of the rapid progress and persistent challenges in the development of wound dressing. Collectively, they demonstrate how innovative biomaterials, natural compounds, and active pharmaceutical ingredients can be combined to create dressings that not only protect, but also actively stimulate tissue repair. From plant-derived compounds and smart polymeric matrices to drug-loaded hydrogels and multifunctional nanofibers, these contributions illustrate the union of material science, pharmacology, and biotechnology in modern wound management. The reviews further consolidate current knowledge and highlight electrospinning, nanostructuring, and biopolymer engineering as transformative approaches for next-generation dressings. The included case report emphasizes the growing importance of understanding biological interactions between wound exudates and dressing materials to optimizing clinical outcomes. Altogether, this Special Issue indicates a field evolving toward personalized, responsive, and multifunctional wound care systems that are capable of accelerating healing while improving patient comfort and quality of life.

Author Contributions: Conceptualization, M.V.G., M.G.A.K., L.P. and C.E.D.-P.; methodology, M.V.G., M.G.A.K., L.P. and C.E.D.-P.; software, M.V.G., M.G.A.K., L.P. and C.E.D.-P.; validation, M.V.G., M.G.A.K., L.P. and C.E.D.-P.; formal analysis, M.V.G., M.G.A.K., L.P. and C.E.D.-P.; investigation, M.V.G., M.G.A.K., L.P. and C.E.D.-P.; resources, M.V.G., M.G.A.K., L.P. and C.E.D.-P.; data curation, M.V.G., M.G.A.K., L.P. and C.E.D.-P.; writing—original draft preparation, M.V.G., M.G.A.K., L.P. and C.E.D.-P.; writing—review and editing, M.V.G., M.G.A.K., L.P. and C.E.D.-P.; visualization, M.V.G., M.G.A.K., L.P. and C.E.D.-P.; supervision, M.V.G., M.G.A.K., L.P. and C.E.D.-P.; project administration, M.V.G., M.G.A.K., L.P. and C.E.D.-P.; funding acquisition, M.V.G., M.G.A.K., L.P. and C.E.D.-P. All authors have read and agreed to the published version of the manuscript.

Acknowledgments: This research was financially supported by "Carol Davila" University of Medicine and Pharmacy Bucharest, Romania, through Contract No. CNFIS-FDI-2025-F-0646.

Conflicts of Interest: The authors declare no conflicts of interest.

List of Contributions:

1. Wong, C.C.; Tomura, K.; Yamamoto, O. Wound Healing Performance in a Moist Environment of Crystalline Glucose/Mannose Film as a New Dressing Material Using a Rat Model: Comparing with Medical-Grade Wound Dressing and Alginate. *Pharmaceuticals* **2023**, *16*, 1532. https://doi.org/10.3390/ph16111532.
2. Alzahrani, N.S.; Aljahdali, B.; Alhosain, A.; Alasmari, A.A.; Amna, T.; Yousef, S.M. *Amaranthus graecizans* L. Mitigates Hyperlipidemia-Induced Nonalcoholic Fatty Liver Disease in Experimental Rats: Future Pharmaceuticals. *Pharmaceuticals* **2025**, *18*, 1196. https://doi.org/10.3390/ph18081196.
3. Asiri, Y.I.; Venkatesan, K. Wound-Healing Potential of Myristica fragrans Essential Oil: A Multi-Targeted Approach Involving Inflammation, Oxidative Stress, and Apoptosis Regulation. *Pharmaceuticals* **2025**, *18*, 880. https://doi.org/10.3390/ph18060880.
4. Hasatsri, S.; Suthi, J.; Siriwut, N.; Charoensappakit, O. Physical Properties and pH Environment of Foam Dressing Containing Eclipta prostrata Leaf Extract and Gelatin. *Pharmaceuticals* **2023**, *16*, 685. https://doi.org/10.3390/ph16050685.
5. Jagiełło, K.; Uchańska, O.; Matyja, K.; Jackowski, M.; Wiatrak, B.; Kubasiewicz-Ross, P.; Karuga-Kuźniewska, E. Supporting the Wound Healing Process—Curcumin, Resveratrol and Baicalin in In Vitro Wound Healing Studies. *Pharmaceuticals* **2023**, *16*, 82. https://doi.org/10.3390/ph16010082.
6. Plugariu, I.-A.; Gradinaru, L.M.; Avadanei, M.; Rosca, I.; Nita, L.E.; Maxim, C.; Bercea, M. Thermosensitive Polyurethane-Based Hydrogels as Potential Vehicles for Meloxicam Delivery. *Pharmaceuticals* **2023**, *16*, 1510. https://doi.org/10.3390/ph16111510.
7. Tudoroiu, E.-E.; Albu Kaya, M.G.; Dinu-Pîrvu, C.E.; Popa, L.; Anuța, V.; Ignat, M.; Visileanu, E.; Kaya, D.A.; Prisada, R.M.; Ghica, M.V. Development of Smart pH-Sensitive Collagen-Hydroxyethylcellulose Films with Naproxen for Burn Wound Healing. *Pharmaceuticals* **2025**, *18*, 689. https://doi.org/10.3390/ph18050689.
8. Kaya, M.G.; Simonca, A.G.; Rau, I.; Coman, A.E.; Marin, M.M.; Popa, L.; Trusca, R.; Dinu-Pirvu, C.-E.; Ghica, M.V. Topical Biocomposites Based on Collagen, Hyaluronic Acid and Metronidazole as Periodontitis Treatment. *Pharmaceuticals* **2024**, *17*, 1336. https://doi.org/10.3390/ph17101336.
9. Aldahish, A.; Shanmugasundaram, N.; Vasudevan, R.; Alqahtani, T.; Alqahtani, S.; Mohammad Asiri, A.; Devanandan, P.; Thamaraikani, T.; Vellapandian, C.; Jayasankar, N. Silk Fibroin Nanofibers: Advancements in Bioactive Dressings through Electrospinning Technology for Diabetic Wound Healing. *Pharmaceuticals* **2024**, *17*, 1305. https://doi.org/10.3390/ph17101305.
10. Sharma, D.; Srivastava, S.; Kumar, S.; Sharma, P.K.; Hassani, R.; Dailah, H.G.; Khalid, A.; Mohan, S. Biodegradable Electrospun Scaffolds as an Emerging Tool for Skin Wound Regeneration: A Comprehensive Review. *Pharmaceuticals* **2023**, *16*, 325. https://doi.org/10.3390/ph16020325.
11. Saberianpour, S.; Melotto, G.; Redhead, L.; Terrazzini, N.; Forss, J.R.; Santin, M. Harnessing the Interactions of Wound Exudate Cells with Dressings Biomaterials for the Control and Prognosis of Healing Pathways. *Pharmaceuticals* **2024**, *17*, 1111. https://doi.org/10.3390/ph17091111.

References

1. Capanema, N.S.V.; Mansur, A.A.P.; de Jesus, A.C.; Carvalho, S.M.; de Oliveira, L.C.; Mansur, H.S. Superabsorbent crosslinked carboxymethyl cellulose-PEG hydrogels for potential wound dressing applications. *Int. J. Biol. Macromol.* **2018**, *106*, 1218–1234. [CrossRef]
2. Martinengo, L.; Olsson, M.; Bajpai, R.; Soljak, M.; Upton, Z.; Schmidtchen, A.; Car, J.; Jarbrink, K. Prevalence of chronic wounds in the general population: Systematic review and meta-analysis of observational studies. *Ann. Epidemiol.* **2019**, *29*, 8–15. [CrossRef]
3. Rodrigues, C.; de Assis, A.M.; Moura, D.J.; Halmenschlager, G.; Saffi, J.; Xavier, L.L.; Fernandes Mda, C.; Wink, M.R. New therapy of skin repair combining adipose-derived mesenchymal stem cells with sodium carboxymethylcellulose scaffold in a pre-clinical rat model. *PLoS ONE* **2014**, *9*, e96241. [CrossRef]
4. Okoye, E.; Okolie, T. Development and in vitro characterization of ciprofloxacin loaded polymeric films for wound dressing. *Int. J. Health Allied Sci.* **2015**, *4*, 234. [CrossRef]
5. Sen, C.K. Human Wound and Its Burden: Updated 2020 Compendium of Estimates. *Adv. Wound Care* **2021**, *10*, 281–292. [CrossRef]
6. Tudoroiu, E.-E.; Dinu-Pîrvu, C.-E.; Albu Kaya, M.G.; Popa, L.; Anuța, V.; Prisada, R.M.; Ghica, M.V. An Overview of Cellulose Derivatives-Based Dressings for Wound-Healing Management. *Pharmaceuticals* **2021**, *14*, 1215. [CrossRef]
7. Hachem, R.; Parikh, U.M.; Reitzel, R.; Rosenblatt, J.; Kaul, A.; Vargas-Cruz, N.; Hill, L.; Moore, L.; Meyer, J.; Chaftari, A.M.; et al. Novel antimicrobial ointment for infected wound healing in an in vitro and in vivo porcine model. *Wound Repair Regen.* **2021**, *29*, 830–842. [CrossRef] [PubMed]
8. Sandri, G.; Bonferoni, M.C.; D'Autilia, F.; Rossi, S.; Ferrari, F.; Grisoli, P.; Sorrenti, M.; Catenacci, L.; Del Fante, C.; Perotti, C.; et al. Wound dressings based on silver sulfadiazine solid lipid nanoparticles for tissue repairing. *Eur. J. Pharm. Biopharm.* **2013**, *84*, 84–90. [CrossRef] [PubMed]
9. Pawar, H.V.; Tetteh, J.; Boateng, J.S. Preparation, optimisation and characterisation of novel wound healing film dressings loaded with streptomycin and diclofenac. *Colloids Surf. B Biointerfaces* **2013**, *102*, 102–110. [CrossRef] [PubMed]
10. Kong, D.N.; Zhang, Q.C.; You, J.; Cheng, Y.Y.; Hong, C.; Chen, Z.H.; Jiang, T.; Hao, T.H. Adhesion loss mechanism based on carboxymethyl cellulose-filled hydrocolloid dressings in physiological wounds environment. *Carbohydr. Polym.* **2020**, *235*, 7. [CrossRef]
11. Yadav, V.; Mittal, A.; Bansal, P.; Singh, S.K. Regulatory approval process for advanced dressings in India: An overview of rules. *J. Wound Care* **2019**, *28*, S32–S42. [CrossRef] [PubMed]
12. Trevisol, T.C.; Fritz, A.R.M.; de Souza, S.; Bierhalz, A.C.K.; Valle, J.A.B. Alginate and carboxymethyl cellulose in monolayer and bilayer films as wound dressings: Effect of the polymer ratio. *J. Appl. Polym. Sci.* **2019**, *136*, 9. [CrossRef]
13. Mishra, S.K.; Mary, D.S.; Kannan, S. Copper incorporated microporous chitosan-polyethylene glycol hydrogels loaded with naproxen for effective drug release and anti-infection wound dressing. *Int. J. Biol. Macromol.* **2017**, *95*, 928–937. [CrossRef]
14. Kamoun, E.A.; Chen, X.; Mohy Eldin, M.S.; Kenawy, E.-R.S. Crosslinked poly(vinyl alcohol) hydrogels for wound dressing applications: A review of remarkably blended polymers. *Arab. J. Chem.* **2015**, *8*, 1–14. [CrossRef]
15. Patil, P.P.; Reagan, M.R.; Bohara, R.A. Silk fibroin and silk-based biomaterial derivatives for ideal wound dressings. *Int. J. Biol. Macromol.* **2020**, *164*, 4613–4627. [CrossRef]
16. Dhivya, S.; Padma, V.V.; Santhini, E. Wound dressings—A review. *BioMedicine* **2015**, *5*, 24–28. [CrossRef] [PubMed]
17. Olatunji, O. Classification of Natural Polymers. In *Natural Polymers*; Springer: Berlin/Heidelberg, Germany, 2016; pp. 1–17.
18. Kulkarni Vishakha, S.; Butte Kishor, D.; Rathod Sudha, S. Natural polymers–A comprehensive review. *Int. J. Res. Pharm. Biomed. Sci.* **2012**, *3*, 1597–1613.
19. Alves, T.F.R.; Morsink, M.; Batain, F.; Chaud, M.V.; Almeida, T.; Fernandes, D.A.; da Silva, C.F.; Souto, E.B.; Severino, P. Applications of Natural, Semi-Synthetic, and Synthetic Polymers in Cosmetic Formulations. *Cosmetics* **2020**, *7*, 75. [CrossRef]
20. Bhatia, S. Natural Polymers vs Synthetic Polymer. In *Natural Polymer Drug Delivery Systems*; Springer: Berlin/Heidelberg, Germany, 2016; pp. 95–118.
21. Tavakoli, J.; Tang, Y. Honey/PVA hybrid wound dressings with controlled release of antibiotics: Structural, physico-mechanical and in-vitro biomedical studies. *Mater. Sci. Eng. C* **2017**, *77*, 318–325. [CrossRef]
22. Yaşayan, G.; Karaca, G.; Akgüner, Z.P.; Bal Öztürk, A. Chitosan/collagen composite films as wound dressings encapsulating allantoin and lidocaine hydrochloride. *Int. J. Polym. Mater. Polym. Biomat.* **2021**, *70*, 623–635. [CrossRef]
23. Gulsun, T.; Inal, M.; Akdag, Y.; Izat, N.; Oner, L.; Sahin, S. The development and characterization of electrospun gelatin nanofibers containing indomethacin and curcumin for accelerated wound healing. *J. Drug Deliv. Sci. Technol.* **2022**, *67*, 103000. [CrossRef]
24. Mogrovejo-Valdivia, A.; Maton, M.; Garcia-Fernandez, M.J.; Tabary, N.; Chai, F.; Neut, C.; Martel, B.; Blanchemain, N. In Vitro Microbiological and Drug Release of Silver/Ibuprofen Loaded Wound Dressing Designed for the Treatment of Chronically Infected Painful Wounds. *Antibiotics* **2021**, *10*, 805. [CrossRef] [PubMed]

25. Zeng, Q.; Qi, X.; Shi, G.; Zhang, M.; Haick, H. Wound Dressing: From Nanomaterials to Diagnostic Dressings and Healing Evaluations. *ACS Nano* **2022**, *16*, 1708–1733. [CrossRef] [PubMed]
26. Namazi, H.; Rakhshaei, R.; Hamishehkar, H.; Kafil, H.S. Antibiotic loaded carboxymethylcellulose/MCM-41 nanocomposite hydrogel films as potential wound dressing. *Int. J. Biol. Macromol.* **2016**, *85*, 327–334. [CrossRef] [PubMed]

pharmaceuticals

MDPI

Review

Biodegradable Electrospun Scaffolds as an Emerging Tool for Skin Wound Regeneration: A Comprehensive Review

Deepika Sharma [1], Shriyansh Srivastava [1,2,*], Sachin Kumar [2], Pramod Kumar Sharma [1], Rym Hassani [3], Hamad Ghaleb Dailah [4], Asaad Khalid [5,6] and Syam Mohan [5,7,8,*]

1 Department of Pharmacy, School of Medical and Allied Sciences, Galgotias University, Greater Noida 203201, India
2 Department of Pharmacology, Delhi Pharmaceutical Sciences and Research University (DPSRU), Sector 3 Pushp Vihar, New Delhi 110017, India
3 Department of Mathematics, University College AlDarb, Jazan University, Jazan 45142, Saudi Arabia
4 Research and Scientific Studies Unit, College of Nursing, Jazan University, Jazan 45142, Saudi Arabia
5 Substance Abuse and Toxicology Research Centre, Jazan University, Jazan 45142, Saudi Arabia
6 Medicinal and Aromatic Plants and Traditional Medicine Research Institute, National Center for Research, Khartoum P.O. Box 2404, Sudan
7 School of Health Sciences, University of Petroleum and Energy Studies, Dehradun 248007, India
8 Center for Transdisciplinary Research, Department of Pharmacology, Saveetha Institute of Medical and Technical Science, Saveetha Dental College, Saveetha University, Chennai 600077, India
* Correspondence: shriyanshsrivastav@gmail.com (S.S.); syammohanm@yahoo.com (S.M.)

Abstract: Skin is designed to protect various tissues, and because it is the largest and first human bodily organ to sustain damage, it has an incredible ability to regenerate. On account of extreme injuries or extensive surface loss, the normal injury recuperating interaction might be inadequate or deficient, bringing about risky and disagreeable circumstances that request the utilization of fixed adjuvants and tissue substitutes. Due to their remarkable biocompatibility, biodegradability, and bioactive abilities, such as antibacterial, immunomodulatory, cell proliferative, and wound mending properties, biodegradable polymers, both synthetic and natural, are experiencing remarkable progress. Furthermore, the ability to convert these polymers into submicrometric filaments has further enhanced their potential (e.g., by means of electrospinning) to impersonate the stringy extracellular grid and permit neo-tissue creation, which is a basic component for delivering a mending milieu. Together with natural biomaterial, synthetic polymers are used to solve stability problems and make scaffolds that can dramatically improve wound healing. Biodegradable polymers, commonly referred to as biopolymers, are increasingly used in other industrial sectors to reduce the environmental impact of material and energy usage as they are fabricated using renewable biological sources. Electrospinning is one of the best ways to fabricate nanofibers and membranes that are very thin and one of the best ways to fabricate continuous nanomaterials with a wide range of biological, chemical, and physical properties. This review paper concludes with a summary of the electrospinning (applied electric field, needle-to-collector distance, and flow rate), solution (solvent, polymer concentration, viscosity, and solution conductivity), and environmental (humidity and temperature) factors that affect the production of nanofibers and the use of bio-based natural and synthetic electrospun scaffolds in wound healing.

Keywords: nanofibers; polymers; scaffolds; wound healing; electrospinning; nanoscaffold; biodegradable polymer

1. Introduction

The skin of the human body is a versatile organ that serves as a natural barrier against environmental elements. The skin is composed of three layers: the epidermis, dermis, and hypodermis, all of which protect the body's internal organs from external threats, whether physical, synthetic, or natural. As the skin plays an important role in the body, any significant damage, including major or severe wounds, must be managed quickly and effectively to prevent further harm [1]. Wound mending has become a significant worldwide general well-being concern for many years. Insufficient skin harm treatment can possibly be deadly. Subsequently, broad exploration in this space has been directed, with an attention on the advancement of successful, helpful methods, and the innovation of novel dressing materials that can advance wound healing [2]. Contingent upon the seriousness and intensity of the injury, a sufficient dressing with viable injury site security and quick skin recovery is clinically vital for speeding up injury recuperation [3]. Covering the injured area with a dressing material that prevents dehydration and contamination has been part of wound care for a long time [4]. Wound recuperating medicines have advanced throughout the past 10 years, from straightforward balms and bandages to cutting edge multifunctional wound dressings. Ideally, a wound dressing should: possess anti-inflammatory characteristics, absorb wound exudates, protect the wound from bacterial infection, shield from external stimuli, induce cell proliferation to expedite healing, and promote tissue regeneration. It should keep the injury site appropriately moist and protect the tissue from further harm. In order to fulfil its role of preventing wound compression, a dressing must possess elasticity in cases where compression is not possible, as well as being composed of a material that is soft, compatible with the body, hypoallergenic, and non-toxic [5]. The use of multipurpose wound dressings accelerate the rate of healing. The electrospinning system has, as of late, acquired fame for the creation of biopolymer-based nanofibrous structures. Electrospinning is a typical, minimal expense and tunable strategy for making super fine filaments with unique properties. Electrospinning innovation has been generally utilized in biomedical materials, for example, tissue designing frameworks, wound dressings, and drug delivery systems. Nanofibers that are spun electrically, with diameters on a nanoscale, are suggested to be great wound dressings and tissue replacements since they look like the extracellular matrix (ECM) [6]. An assortment of regular biopolymers (e.g., cellulose) were electrospun into nanofibers to reproduce the local tissue network for wound mending. Collagen, hyaluronic acid, gelatin, and chitosan were employed to their fullest potential simultaneously. Synthetic bio-based polymers polylactides (PLAs) and polyhydroxyalkanoates (PHAs) are frequently used for the electrospinning of wound dressings. By electrospinning natural and synthetic polymers (derived from biological sources) in coaxial, multi-nozzle, or blend configurations, wound dressing mechanical degradation and/or morphological properties can be tailored [7]. This review aims to highlight and describe the recent developments in the electrospinning of various synthetic and natural biopolymers, emphasizing their applications in wound healing. An overview of the four stages of wound healing and the electrospinning process and its effects on fiber morphology are provided. Additionally, a summary of newly developed multifunctional electrospun structures for wound healing, including cellulose, chitosan, PHAs, and PLA, PCL, PES, PS, PAA, and thermoresponsive polymers such as Poly(N-isopropylacrylamide) (pNIPAAm) and poly(N-vinlycaprolactam) (PVCL), are presented and discussed. The review's final section discusses the potential uses of electrospun biopolymer fibers for treating wounds. To locate relevant material, we selected keywords such as nanofibers, polymers, scaffolds, wound healing, electrospinning, nanoscaffold, and biodegradable polymer. The search for these terms was conducted in several relevant databases, including Google Scholar, PubMed, and Scopus. The range of research materials examined encompassed research articles, review articles, book chapters, and conference abstracts published between 2017 and 2023, resulting in a total of 147 published materials, as shown in Figure 1. The literature without specific and detailed data pertaining to the topic was excluded from this review.

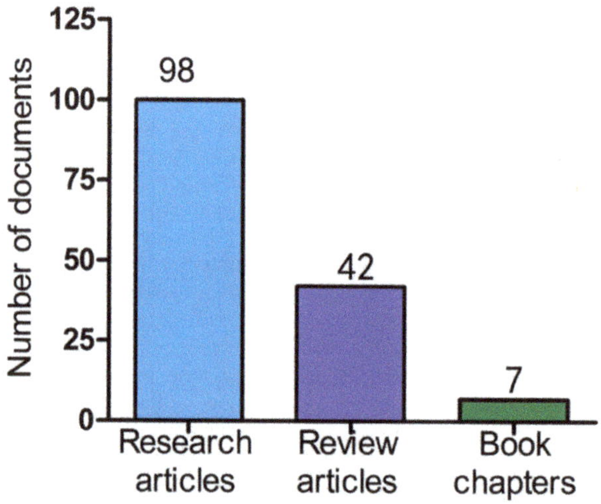

Figure 1. Total number of documents screened for review manuscript preparation. Documents search has been performed using keywords such as nanofibers, polymers, scaffolds, wound healing, electrospinning, nanoscaffold, and biodegradable polymer.

2. An Overview of Wounds and Their Consequences

Various sources can lead to wounds, including surgery, trauma, external pressures, abrasions, and illnesses such as diabetes and cardiovascular diseases. Depending on the cause and the severity of the injury, these wounds can be classified as either acute or chronic [8]. An organized and appropriate repair process is typically followed by an acute wound, leading to the long-term restoration of anatomical and functional integrity. Chronic wounds, on the other hand, are unable to reach ideal anatomical and functional integrity. The healing process may be altered based on the characteristics of the patient and the environment, such as the type, intensity, and state of the injury, in addition to potential health conditions, such as vascular, metabolic, and autoimmune diseases, and the use of medications [9]. A wound that has been healed minimally is identified by the re-establishment of its anatomical makeup, yet without ongoing functional results; as a result, it can reappear. A perfectly healed wound is when the region returns to its original anatomy, performance, and outward appearance after an injury. A wound that has been fully healed is set apart from these two states by the formation of lasting anatomical and functional continuity. Numerous additional elements, including oxygen, infection, swelling, inflammation, trauma, and the body's own system, can be used to evaluate a wound's degree of healing. All of these characteristics can reveal information about the cause, pathophysiology, and state of a wound [10].

In conclusion, it is essential to think about how injuries shape the host, as patient health is essential in deciding how systemic components shape the wound. Since the mending procedure is ever-changing and requests a consistent, organized, and steady assessment, including continuous re-evaluation of wound range, type, and seriousness, it can be hard to gauge the recuperating process. Persistent wounds reduce the quality of life, and the cost of care is seen in morbidity and even mortality, as well as the psychological cost, and the lengthened hospital stay. These factors have led to wounds being referred to as a "Silent Epidemic" [11]. Most financial costs are a result of employing medical personnel; hospital stays, both in terms of length and expense; as well as the selection of materials and treatments. For all of these reasons, creating new technologies aimed at enhancing the healing process is challenging [12].

2.1. Chronic and Acute Wound Healing

The normal wound-healing process for acute injuries (such as those caused by trauma or surgery) creates an orderly and predictable pattern of tissue repair [13]. In comparison, the management of chronic wounds is chaotic, and they can primarily be classified as vascular ulcers (encompassing venous and arterial ulcers), diabetic ulcers, and pressure ulcers [14]. Chronic wounds that become inflamed for long periods of time lead to the growth of biofilm, the gathering of microorganisms, as well as the release of platelet-derived materials such as TGF-β and molecules from the extracellular matrix. The production of inflammatory cytokines, such as TNF-α and IL-1, over a prolonged period of time, causes a high amount of protease to be present in the wounded area. This amount surpasses the number of inhibitors, resulting in the breakdown of the extracellular matrix and fueling the inflammatory and proliferative phases of healing [15]. Chronic injuries also include phenotypic flaws in the cells and The accumulation of inflammatory cells in the wound bed of a chronic wound leads to an increase in the concentration of reactive oxygen species (ROS), causing damage to Extracellular Matrix (ECM) proteins and leading to the premature aging of the cells [16]. Chronic injuries also include phenotypic flaws in the cells and dermis, such as decreased growth factor receptor density and mitogen potential, which prevent local cells from properly responding to signals that promote wound healing [17].

2.2. Progression of Healing a Wound

The human body's proceeding of wound healing is made up of four phases that are tightly linked and overlap with one another, the steps are: hemostasis, inflammation, proliferation, and remodeling [10].

2.2.1. Hemostasis

Platelet adhesion and blood coagulation are the primary mechanisms for attaining hemostasis [18]. Clotting begins with tissue factors, which are typically away from the circulatory system. When damage happens to the vascular system, the tissue factors connect with factor VII, allowing the tissue factor-producing cells, such as adventitial fibroblasts, to be included in the blood clotting process. In turn, factors IX and X are activated by the TF: factor VII complex. The extrinsic pathway is the name provided to this process that activates factor X since it takes place outside the endothelium [19]. A minimal quantity of prothrombin is changed into thrombin when coagulation factor X (Xa) binds with its cofactor (factor Va). Platelet activation, a principal purpose of the initially transformed thrombin, prepares the path for the intrinsic route. The intrinsic pathway also activates factor X and is a concurrent and supportive mechanism. Once detached from factor VIII, the von Willebrand factor (vWf) helps further bind platelets to the wounded area [19]. Once the activated platelets connect with factors V, VIII, and IX, factor Xa is generated and added to the prothrombinase on the platelet's surface, comprising of factors Xa and Va, which leads to a high level of thrombin and hastens the formation of the fibrin clot. The intrinsic and extrinsic pathways then come together, causing the production of fibrin subunits that link up, forming strands that bind the platelets and secure the plug in position [20]. The protein C/protein S/thrombomodulin (TM) system on endothelial cells is capable of deactivating factors Va and VIIIa, thus limiting clot formation to the damaged region. When platelets aggregate and degranulate, they release a range of substances, including platelet-derived growth factor (PDGF), transforming growth factor-β (TGFβ), transforming growth factor-α (TGFα), basic fibroblast growth factor (FGF), and insulin-like growth factor-I (IGF-I), which activate the inflammatory process. This is performed by employing chemotaxis, allowing monocytes and neutrophils to move from the blood vessels to the injury site [21]. Figure 2 depicts the various stages of wound healing.

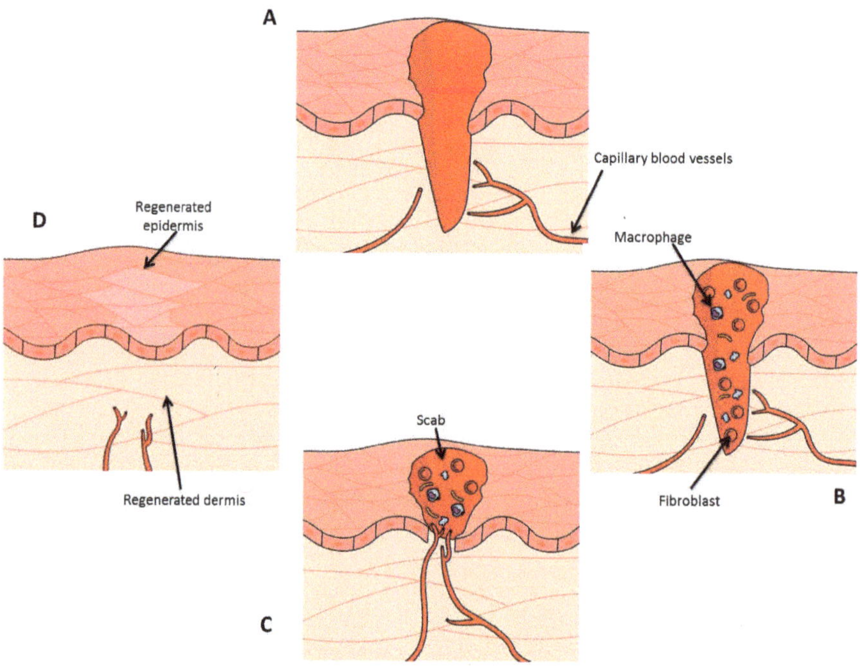

Figure 2. This figure depicts the four stages of wound healing, which are (**A**) hemostasis, (**B**) inflammation, (**C**) proliferation, and (**D**) extracellular matrix remodeling. During wound healing, fibroblasts (the body's connective tissue cells) and macrophages, which defend against infection, play an enormous role.

2.2.2. Inflammation

Following clot formation and blood loss regulation, different chemical mediators control the inflammatory phase. Cyclooxygenase 2 (COX-2) activates endothelial cells to produce prostaglandins, resulting in vasodilation, the breaking apart of platelets, and the formation of leukotrienes [22]. The process of exuding and cleaning up begins when the grouped platelets burst open and send out powerful chemo-attractants that draw in neutrophils, macrophages, and lymphocytes [10]. Neutrophils, which are drawn to the fibrin matrix by PDGF and other cytokines, are frequently the first cells to migrate. Bacteria, foreign matter, and cell debris are all phagocytosed by neutrophils. Neutrophils utilize proteolytic enzymes and reactive free oxygen radicals to clear away bacteria and any other detritus at the injury site. Furthermore, they discharge interleukin-1, interleukin-6, and tumor necrosis factor-alpha, which serve to galvanize fibroblasts and epithelial cells [21]. Neutrophils are either physically sloughed off or phagocytosed by macrophages [23]. The populace of inflamed cells gradually shifts to one that is dominated by monocytes over the next two to three days. These cells are then converted into macrophages, which take in bacterial leftovers and tissue while also producing numerous growth factors. The start of the expansion period of healing is contingent on the transformation of monocytes into macrophages. Macrophages release collagenases to clean the wound, in addition to IL-1 and IL-6. These macrophages also emit PDGF, TGFβ, TGFα, FGF, IGF-1, and TNFα. These growth factors and cytokines are necessary for the stimulation of keratinocytes, the recruitment and activation of fibroblasts, and the encouragement of angiogenesis [24].

2.2.3. Proliferation

This phase of wound recovery includes the formation of granulation tissue, angiogenesis, and the return of structural functionality. Fibroblasts are the main cells responsible for the development of new blood vessels and collagen production in the dermis, transforming the blood clot into granulation tissue, which supplies structural and nourishing support for the recovery of the outer layers. Additionally, keratinocytes migrate and divide as they expand the newly created epithelial covering that makes up the different layers of the epidermis toward the wound's edge [25]. The gradient in chemotactic growth factor cytokines and chemokines concentration controls the fibroblasts' direction of migration. Two factors that influence the behavior of fibroblasts are PDGF and TGF-β. PDGF induces the multiplication, chemotaxis, and secretion of collagenase in fibroblasts, while TGF-β triggers the transcription of collagen, proteoglycan, and fibronectin genes, as well as the production of tissue inhibitors of metalloproteinases (TIMPs). As they progress, fibroblasts rearrange their shape by stretching out cytoplasmic projections to new binding sites, which they use to detach themselves from the ECM and the provisional matrix in the clot and move ahead using their cytoskeleton network. Additionally, fibroblasts manufacture and deposit collagen, proteoglycans, and other components of granulation tissue [21]. VEGF has a specific role in the production of new capillaries from existing small blood vessels, a process known as angiogenesis [21]. The body utilizes re-epithelization, a course of action spurred by inflammatory cytokines to restore a protective layer against fluid leakage and bacterial infiltration. Myofibroblasts, which are activated by macrophages during the re-epithelization process, help to contract the wound by working on actin and myosin. The consequence of cell bodies coming together to diminish the amount of tissue that requires healing is wound contraction, which reduces the size of the scar [25].

When growth factors EGF, KGF, and TGFα bind to receptors on the basal epithelial cells, these cells migrate and proliferate. This causes the desmosomes and hemidesmosomes, which connect the basal epithelial cells to their neighboring cells and basement membrane to disperse, thus creating a space between them and allowing them to move. The cuboidal basal epithelial cells transform into a flat shape and travel in a single layer across the collagen fibers of the new granulation tissue.

2.2.4. Remodeling

During the remodeling phase, the granulation tissue slowly changes into scar tissue. Scar tissue has an abundance of collagen fibers and is not as cellular or full of blood vessels as regular tissue [26]. The collagen initially laid down is less dense than that of healthy skin, with its fibers running parallel to the skin. As lysine residues become more hydroxylated and glycosylated, the collagen in the granulation tissue becomes less thick. This type I collagen is thicker and follows the lines of relaxed skin tension, helping to bolster the repair tissue's strength [24]. The wound bed includes cells that generate proteolytic enzymes such as MMPs that can destroy entire fibrillar collagen molecules, damage collagen, and degrade proteoglycans. Neutrophilelastase, a serine protease, can break down almost any type of protein. TIMPs have the ability to restrain MMPs, while α1-protease inhibitors and α2 macroglobulin can reduce serine protease activity. Fibroblasts continually produce collagen, forming larger bundles bolstered by covalent crosslinks that develop over time [21].

Despite the breakdown and production of organized collagen, as well as the addition of other proteins, collagen synthesis goes on for approximately a month.

3. Electrospinning Is an Emerging Way to Create Polymer Nanofibrous Structures for Aiding in Wound Healing

Electrospinning allows for the development of systems of nanosized fibers that are similar to the original structure of the ECM, which helps the cells to carry out their regular activities such as adhesion and growth [27]. The principle behind creating fibers is to employ electrostatic force, which results in the fiber being spun from the solution. In order to achieve charging potential, a high voltage is briefly applied to the fluid reservoir. As depicted in Figure 3, a syringe linked to a pump is used to insert the spinning solution, which then creates a pendant drop at the spinneret's end with gentle pressure. The droplet is transformed into the Taylor cone, a hemispherical shape, by the action of this electric force. A steady jet can form depending on the viscosity and surface tension of the fluid. An elongated fiber structure develops on the collector when the electrostatic force is greater than the surface tension. As the solvent approaches the collector's surface, it evaporates. Due to their high surface-to-volume ratio and tiny pores, electrospun fibrous networks can effectively cause hemostasis without the utilization of a hemostatic agent. Exudates are effectively consumed by nanofibers, which provide a soggy climate for cell development. The porosity part of these designs, with their small pores, restricts bacterial contamination, provides high penetrability, and shields injured tissue from drying out. One more key component of the electrospinning method is the capacity and adaptability to embed drugs and other bioactive synthetic substances into nanofibers, for example, development factors, anti-inflammatory agents, nanoparticles, and antimicrobials [28]. Figure 3 depicts the electrospinning process setups.

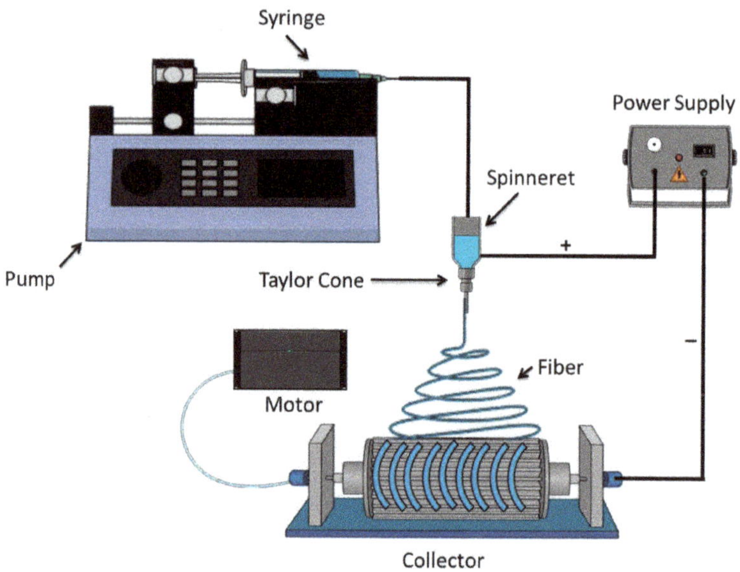

Figure 3. Electrospinning process setups.

4. The Influence of Different Factors on Electrospinning Is Investigated

The electrospinning process is influenced by a number of factors. The factors can be divided into three groups: solution, environmental, and electrospinning parameters. Examples of the electrospinning parameters are voltage, electric field, the gap between the needle and the collector, flow rate, and needle diameter. As for the solution parameters, these include the solvent, polymer concentration, viscosity, and solution conductivity. Temperature and relative humidity are included in the environmental parameters. Table 1 represents the consequences of various electrospinning factors on fiber morphology.

4.1. *Effect of Applied Voltage*

Generally, when the voltage reaches a certain level, a current running through a metal needle from a high-voltage energy source causes a round droplet to change shape into a Taylor cone and create tiny nanofibers [29]. It is thought that the stretching of the polymer solution due to the electric repulsion within the polymer jet is what causes the production of nanofibers with a smaller diameter when the voltage is increased [30]. Utilizing PEO/water combinations, Deitzel et al. [31] reported that beads formed as the applied voltage increased. Meechaisue et al. [31] and Zong et al. [31] reported similar outcomes as well. It was concluded that the diameter of the nanofibrous scaffolds increased as the voltage increased. This was due to the jet length increasing with the higher voltage [32].

4.2. *Effect of Solution Flow Rate*

The flow of the polymeric solution through the metallic needle tip determines the morphology of the electrospun nanofibers. Beyond a certain point, increasing the flow rate results in the formation of beads in addition to an increase in pore size and fiber diameter (caused by the nanofiber jet's failure to completely dry during its flight between the needle tip and metallic collector) [33]. For instance, when the flow rate was increased to 0.10 mL/min for polystyrene, beads began to form. However, when the rate of flow was lowered to 0.07 mL/min, nanofibers were produced with no beads. Additionally, the density of the surface charge can cause imperfections in the nanofiber structure. If the surface charge density changes, the nanofiber's morphology might too. For instance, a direct relationship between flow rate and electric current was discovered by Theron, S et al. They investigated the effects of flow rate and surface charge density using a variety of polymers, including PEO, polyacrylic acid (PAA), polyvinyl alcohol (PVA), polyurethane, and polycaprolactone (PCL). They discovered that for PEO electrospun nanofibers can combine as they approach the collector, resulting from a boost in the flow rate, which leads to a higher electric current and a decrease in the surface charge density [34].

4.3. *Influence of the Needle-to-Collector Distance and Needle Diameter*

The morphology of an electrospun nanofiber is largely dependent on the distance between the metallic needle tip and collector. The distance between the metallic needle tip and collector varies with the polymer system in a manner similar to that of the applied electric field, viscosity, and flow rate. The distance can have a big impact on the nanofiber morphology, as it is affected by the deposition time, evaporation rate, and instability interval of the whipping process [35]. Therefore, in order to prepare uniform electrospun nanofibers, a critical distance must be maintained [36].

4.4. *Effects of Polymer Concentration and Solution Viscosity*

The combination of surface tension and an applied electric field breaks down the entangled polymer chains into smaller pieces, which prevents them from reaching the collector electrode due to the low concentration of the polymeric solution [37]. These pieces result in the development of beads or beaded nanofibers. As the concentration of the polymeric solution increases, the viscosity of the solution rises, resulting in an increase in the entanglement between the polymer chains. Surface tension is overcome by these chain entanglements, which leads to uniform electrospun nanofibers without beads. When the concentration of the solution surpasses the critical value, the flow of the liquid through the needle tip is impeded, leading to the production of beaded nanofibers.

Zong et al. observed that the form of the beads shifts as the viscosity increases while investigating PDLA and PLLA [38]. Doshi et al. also reported on the impact of concentration and viscosity on the morphology of the nanofibers. They discovered that 800–4000 pascal seconds (Pa.s) is the ideal viscosity for the creation of electrospun nanofibers while working with PEO [39].

4.5. *Effect of Electrical Conductivity*

The Taylor cone formation is influenced by electrical conductivity, which also helps control the nanofibers' diameter. Because the surface of the droplet is not sufficiently charged to form a Taylor cone in a solution with lower conductivity, electrospinning does not occur. When the electrical conductivity of the solution reaches a critical level, the Taylor cone forms and the diameter of the fiber also decreases [40].

Conductivity stops the Taylor cone formation and electrospinning above a critical point. The electrospinning procedure begins once there are enough free charges in the conductive polymer mixture to create a Taylor cone on the fluid's surface. Salt addition affects electrospinning in two ways: (i) it raises the ion number in the mixture, therefore growing the surface charge density of the liquid and the electrostatic power generated by the electric field, and (ii) it enhances the conductivity of the solution, thereby lessening the tangential electric field along the surface of the fluid. The effect of salt on the diameter of nanofibers has been studied by numerous researchers. For instance, KH_2PO_4, NaH_2PO_4, and NaCl in 1% w/v were studied by Zong et al. to see how they affected the diameter of polymer nanofibers (D,L-lactic acid). They observed that the nanofibers were smoother, more beaded, and had a smaller diameter than the pristine nanofibers when they added salt to the polymer solution one at a time.

4.6. Role of Solvent in Electrospinning

Researchers looked into the ways in which the solvent and solvent combination impacted the shape of nanofibers [41] and they came to the conclusion that the solvent has an impact on the polymer system in a manner similar to applied voltage [42]. The solvent also plays an essential role in the manufacture of highly porous nanofibers.

When a polymer is dissolved in two solvents, one of them may act as a non-solvent. The creation of highly porous electrospun nanofibers results from the phase separation caused by the different evaporation rates of the solvent and non-solvent [30]. Y. Zhang et al. [43] reported similar outcomes as well. Change in the proportions of tetrahydrofuran (THF) and dimethylformamide (DMF), according to Megelski et al. created porous nanofibers [33]. Along with the solvent's volatility, its conductivity and dipole moment are crucial factors to consider.

Jarusuwannapoom et al. conducted an experiment involving eighteen different solvents to measure conductivity and dipole moment. Ultimately, it was determined that ethyl acetate, DMF, THF, methyl ethyl ketone, and 1,2-dichloroethane can be utilized in the electrospinning of polystyrene polymeric solution due to their comparatively higher electrical conductivity and dipole moment [44].

4.7. Effect of Humidity and Temperature

Recently, it was reported that environmental (ambient) factors such as relative humidity and temperature also impact the nanofibers' diameter and morphology in addition to electrospinning and solution parameters [45]. Pelipenko et al. used PVA and PEO to study how the diameter of nanofibers changed as the humidity changed. They noticed that as humidity increased from 4% to 60%, the diameter of the nanofibers decreased from 667 nm to 161 nm (PVA) and 252 nm to 75 nm (PEO). Park and Lee also observed that the average diameter of PEO nanofibers reduces in relation to an increase in humidity, which counterbalances the effects of temperature on the diameter [32]. Temperature alters the average diameter of the nanofibers in two opposing ways. Firstly, it speeds up solvent evaporation; secondly, it reduces solution viscosity. The mean fiber diameter decreases as a consequence of both the increased dissolution and the decreased solution viscosity, which operate through two different mechanisms. Vrieze et al. reported a similar observation while working with poly(vinylpyrrolidone) (PVP) and cellulose acetate (CA) [46].

Table 1. Effects of main electrospinning factors (solution, processing and ambient) on fiber morphology.

Parameters	Effect on Fiber Morphology	References
Viscosity	A thicker fiber diameter is caused by a thicker consistency of the liquid. There is no any continuous fiber formation if the viscosity is very low, and it is challenging to expel the jet from the needle tip if it is too high.	[47]
Polymer concentration	Increase in fiber diameter with an increase in concentration.	[48]
Molecular weight of polymer	Reduction in the number of beads and droplets with an increase in molecular weight.	[49]
Electrical Conductivity	Decrease in fiber diameter with an increase in conductivity.	[50]
Applied voltage	Decrease in fiber diameter with an increase in voltage.	[51]
Distance between tip and collector	Generation of beads with too small and too large distances, a minimum distance required for uniform fibers.	[52]
Feed rate/Flow rate	Decrease in fiber diameter with a decrease in flow rate, generation of beads with too high flow rate.	[53]
Humidity	High humidity results in circular pores on the fibers.	[54]
Temperature	Increase in temperature results in a decrease in fiber diameter.	[54]

5. Wound Dressings with Multiple Functions

Research has been conducted in recent years to develop dressings with a variety of capabilities that fulfill all the requirements for successful wound healing. Electrospinning, a scope of regular or engineered polymers and including drugs, nanoparticles, and bioactive mixtures, can be utilized to make multifunctional composite frameworks.

5.1. Antibacterial Activity of Electrospun Nanofibers for Wound Dressing

Antibacterial treatments for wound recuperation are a well-known research region since wound contaminations are a major worldwide concern. To limit the adverse consequences of contaminations in the injury locale, it is basic to utilize an injury dressing that can both blockade bacterial infiltration and microbial colonization into the injury site while likewise encouraging skin recovery. Most antibacterial nanofibers are fabricated by electrospinning antibacterial mixtures into the filaments. Anti-infection agents, metallic nanoparticles, and compounds obtained from regular concentrates have all been joined to work on the antibacterial properties of electrospun nanofibers. Metallic nanomaterials, for example, such as zinc oxide, silver, iron oxide, and gold nanoparticles (AgNPs), are notable for their capacity to mend wounds [55].

They can be utilized in the creation of wound dressings due to their capacity to combat human pathogens. Due to this, researchers have recently become very interested in metallic nanoparticles. Particularly fascinating are silver nanoparticles. They have a high degree of toxicity and a broad area, making them more likely to come into contact with pathogens [56]. Silver nanoparticles have been commonly used for the production of antimicrobial materials [57]. Incorporating metal nanoparticles and metal oxide into the polymeric membrane structure is one of the greatest ways to fabricate dressings with antibacterial properties. Examples of materials that have a wide pore size, great gas flow-through capability, and a high ratio of surface area to the volume include hydrogels, nanocomposites, and nanofibers. An overview of current nanoparticles and nanomaterials-based wound dressings is shown in Table 2.

The ideal approach for developing materials for wound healing appears to be the combination of hydrogels, nanocomposites, or nanofibers with nanoparticles. Multiple methods of incorporating Ag nanoparticles into the polymer structure can be achieved through electrospinning, chemical alteration, and the creation of hydrogels [58].

Bioactive wound dressings often have their antimicrobial properties increased with the addition of silver nanoparticles [59]. Silver nanoparticles offer several advantages for wound healing, such as low toxicity to the body, an antibacterial effect, and the prevention of drug resistance [60].

Ganesh et al. developed PVA–chitosan composite electrospun nanofibers with co-encapsulated Ag nanoparticles and sulfanilamide to have a synergistic wound-healing effect. In order to verify that the physicochemical characteristics of Ag nanoparticle-loaded nanofibers were successfully formulated, X-ray diffraction analysis and Fourier transform infrared spectroscopy were used. The results from SEM images indicate that the nanofibers have a continuous and smooth structure with an average diameter of 150 nm, making them suitable for encapsulating silver nanoparticles for the treatment of microbially infected wound healing. In addition, the swelling analysis showed that the amount of Ag nanoparticles and sulphanilamide had an effect on how much the PVA–chitosan nanofibers swelled. To prevent the nanofibers from absorbing water and swelling, the Ag nanoparticles and sulphanilamide were bound to the polymer matrix using hydrogen bonds [61]. Research on antibacterial activity showed that the zone of inhibition against *Staphylococcus aureus*, *Escherichia coli*, and *Pseudomonas aeruginosa* was notably increased when PVA–chitosan nanofibers were combined with Ag nanoparticles and sulphanilamide in comparison with the plain nanofiber. This implies that the antimicrobial effect of the scaffold was improved by the combination of Ag nanoparticles and sulphanilamide. In vivo results using a rat model showed that the PVA–chitosan nanofibers and the co-loaded nanofibers had similar results, both of which reached $90.76 \pm 4.3\%$ after seven days. In contrast, the control group had a wound closure rate of $55.26 \pm 3.5\%$ after 20 days. Alipour et al. developed PVA–pectin-based nanofibers with Ag nanoparticles loaded into them for use in the treatment of wounds. The creation of PVA–pectin nanofibers was confirmed by the use of energy dispersive X-ray analysis (EDS), XRD analysis, and FTIR spectra analysis. Testing of the fibers' mechanical properties, such as elongation at break ($260.5 \pm 8.2\%$), Young's modulus (7.7 ± 0.21 Mpa), and tensile strength (63.4 ± 3.3 Mpa), showed good results. Furthermore, the in vitro cytotoxicity evaluation of the polymeric nanofibers using the MTT assay revealed that HSF-PI 18 fibroblast cells had a high rate of viability and demonstrated strong antibacterial effects against *Escherichia coli*, *Pseudomonas aeruginosa*, and *Staphylococcus aureus strains*.

Lee et al. designed nanofibers fabricated of chitosan, with silver nanoparticles entrapped within, for the fast recovery of bacteria-infected wounds. The SEM images illustrated that the mean fiber diameters for the plain nanofibers and nanoparticle-loaded nanofibers were 460 ± 80 nm and 126 ± 28 nm, respectively. The in vitro experiments of the nanofibers demonstrated a sizeable inhibition area against Methicillin-resistant *Staphylococcus aureus* and *P. aeruginosa*, suggesting that the chitosan-based nanofibers coated with Ag nanoparticles may be a suitable treatment for contaminated wounds [62].

Table 2. An overview of recent nanoparticles and nanomaterials-based wound dressings.

Electrospun Material	Nanoparticle	Bacterial Species	Composite Nanofiber Diameter	Electrospinning Parameter	Reference
The polyethylene oxide/Graphene oxide was electrospun with peppermint oil	CeO_2	*S. aureus* and *E. coli*	310–365 nm	Electrospinning was conducted 15 cm away from the source and with a voltage of 15 kV, while the feeding rate remained at 1 mL per hour.	[63]
Nanofibrous scaffolds from Gum Arabic, polycaprolactone, and polyvinyl alcohol	Ag (10–100 nm)	*S. aureus, P. aeruginosa, E. coli*, and fungus *Candida albicans*	150–250 nm	A 10 mL syringe that held the ready-fabricated polymeric solution was filled with it, and a syringe pump was used to deliver it at a flow rate of 0.5 mL/h. The voltage that was used was 18 kV, and the distance between the tip and the collector was 150 mm.	[64]
Electrospun Chitosan/Gelatin	Fe_3O_4	*S. aureus* and *E. coli*	307–435 nm	The following electrospinning parameters were set: 0.8 mL/h feeding rate; 15 kV voltage; and 15 cm distance between the needle tip and collector.	[65]
Polyethylene Oxide/Carboxymethyl Chitosan Nanofibers	Ag (12–18 nm)	*S. aureus, P. aeruginosa, E. coli*, and fungus *Candida albicans*	50–300 nm	The composite fiber membranes were fabricated as follows: 40% relative humidity, a 20 cm span between needle-to-collector, and a 20 kV applied spinning voltage.	[58]
Polyvinyl alcohol–chitosan composite electrospun nanofibers	Ag	*S. aureus, P. aeruginosa*, and *E. coli*	150 nm	At room temperature and relative humidity of 45.5%, the electrospinning procedure was completed. The collector was placed 15 cm from the needle tip, voltage (15 kV) was used. A single syringe piston pump was used to regulate the solution feed rate at 0.5 mL/min.	[61]
Electrospun chitosan nanofibers	Ag	*S. aureus*, and *P. aeruginosa*	The average fiber diameters of CTS and CTS/AgNPs nanofibers were 460 ± 80 nm, 126 ± 28 nm, 238 ± 46 nm, 343 337 ± 49 nm and 349 ± 56 nm for AgNPs contents of 0, 4, 2, 1.3, and 0.7 wt.%, respectively	The polymer solution was put into a syringe with a Luer lock and 22 G metal blunt needle. A high-voltage DC power supply was used to electro-spin it on an aluminum foil covered rotating mandrel at 23 kV with a 1 mL/h feed rate and a needle tip-to-collector distance was 15 cm.	[62]
Ultrafine Cellulose Acetate Fibers	Ag	*S. aureus, E. coli, K. pneumoniae*, and *P. aeruginosa*	The average diameters of the cellulose acetate fibers electrospun with 0.05 and 0.5 wt.% AgNO3 were 3.3 and 6.9 nm, respectively	Distance of 10 cm from the needle tip to the ground electrode and a flow rate of 3 mL/h, CA solutions electrospun at a voltage of 17 kV.	[66]
Electrospun PVA Nanofibrous Membranes Impregnated Cellulosic Fibers	Ag	*S. aureus*	169 nm	the prepared electrospinning solution was placed in a 10 mL needle tube, and 17 G needles were installed. The spinning distance was adjusted to 15 cm. Voltage was supplied between the needle tip (+14.0 kV) and the roller collector (−3.50 kV) covered with aluminum foil. The collector speed of 80 r/min was chosen. The temperature and relative humidity were kept at (25 ± 5) °C and 30% ± 5%, respectively.	[67]

5.2. Electrospun Wound Dressings Loaded with Bioactive Molecules

Cells (such as neutrophils, macrophages, and fibroblasts), growth factors, and cytokines interact in a complex manner during the various stages of wound healing [68]. To improve this interaction, various biologically active molecules have been incorporated into electrospun membranes by researchers [69]. The wound-healing process needs to be managed with the precise and directed liberation of natural substances (such as growth factors, vitamins, and anti-inflammatory molecules) at the wound site [70]. Figure 4 represents the various bioactive molecules impregnated into nanofibrous scaffold and their functions in the wound-healing process.

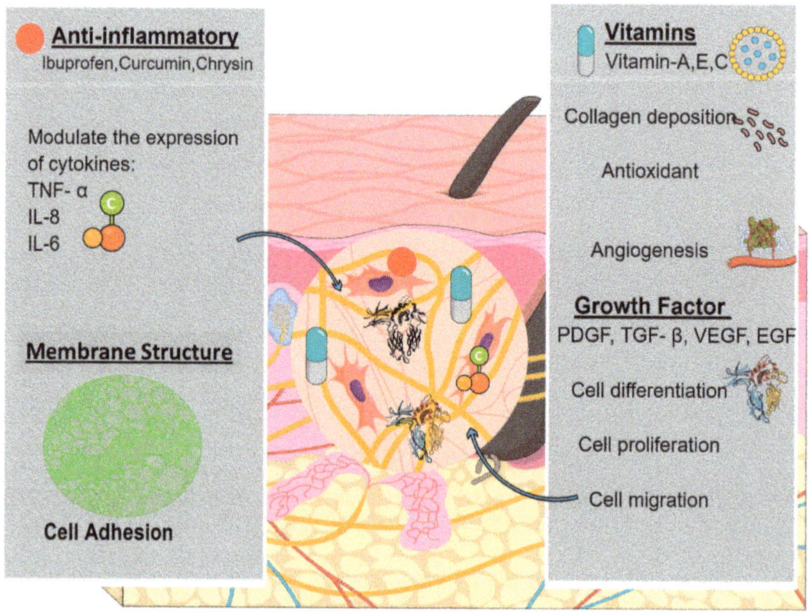

Figure 4. Represents the various bioactive molecules impregnated into nanofibrous scaffolds and their function in wound-healing process.

5.2.1. Growth Factors and Cytokines

GFs are physiologically active polypeptides that regulate cell proliferation, migration, differentiation, metabolism and proliferation during the healing process of wounds [71]. The recuperating system for wounds is constrained by a large number of development variables and cytokines, for example transforming development factor-β (TGF-β), fibroblast development factor (FGF), epidermal development factor (EGF), platelet inferred development factor (PDGF), and vascular endothelial development factor (VEGF) [72]. Fragments such as TGF-β, IL-1, IL-6, PDGF, EGF, and VEGF are all essential for the formation of granulation tissue, control of the inflammatory process, and the promotion of angiogenesis. In order to improve skin regeneration, Norouzi et al. [73] looked into the manufacture of core–shell nanofibrous membranes fabricated of gelatin and poly (lactic-co-glycolic) acid (PLGA) using multi-jet electrospinning. These membranes demonstrated the presence of gelatin and PLGA-EGF nanofibers with diameters that range from 315 nm to 465 nm and 130 nm to 220 nm, respectively. The swelling capacity of the membranes was improved by the combination of PLGA and gelatin nanofibers, with the swelling ratio rising from 23 ± 4% for pure PLGA fibers to 130 ± 10% for PLGA/gelatin nanofibrous membranes. In addition, after a beginning burst rescue, the EGF rescue from these membranes occurred over the course of a 9-day sustained release. Additionally, these membranes were able to increase collagen type I and III expressions, cell proliferation, adhesion, and blood clotting.

Jin, G et al. used two distinct techniques to include multiple epidermal induction factors in to gelatin/poly (l-lactic acid)-co-poly(caprolactone) (PLLCL) nanofibers: Four different types of nanofibers were prepared using the blend electrospinning approach, with diameters of 456 ± 62 nm, 382 ± 100 nm, 299 ± 46 nm, and 366 ± 125 nm. The gelatin/PLLCL/EIF (b) nanofibers had a burst release of EGF over the first three days and then stabilized, with a release of 77.8% after 15 days. On the other hand, the gelatin/PLLCL/EIF (cs) nanofibers had a more sustained diffusion of EGF, with a cumulative release of 50.9% after 15 days [74]. This controlled release had a positive effect on ADSCs, leading to a 43.6% increase in cell multiplication on the gelatin/PLLCL/EIF (cs) nanofibers compared with the gelatin/PLLCL/EIF (b) nanofibers. Furthermore, the rates of cell multiplication on the gelatin/PLLCL/EIF (cs) and gelatin/PLLCL/EIF (b) nanofibers were 560% and 404%, respectively, between days 5 and 15.

5.2.2. Vitamins

Vitamins A, C, and E to the injured area can accelerate the healing process [75]. Vitamin A encourages the production of macrophages and monocytes at the wound site, as well as stimulating collagen production and re-epithelialization [76]. The ability of Vitamin E to promote angiogenesis, lessen scarring, and have antioxidant and anti-inflammatory effects also helps to speed up wound injury [77].

Sheng et al. looked at adding the PEGylated derivative of Vitamin E (TPGS), i.e., D-α-Tocopheryl polyethylene glycol 1000 succinate to Silk fibroin (SF) nanofibers in order to hasten the healing of wounds [78]. The membranes produced TPGS in an initial burst during the initial half hour after production, after which it gradually diffused over the following three days. Furthermore, the L929 cells were able to survive and proliferate on the surface of nanofibers infused with TPGS (2, 4, and 8% w/w) and SF.

In 2018, Kheradvar et al. created SF_PVA_AV nanofibers with starch nanoparticles that had been loaded with Vitamin E (VE-SNPs) [79]. The VE-SNPs generated had a mean diameter of 44.7 nm, a 91.63% encapsulation efficiency, and a round shape morphology. The SF_PVA_AV nanofibers had a diameter of 298.23 ± 6.92 nm. These nanofibers released Vit E rapidly in the first 4 h and then had a sustained release over the duration of 144 h. Moreover, the antioxidant activity increased by 34.7 ± 2.05% (for 1 mg) and 66.27 ± 3.7% (for 5 mg) due to the VE-SNPs loading. Testing showed that the electrospun membranes were biocompatible as they can help with fibroblast adhesion, spreading, and proliferation.

Vit C was incorporated into SF nanofibrous matrices by Fan and their collaborators [80]. It was found that when the quantity of Vitamin C in SF nanofibers was augmented, the average size of the fibers went up from 362 ± 121 nm (with 1 wt.% Vit C) to 416 ± 133 nm and then 506 ± 68 nm (with 3 wt.% Vitamin C).

The SF nanofibers show a burst of Vit C rescue in the initial 20 min before leveling out after 250 min (60% for 1 wt.% Vitamin C and 70% for 3 wt.% Vitamin C). The incorporation of Vit C caused the key functional genes (Col1a1, Gpx1, and Cat) in the membranes to be expressed at a higher level, resulting in more viable cells.

5.2.3. Anti-Inflammatory Agents

The first anti-inflammatory molecule to be introduced into electrospun nanofibers was curcumin [81]. Curcumin can suppress the inflammatory enzymes cyclo-oxygenase (COX)-2 and lipoxygenase (LOX) as well as inhibit the release of two inflammatory cytokines (Interleukin (IL)-8 and tumor necrosis factor (TNF)-α released by monocytes and macrophages [82]. Merrell et al. conducted research on PCL nanofibers loaded with curcumin for use as wound dressings. The diameters of the nanofibers shifted from 300–400 nm (for PCL nanofibers) to 200–800 nm (for PCL/curcumin nanofibers) when 3% and 17% of curcumin were incorporated [83]. The nanofibers were capable of releasing curcumin for three days, which had a protective effect on HFF-1 cells exposed to hydrogen peroxide and decreased the pro-inflammatory response of lipopolysaccharide-stimulated mouse peritoneal macrophages. The IL-6 expression dropped from around 1220 pg/mL to around 600 and 400 pg/mL for cells treated with PCL nanofibers loaded with 3% and 17% curcumin, respectively. By day 10, mice treated with PCL nanofibers containing curcumin had nearly 80% wound closure, significantly higher than the 60% seen for mice treated with PCL nanofibers only. Due to its anti-inflammatory effects, chrysin, a natural flavonoid found in a variety of plant extracts have also been added to nanofiber-based wound dressings [84]. Deldar and his team blended chrysin into PCL/poly(ethylene glycol) (PEG) nanofibrous meshes to create a wound dressing with anti-inflammatory and antioxidant characteristics. This is because chrysin is known to impede nitric oxide (NO) synthase, the manufacture of NO, and the release of TNF-α and IL-1β, as well as reducing lipopolysaccharide-activated COX-2 expression [85].

Mohiti-Asli and their fellow researchers incorporated ibuprofen into PLA nanofibers to promote the mending of third-degree wounds [86]. The presence of ibuprofen in the production of nanoscaffolds led to an increase in their diameters, with values of 329.11 $\pm$ 249.62 nm, 478.31 $\pm$ 167.61 nm, and 585.38 $\pm$ 131.51 nm for 10%, 20%, and 30% of ibuprofen, respectively. These nanofibrous mats were noted to be helpful in facilitating cell attachment, especially the PLA nanofibrous mat containing 20% ibuprofen. In addition, the PLA nanofibrous mat with 20% IBP was found to be capable of degrading when applied to third-degree wounds in mice, resulting in a 60% wound contraction after 14 days. Table 3 outlines a selection of growth factors, vitamins, and anti-inflammatory agents that can be included in electrospun meshes for wound healing.

Table 3. List of different growth hormones, vitamins, and anti-inflammatory agents that can be integrated into electrospun fabrics for treating wounds.

Growth Factor	Polymer	Technique Used	Fiber Diameter	Release Profile	Main Findings	Reference
Epidermal growth factor (EGF)	Gelatin and a combination of lactic acid and glycolic acid (PLGA)	Emulsion electrospinning	• Diameter of Polylactic glycolic acid: 630 ± 80 nm • Diameter of Gelatin: 175 ± 45 nm • Diameter of Polylactic glycolic acid /Epidermal growth factor/gelatin: 390 ± 75 nm	The EGF release profile shows a rapid release on day 1, and continuous release throughout the course of nine days (total EGF release was 4.2 ± 0.2 ng/mL).	The MTT experiment revealed that fi fibroblast proliferation was greater on PLGA/EGF/gelatin membranes.	[73]
EGF, insulin, hydrocortisone, and retinoic acid	Gelatin/ PLLCL	Blend electrospinning: gelatin/PLLCL (b) Co-axial electrospinning: gelatin/PLLCL (cs)	• Diameter of PLLCL: 456 ± 62 nm • Diameter of Gelatin/PLLCL: 382 ± 100 nm • Diameter of gelatin/PLLCL/EIF (b): 299 ± 46 nm • Diameter of gelatin/PLLCL/EIF (cs): 366 ± 125 nm	• Gelatin/PLLCL/EIF (b): approximately 77.8% of Epidermal Growth Factor had been released after 15 days. • Gelatin/PLLCL/EIF (cs): approximately 50.9% of EGF released after 15 days.	The ASCs (adipose-derived stem cells) multiplied to a greater extent (43.6%) when in a combination of gelatin/PLLCL/EIF (cs) than when in gelatin/PLLCL/EIF alone. (b) The proportion of differentiated epidermal cells was 62.2% and 43.0% for gelatin/PLLCL/EIF (cs) and gelatin/PLLCL/EIF (b) membranes, respectively.	[74]
Vitamins	Polymer	Technique used	Fiber diameter	Encapsulation efficiency	Main conclusions	Reference
Vitamin E	SF	Blend electrospinning	• Silk Fibroin/Vit E (2%) average diameter: 722.52 ± 300 nm • Silk Fibroin/Vit E (4%) average diameter: 387.9 ± 114 nm • Silk Fibroin/Vit E (8%) average diameter: 384.3 ± 161 nm	• Silk fibroin/Vitamin E (2%): 65.82%. • Silk fibroin/Vitamin E (4%): 78.59%. • Silk fibroin/Vitamin E (8%): 70.02%.	In the initial 30 min, there was a rapid release of the drug observed from Vit E, which was then followed by a gradual release over the next 72 h. Moreover, supplementing L929 cells with Vitamin E allowed them to adhere better and grow faster.	[78]
Vitamin E	SF/PVA/AV	Vit E loaded into starch nanoparticles and blend with electrospinning solution	• SF/PVA/AV: 298.23 ± 6.92 nm	Vitamin E into starch nanoparticles was 91.63%.	Vitamin E released quickly at first, then slowly over the course of 144 h; The higher Vit E level led to enhanced antioxidant activity. In contact with electrospun membranes, the fibroblasts cells continued to be functional, adhering and dividing.	[79]

Table 3. *Cont.*

Growth Factor	Polymer	Technique Used	Fiber Diameter	Release Profile	Main Findings	Reference
Vit C	Silk Fibroin	Blend electrospinning	• Silk Fibroin: 362 ± 121 nm • Silk fibroin/Vitamin C (1%): 416 ± 133 nm • Silk Fibroin/Vitamin C (3%): 506 ± 68 nm	NA	A burst peak was visible in the Vit C release profile from SF nanofibers during the first 20 min. Vitamin C had a positive effect on the viability of fibroblasts, as well as boosting the mRNA levels of key genes such as Col1a1, Gpx1, and Cat.	[80]
Anti-inflammatory molecule	Polymer	Technique used	Fiber diameter	Release profile	Main findings	Reference
Curcumin	Polycaprolactone	Blend electrospinning	• Polycaprolactone: 300–400 nm • Polycaprolactone/curcumin: 200–800 nm	• Polycaprolactone or curcumin (17%): 35 microgram was released on 3rd day. • PCL/curcumin (3%): 20 microgram was released on 3rd day.	The antioxidant qualities of fibers loaded with curcumin were further demonstrated by the Oxygen Radical Absorbance Capacity (ORAC) assay. The membranes had a cytoprotective effect on human fibroblast cells and were biocompatible. In vivo tests conducted in a living organism demonstrated that PCL/curcumin nanofibers had the capacity to accelerate the recovery of injuries in a diabetic mouse model.	[83]
Chrysin (Chr)	PCL/PEG	Blend electrospinning	• Polycaprolactone/poly (ethylene glycol): 300–400 nm • Polycaprolactone/poly (ethylene glycol)/Chrysin: 250–650	• Polycaprolactone/poly(ethylene glycol)/Chrysin (5%): 25 micrograms of Chrysin was released after 3 days. • Polycaprolactone/poly (ethylene glycol/Chrysin (15%): 96%): 43 micrograms of Chrysin was released after 3 days.	It was demonstrated that the nanofibers, which had antioxidant properties and were biocompatible, had cytoprotective effects on human fibroblast cells when they were loaded with Chrysin. The reduced levels of IL-6, IL-1β, tumor necrosis factor-α, and NO in macrophages showed the anti-inflammatory capabilities of Chrysin-filled nanofibrous mats.	[85]
Ibuprofen	PLA	Blend electrospinning	• Poly lactic acid/ibuprofen (10%): 329.11± 249.62 nm • Poly lactic acid/ibuprofen (20%): 478.31 ± 167.61 nm • Poly lactic acid/ibuprofen (30%): 585.38 ± 131.51 nm	0.25 milligrams of ibuprofen was released from poly lactic acid/ibuprofen (30%) nanofibers after 336 h.	The nanofibers with 20 wt.% IBP had the highest cell viability and proliferation. The addition of IBP to PLA nanofibers encouraged the growth and viability of both HEK and HDF.	[87]

6. Wound Healing Using Bio-Based Electrospun Fibers

Bio-based polymers are regular macromolecules fabricated by carrying on with living things (generally called biopolymers). Plants (cellulose, lignin), animals (collagen, chitin, chitosan), microorganisms (bacterial cellulose, PHA), and biotechnological processes are wellsprings of biopolymers. By virtue of their specific credits, they have displayed promising results in biomedical applications; for instance, drug movement, tissue planning, and wound patching are listed in Figure 5.

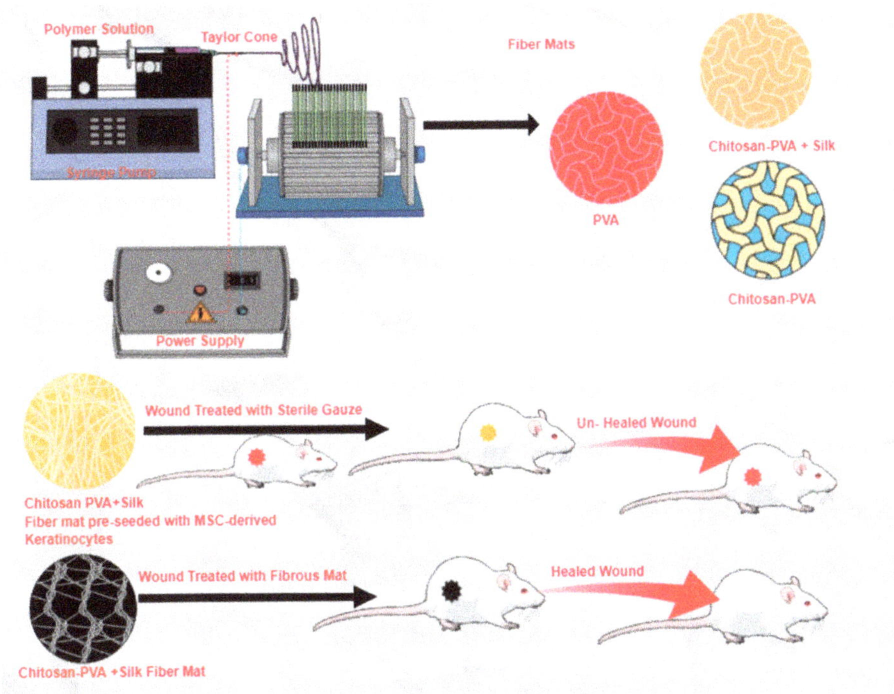

Figure 5. Electrospun Chitosan–PVA-Silk nanofibers mat for wound healing.

Biopolymers, in their unadulterated structure or in a mix with different polymers, can be framed into stringy platforms, making them an engaging contender for skin substitution. Various electrospun biopolymer dressings with different functions and wound type targets are listed in Table 4.

Table 4. Different electrospun biopolymer dressings with different functions and wound type targets.

Electrospun Mesh	Incorporated Therapeutics	Function and Wound Type	References
Chitosan/Poly (l-lactide)	Graphene oxide	Antimicrobial action in infected chronic injuries.	[88]
Chitosan/keratin/polycaprolactone	Aloe vera extract	Burn and acute wounds can be aided by properties that are anti-inflammatory, antibacterial, antiviral, and antioxidant.	[7]
Polyhydroxyalkanoates	Dodecyl trimethylammonium chloride biocide	The antioxidant, anti-inflammatory, and anti-infective qualities of certain substances can provide a boost to cell reinforcement and angiogenic properties for diabetic injuries, resulting in antimicrobial effects for chronic wounds.	[89]
Polydopamine or polylactic glycolic acid	Fibroblast growth factor and ponericin G1 are both present	The skin tissue regeneration process has antibacterial and cell growth-promoting properties.	[90]
Chitosan/Polyvinyl alcohol	Nanobioglass	For chronic injuries, biocompatibility, antimicrobial action, and recovery advancement.	[91]
PLGA	Ciprofloxacin	Antibacterial and skin tissue regenerative effects that encourage cell growth	[90]
PLA	Doxycycline	Antibacterial activity, chronic wounds.	[92]
PHBV/cellulose	Zinc Oxide nanocrystals	Antibacterial activity in wounds that are both acute and infected.	[93]
PLLA	Curcumin	Antioxidant, anti-inflammatory effects.	[94]
CA/polyester urethane	Polyhexamethylene biguanide	Antimicrobial activity.	[95]

6.1. Biomaterials for Wound Healing: Cellulose Electrospun Nanofibers

Cellulose, is a naturally occurring biopolymer that is friendly to the environment and biocompatible and biodegradable, and has multiple biomedical uses such as constructing scaffolds for tissue regeneration, wound dressings, artificial tissue and skin, managing drug release, cleaning blood, and creating materials for cell cultures [96]. Similar research was performed on bacterial cellulose-based scaffolds to see if they can be used in pre-clinical and clinical trials, such as for wound dressings for skin lesions [97]. A patient with second-degree burns on his face was provided Nanocell®, a bacterial cellulose-based scaffold, in order to facilitate the healing process without the need to apply additional bandages to the wound sites. After two weeks, the facial burns were completely repaired without any allergic or skin-irritating reactions, demonstrating the effectiveness of bacterial cellulose dressings for treating burned skin. Electrospinning is a novel technology that can be utilized to produce cellulose nanofibers, various polymer/cellulose mixtures, or blends of cellulose with nanoparticles that possess increased functional qualities, such as antimicrobial features to prevent wound site infection [98].

Nonwoven nanofibers with extensive surface areas and closely interlinked pores are especially useful for treating wounds as they are able to absorb large quantities of exudate and promote effective gas exchange [99]. Additionally, cellulose scaffolds can carry a range of bioactive compounds, such as molecules that reduce inflammation and kill bacteria [100]. Roy et al. [101] confirmed the potency of bamboo-incorporated paclitaxel-infused cellulose electrospun fibers in the treatment of skin cancer and wound recovery. Song et al. conducted an experiment where the surfaces of cellulose, carboxymethylated cellulose (CMC), and ribbon-shaped CA electrospun fibers were modified with Ag nanoparticles at various pH levels [102]. The antimicrobial characteristics and application potential of CMC fibers were amplified by the addition of silver nanoparticles which were arranged in the following order at the same pH levels: CMC > cellulose > CA.

6.2. Chitosan Electrospun Nanofibers for Wound Healing

Chitin and its deacetylated version, chitosan, have antibacterial, biocompatible, and hemostatic characteristics, which can be used to heal injuries [103]. Chitosan has antibacterial action in its capacity as a feeble polybase because of the presence of countless amino gatherings on its chain. The favourable to incendiary properties of chitosan have been proposed to assume a significant part in injury recuperating. Chitosan initiates macrophages, which helps with the recuperating of wounds. Moreover, chitosan can cause polymorphonuclear neutrophils (PMNs) to relocate during the beginning phases of wound mending, bringing about the arrangement of granulation tissue. Jayakumar et al. showed that chitosan has the capacity to stimulate the regeneration of the skin's granular layer and re-epithelialization [104].

Furthermore, due to its strong bond with the injury and its capability to interact with negatively charged red blood cells, chitosan is able to successfully halt bleeding [105]. Min et al. fabricated chitin and chitosan nanoscaffolds for wound dressing by using electrospinning with 1,1,1,3,3,3-hexafluoro-2-propanol as the spinning solvent. The pro-inflammatory properties of chitosan have been recommended to assume a significant part in injury recuperating. Chitosan enacts macrophages, which support the mending of wounds. Moreover, chitosan can cause polymorphonuclear neutrophils (PMNs) to relocate during the beginning phases of wound mending, bringing about the development of granulation tissue.

Chitosan compounds containing quaternary ammonium bunches have been demonstrated to be antibacterial and antifungal. The cytoplasmic film of the bacterial cell is normally perceived as the objective area of these cationic polymers. Wound dressings can be produced using miniature and nanoscale nanofibrous materials. Chen and partners portrayed a nanofibrous layer fabricated of chitosan and collagen that has been displayed to work on injury recuperation. The film was found to advance injury recuperation, cell relocation, and expansion. Noh et al. investigated the cytocompatibility of chitin nanofibers.

The three-layered properties of these materials and their high surface area to volume ratios may be responsible for this, as they are perfect for cell attachment, advancement, and multiplication. In one review, to fabricate composite fibers, PEO/chitosan arrangements and polycaprolactone (PCL)/olive oil arrangements were electrospun together. Olive oil, chitosan, PCL, and PEO composite nanofibers were successfully created using the electrospinning process. By employing SEM and FTIR, the structure and shape of electrospun nanofibers were determined. The response surface methodology and Box-Behnken design were utilized to identify the relationship between the parameters of the process and the diameter of electrospun nanofibers, with the predicted minimum value of diameter being 88 nm when voltage, TCD, and flow rate were used at three levels (21.2 kV, flowrate of 0.2 mL hr^{-1}, and tip to collector distance of 14.3 cm). These data were consistent with the experimental data of 86 nm. It was established that the optimal weight percentage of olive oil was 2% through the integration of different weight percentages of olive oil into electrospun nanofibers. After a one-day study, 58.1% of the total olive oil encapsulation was released, according to the in vitro release behavior of olive oil from PEO/chitosan/PCL/olive oil scaffolds. It was observed that cell attachment of the created nanofibrous scaffolds was satisfactory, with cell proliferation and a non-toxic behavior being demonstrated by the cytotoxicity results [106].

6.3. Effectiveness of Electrospun PLA Nanofibrous Scaffolds in Wound Healing

Polylactic acid (PLA) is a biopolymer that is created from a mixture of synthetic elements. Its components, such as maize starch, sugar, and rice are easy to obtain and are used in the process of ring-opening or lactic acid condensation polymerization to form the PLA monomer, which is 2-hydroxypropionic acid. There are three isomers of PLA: poly(d-lactide), racemic poly(dl-lactide), and poly(l-lactide) [107]. PLA is a thermoplastic polyester with thermomechanical properties that is both biocompatible and biodegradable, as well as able to be absorbed by living organisms. Alves et al. demonstrated that PLA electrospun membranes can be used effectively as drug delivery systems for sustained release applications in the formation of wound dressings [108]. The efficiency of dexamethasone acetate (DEX) and betamethasone being released was tested using physical adsorption and mix electrospinning techniques through PLA electrospun strands. The effects of the drugs on the morphological and mechanical properties of the PLA fibers were investigated. When the pharmaceuticals were mixed with the PLA solution and electrospun, the drug-loaded fibers had a more consistent release profile over the initial five hours than when the drugs were simply attached to the PLA electrospun membranes. Moradkhannejhad et al. investigated how PLA electrospun nanofibers loaded with curcumin can have their hydrophobicity changed by adding PEG with different molecular weights and concentrations [109].

Yang, C et al. employed coaxial electrospinning to create a (PGS)/PLLA fibrous scaffold with a PGS core and a PLLA shell. This type of structure showed enhanced cell proliferation and less inflammation than a pure PLLA scaffold. Additionally, when the poly glycerol sebacate or CUR or PEG nanofibers were incubated in PBS, an increase in weight loss values was observed when both the concentration and molecular weight of PEG were adjusted. The electrospun CUR-loaded PEG or PLA membranes were able to adjust the hydrophilicity and hydrophobicity of the medium, thus providing favourable conditions for cell growth as well as improved drug delivery. The porous shell surface shape of the generated fibers highlighted their exceptional ability to repair skin injured tissues [107]. Augustine et al. used coaxial electrospinning to create wound-healing nanofibers that consisted of core–shell fibers. Yang, C et al. utilized this method to create a core–shell structured PLLA/chitosan nanofibrous scaffold. GO nanosheets were then coated on the core PLLA-shell chitosan nanofibers to create a synergistic microenvironment for fast wound recovery [110]. This increased the membrane's hydrophilicity. Chitosan/PLLA nanofibrous scaffolds with GO coating showed promising antibacterial activity and stimulated the growth of pig iliac endothelial cells. In rats, GO-coated chitosan/PLLA nanoscaffolds provided a positive effect on wound healing [111].

6.4. Utilization of Electrospun PHA Nanofibrous Scaffolds in Wound Healing

PHAs are a type of biopolyester thermoplastic [112]. Many bacteria create them as a substitute source of nutrition (carbon) when growth is not steady.

Shishatskaya et al. [113] used poly (3-hydroxybutyrate-co-4-hydroxybutyrate) due to its low crystallinity and good elasticity, which is considered one of the best PHAs for producing electrospun fibers for wound-healing applications. They found that the presence of fibroblasts had a significant influence on the quantity of hyperemia and purulent exudate, and concluded that composite fibers were a better choice for wound-healing applications. It was determined that wound healing under the cell-loaded poly (3-hydroxybutyrate-co-4-hydroxybutyrate) membrane was 1.4 times faster than wound healing under the cell-free membrane and 3.5 times faster than wound healing under the eschar membrane (control) [114]. Over the last three decades, PHA has been shown in numerous studies to have a variety of benefits over other biomaterials in medical applications, including biocompatibility, mechanical stability, strength, and biodegradability under physiological conditions with non-toxic degradation products. It was discovered that some PHA breakdown products have potential use in the pharmaceutical industry and have demonstrated a growth-suppressing effect on bacteria [115].

The cell-loaded membrane group regained all its areas after two weeks, while the pure poly (3-hydroxybutyrate-co-4-hydroxybutyrate) meshes in the control groups had 90% and 70% area reductions, respectively.

The application of electrospun fibrous meshes containing keratin and 3-hydroxybutyrate-co-3-hydroxyvalerate (PHBV) for wound dressing purposes was investigated [116]. Azimi et al. used electrospinning to manufacture a combination of poly (3-hydroxybutyrate)/poly(3-hydroxyoctanoate-co-3-hydroxydecanoate) [P(3HB)/P(3HO-co-3HD)]. Additionally, they decorated the fiber meshes with chi-tin-lignin/glycyrrhizin acid (CLA) complexes through electrospray [117]. CLA complexes are organic molecules on a microscopic scale that have been demonstrated to be useful for enhancing the skin's properties when tested on an artificial skin sample [118].

Kandhasamy et al. designed a composite scaffold with a PHB/gelatin/ostholamide blend coating of collagen, which displayed strong anti-inflammatory action, and which is an encouraging indication for wound relief applications. The incorporation of ostholamide into the scaffold provided increased mechanical stability, a slow enzymatic breakdown rate, and successful anti-bacterial action against *Pseudomonas aeruginosa and Staphylococcus aureus* [119]. The NIH 3T3 fibroblast proliferation experiments in both in vivo and in vitro settings proved to be very compatible as seen in successful wound relief in Wistar rats. After fifteen days, the PHB or gelatin or ostholamide (OSA) or collagen scaffold had entirely closed the wound, while the PHB or gelatin or OSA or collagen scaffold, the pure collagen scaffold, and the cotton gauze positive control had all reduced the wound size by 75%, 65%, and 45%, respectively.

6.5. Evaluation of Electrospun PCL Nanofibrous Scaffolds in Wound Healing

Polycaprolactone (PCL) is the most in-demand material due to its semi-crystalline nature and its ability to be adjusted in terms of mechanical properties and solubility in a variety of solvents. This makes it a great option for combining with other polymers. Additionally, compared with other polyesters, PCL breaks down at a slower rate, making it beneficial for certain purposes [120]. The degradation products of PCL are naturally non-toxic, making it a suitable component for skin regeneration therapies. It is often combined with natural polymers such as collagen before electrospinning, or collagen is deposited on the PCL nanofibers. Additionally, PCL has been mixed with gelatin, derived from collagen, and gelatin has been used as the core polymer in core–shell PCL/gelatin nanofibers. Double-nozzle electrospinning has been used to produce separate gelatin and PCL nanofibers, generating two distinct types of nanofibers which can be mixed or layered in the scaffolds [121]. Compared with the other structures, multilayered and blended ones were discovered to be most suitable for the majority of native skin needs. These include whey keratin, protein, chitosan, hyaluronic acid, and fibrinogen [122]. Gum Arabic and Zein (a corn protein) are both utilized as food additives [123]. In addition to PCL, other natural polymers were used to modify the nanofibers. The electrospinning solution combined PCL with these organic polymers, and growth factors such as epidermal growth factor were immobilized onto PCL/collagen or PCL/gelatin nanofibers [124]. TGF-β1 has been incorporated into PCL/collagen electrospinning solutions in the past to alter PCL nanofibrous scaffolds. In this study, alaptide or l-arginine was included in PCL electrospun nanofibrous membranes. Back in the 1980s, Kasafirek et al. at the Research Institute for Pharmacy and Biochemistry in Prague, Czechoslovakia, synthesized alaptide, a spirocyclic dipeptide, which was created to act as an analogue of the melanocyte-stimulating hormone release-inhibiting factor [125].

Alaptide showed considerable promise for enhancing transdermal drug absorption and for repairing harmed tissue [126]. Arginine acts as a precursor for nitric oxide, which is correlated with wound healing. This substance aids the growth, resistance to cell death, and immunity of fibroblasts, which are integral to the healing of wounds [127] and promoted the healing of wounds by forming new skin cells and increasing blood flow.

6.6. Utilization of PES Electrospun Fibers in Wound Healing

Kanji et al. [128] demonstrated that human umbilical cord blood-derived CD34+ cells expanded on Polyether sulfone nanofibers can be effectively used to treat diabetic wounds, speeding up wound closure and improving re-epithelialization and neovascularization. Additionally, the use of CD34+ cells was found to reduce the pro-inflammatory activity of NF-κB and TNF-α, IL-1β, and IL-6, and to prevent MMP-1 from being expressed at a high level. It appears that PES nanofibrous membranes created using electrospinning can be employed as a fresh approach to wound healing, as they have higher absorption capabilities, more matured fibroblast production, and more collagen deposition than other commercial wound treatments.

6.7. Wound Healing Using PS Electrospun Fibers

In its non-crystalline form, polystyrene is a transparent and colorless solid that is fragile, rigid, and has high electrical insulation and minimal dielectric loss. To create a wound dressing, polystyrene was spun with poly caprolactone and chamomile extract, which contains phenolics and flavonoids such as apigenin which is known to have strong wound-healing capabilities [129]. Skin cells were grown in bioreactors that had motion and on electrospun polystyrene nanofibrous scaffolds which were situated at the air/liquid interface [130].

6.8. Application of PAA Electrospun Fibers in Wound Healing

Using poly(acrylic acid) nanofibers combined with reduced graphene oxide, photothermal activation of the nanofibers was used to modulate antibiotic distribution [131]. Another study concluded that electrospun nanofibers fabricated of poly(acrylic acid) and a synthetic biodegradable elastomer called poly(1,8-octanediol-co-citric acid) had intrinsic antibacterial activity and could be used to deliver physiologically relevant growth factor concentrations topically [132].

6.9. Application of Thermoresponsive Electrospun Fibers in Wound Healing

The physical and chemical characteristics of the thermoresponsive polymer used in the fabrication of scaffolds combined with the biological host's regulatory mechanisms are influential in the behavior and function of the scaffolds. Taking advantage of these biological reactions, these scaffolds and the biomaterials that compose them can be used to create novel drug delivery systems that can be used to hasten the wound-healing process, manage the scarring process, and moderate the inflammatory response [133]. Bioactive thermoresponsive nanofiber mats have been created to aid in the treatment of wounds. Various polyblend nanofiber formulations are formed by combining PNIPAAm, PCL, and egg albumin with various concentrations of gatifloxacin hydrochloride (0–20%). These nanofibers exhibit rapid drug release within the first 10 h and sustained release over 696 h. In order to test the antibacterial capabilities of these gati-loaded nanofibers, they are evaluated against the Gram-positive pathogen *Staphylococcus aureus*, which is commonly present in wounds. In the presence of Gati-loaded scaffolds, a decrease in bacterial growth is evident, and the antibacterial properties become more potent as the concentration of Gati rises. In a study involving a rat model, the capacity of nanofibers to stimulate wound healing in vivo was evaluated. The wounds treated with 15% Gati-loaded nanofibers experienced significantly rapid healing than the wounds in control; after 21 days, 95% of the wounds had healed, while only 45% of the wounds in control had been healed. The results of this study demonstrate the capability of thermoresponsive scaffolds in wound healing. Karri et al. [134] created a new nanohybrid scaffold by combining curcumin with chitosan nanoparticles and then embedding it into a collagen scaffold to enhance tissue expansion. According to this study, a combination of curcumin, chitosan, and collagen created using coaxial electrospinning showed excellent healing in diabetes. This combination of drugs, known as a core–shell nanofibrous bioactive insulin-loaded PLGA scaffold created by Lee et al., was able to release a synthetic hormone over a four-week period, aiding in the healing of diabetic wounds [135]. Table 5 shows the various electrospun scaffolds used in the healing of wounds.

Table 5. Summary of various electrospun scaffolds in wound healing.

Electrospun Scaffolds	Main Findings	References
Electrospun fibers fabricated from a combination of Paclitaxel and (2-hydroxyethyl methacrylate)/bamboo cellulose were created.	This structure can be used to combat skin cancer and increase wound recovery.	[101]
Cellulose that has been carboxymethylated and CA electrospun fibers that are shaped like ribbons and contain silver nanoparticles.	The addition of silver nanoparticles improved the antibacterial and healing abilities of CMC fibers.	[102]
Nanofibrous networks fabricated of chitin and chitosan can be created by utilizing 1,1,1,3,3,3-hexafluoro-2-propanol as a spinning solvent.	Chitosan stimulates macrophages to aid in wound repair, causing polymorphonuclear neutrophils to move to the wound site at the initial time of healing.	[136]
PEO/chitosan/PCL/oliveoil (Composite fibers).	Composite fibers exhibited antibacterial action *S. aureus* and *E. coli*, a 0.6-fold decrease in edema, facilitated cell growth, and proliferation.	[106]
A fibrous mesh composed of both poly (glycerol sebacate) and poly L-lactic acid was created via coaxial electrospinning.	Exhibited cell proliferation, with a lower inflammatory response, re-establish pores and skin wound tissues.	[107]
Collagen-coated PHB/gelatin/ostholamide (OSA) Electrospun Nanofiber mesh	Nanofiber mesh shows excellent mechanical stability, reliable enzymatic breakdown, and effective antibacterial development towards *Pseudomonas aeruginosa* and *Staphylococcus aureus*.	[119]
Electrosprayed fiber networks composed of poly(3-hydroxybutyrate)/poly(3-hydroxyoctanoate-co-3-hydroxydecanoate) with a complex of chitin-lignin/glycyrrhizin acid.	CLA complexes useful bio-based mixtures for functionalizing pores and skin contact substrates in an in vitro skin model and helpful in wound healing.	[117]
PCL-gelatin electrospun nanoscaffolds incorporated with quercetin and ciprofoxacin hydrochloride (CH).	The full thickness wound was healed in 16 days.	[137]
Electrospun nanofibers containing Polyacrylic acid, and a synthetic biodegradable elastomer called poly(1,8-octanediol-co-citric acid).	Excellent antibacterial activity and delivery of physiologically relevant growth factor concentrations topically.	[132]
Electrospun mesh of polystyrene incorporated with p chamomile extract and poly(caprolactone).	Excellent wound-healing properties.	[129]

7. Current Commercial Electrospun Wound Dressing

Pathon, TPP-fibers (TecophilicTM), SurgiCLOT, and SpinCareTM are all products that can be used to dress a wound. Table 6 outlines the various commercial electrospun products that can be employed for wound healing. SpinCareTM is a portable electrospinning tool that is often utilized for wound management. SurgiCLOT is a bio-based and polysaccharide wound dressing that is derived from dextran [138]. Glucose-connected polymers encompass dextran, which can be extracted from sucrose through the use of particular lactic acid bacteria such as *Lactobacillus* spp., *Leuconostoc mesenteroides*, and *Streptococcus mutans* [139]. Due to dextran's resistance to both cell adhesion and protein adsorption, hydrogels fabricated from this polysaccharide make excellent scaffolds for soft tissue engineering applications. This biopolymer, which is sometimes referred to as a type of synthetic polymer called polyurethane, is used in clinics because of its antiplatelet characteristics. However, one unique quality of polyurethanes is that they can have natural sources for their monomers. Vegetable oils, such as canola, castor, and olive oils, are the main source of polyols in nature. Therefore, it is possible to anticipate that green polyurethanes will eventually be used in biomedical products. The chemistry of the polyurethane and the method of degradation both have a notable effect on the resulting by-products. Three distinct processes involved in the biological degradation of polyurethanes in the natural environment: hydrolytic, enzymatic, and oxidative.

Table 6. Various electrospun commercial wound dressings.

Product	Polymer	Device	References
Pathon	Polyurethane	Composite mesh, NO drug deliver	[140]
SurgiCLOT®	Dextran	Fibrin Sealant Patch	[141]
SpinCare™	Various electrospinnable polymers	Portable electrospinning wound dressing device	[142]
Tecophilic™	Polyurethane-PEG	Photosensitizing-loaded mesh	[143]

8. Chronic Diabetic Wound Healing Based on Electrospun Nanofibers

Augustine and other researchers presented the formation of a novel cerium oxide nanoparticle composed of an electrospun poly (3-hydroxybutyrate-co-3-hydroxy valerate) membrane [144]. Wound-healing studies in diabetic rats concluded that poly (3-hydroxybutyrate-co-3-hydroxy valerate membranes combined with 1% cerium oxide nanoparticle were completely compatible with cells, making them potential biomaterials for treating the diabetic wound. Lee et al. developed core–shell nanofiber scaffolds that incorporated polylactic glycolic acid and insulin solutions, allowing for a managed release of insulin for four weeks [135]. These scaffolds had more hydrophilic properties than blended nanofibrous scaffolds and were able to retain more water and found to improve diabetic wound, decrease the quantity of type I collagen in vitro, and increase the amount of transforming growth factor-beta (TGF-β) in vivo. Chen et al. created composite nanofiber, containing Polyvinyl alcohol and Chitosan. This composite also had hemostatic and antibacterial qualities and greater mechanical strength [91]. A three-layer synthetic scaffold was created, with chitosan as the first layer, a combination of chitosan and polyvinyl alcohol as the second layer electrospun, and nanobioglass (with up to 40% PVA) as the third layer electrospun. These composite nanofiber mats showed great cytocompatibility with fibroblasts in vitro. On its own, Polyvinyl alcohol can lower the pH of a wound site (5.8–6.2), which can slow down cell growth. However, the addition of chitosan helps to keep the pH level around 6.5, allowing for faster wound healing with less cell damage. In diabetic mice, the resulting composite nanofiber membrane significantly boosted the wound closure rate by reducing inflammation, neovascularization, and increasing the collagen synthesis. The combination of poly (lactic-co-glycolic acid) and collagen in hexafluoro-2-propanol as the solvent enabled the electrospinning technique to form nanofibers. Moreover, this created a humid atmosphere which encouraged cell movement. Research in diabetic mice has demonstrated that metformin can activate the AMPK/eNOS pathway by enhancing the angiogenesis of endothelial progenitor cells [145]. When the PLGA-collagen nanofiber is blended, it brings about a diminishment in the fiber diameter, a rise in the water contact angle, and a higher absorption of water by the nanofibers. Animals with diabetes that had the PLGA-collagen-Met nanofiber treatment showed almost 95% closure of the wound in comparison with those only receiving gauze treatment, which had 73% wound closure [146]. Kargozar et al. examined that the combination of gum tragacanth, poly caprolactone, and polyvinyl alcohol created nanofiber mats with a ninefold higher tensile strength than mats composed of polycaprolactone and gum tragacanth alone, reaching 2.7 MPa in comparison with 0.3 MPa [147]. A rise in the amount of polyvinyl alcohol and gum tragacanth caused a decrease in nanofiber diameter, leading to improved cytocompatibility and accelerated healing of wounds in diabetic rats due to a decrease in polycaprolactone hydrophobicity.

9. Conclusions and Future Prospectives

Nanofibers-based wound dressings have more potential and effectiveness than conventional wound dressings. The wound-healing process is considered to be incredibly complex since it is crucial for maintaining homeostasis. Biomimetic dressings can be fabricated by electrospinning with improved biological activity to promote tissue regeneration, but only a limited number of materials have proved suitable. An emerging field of study reveals the cellular and molecular control mechanisms that regulate the inflammatory response during wound healing, providing an important contribution to pathological tissue repair, as well as theoretical support for electrospinning-based wound-healing regulation. The use of electrospun materials, drugs, or cells to directly stimulate physiological repair has become a promising research field at the molecular level. It may be technically challenging to do so on a molecular level, but it seems possible to mimic the ECM by combining the biological properties of natural polymeric materials with nanoscale structures, thereby stimulating cell migration and proliferation, controlling inflammation, and speeding up wound healing. Electrospun membranes help with cell adhesion, proliferation, and differentiation, and can help prevent or decrease skin infections. In the future, wound-healing scaffolds include theranostic materials that combine interactive and bioactive means together with therapeutic and diagnostic functionality into a single scaffold. It is envisioned that new technologies integrate target biomarkers into scaffolds to monitor wound healing. In addition to excellent antimicrobial, angiogenic, antiproliferative, anti-inflammatory properties, and nanofibers impregnated with biological macromolecules also exhibit greater biocompatibility and biodegradability, as well as high surface-to-volume ratios. However, there are few shortcomings of electrospun nanofibers in the field of wound healing. Therefore, the future challenges can be addressed as follows: (i) By using multiaxial electrospinning setups with multiple needles/needleless spinning techniques, the yield of nanofiber fabrication can be enhanced in industrial and large-scale settings. (ii) Biocompatible nanofibers are required to obtain the best possible morphology, composition, pore size, and diameter for efficient market-scale technology transfer. (iii) Solving the environmental issues and safety matters in solvent evaporation during the spinning process: solvent recovery systems or green chemistry techniques for melt electrospinning. In the near future, the combination of multiple nanofiber production processes and surface modification strategies, such as heat and plasma treatment, will allow the nanofiber's physiochemical properties to be improved. Furthermore, the creation of pH, temperature, light, electrical, or magnetic field responsive nanofibers will allow for the regulated or multi-stage release of biological molecules at the wound site. Clinical trials must be conducted in order to commercialize drug delivery systems based on electrospun membranes intended for skin regeneration and to enhance the quality of life for patients.

Author Contributions: Conceptualization, D.S.; data curation, S.S., S.K. and P.K.S.; writing—original draft preparation, S.S., S.K., P.K.S., R.H., H.G.D. and A.K.; writing—review and editing, S.S., S.K., P.K.S., R.H., H.G.D., A.K. and S.M.; supervision, S.S., D.S. and S.M. All authors have read and agreed to the published version of the manuscript.

Funding: This research was funded by Deputyship for Research and Innovation, Ministry of Education in Saudi Arabia through the project number ISP22-10.

Institutional Review Board Statement: No applicable.

Informed Consent Statement: No applicable.

Data Availability Statement: Data sharing is not applicable.

Acknowledgments: The authors extend their appreciation to the Deputyship for Research and Innovation, Ministry of Education in Saudi Arabia for funding this research work through the project number ISP22-10.

Conflicts of Interest: The authors declare no conflict of interest.

References

1. Adeli, H.; Khorasani, M.T.; Parvazinia, M. Wound dressing based on electrospun PVA/chitosan/starch nanofibrous mats: Fabrication, antibacterial and cytocompatibility evaluation and in vitro healing assay. *Int. J. Biol. Macromol.* **2019**, *122*, 238–254. [CrossRef] [PubMed]
2. Fang, Y.; Zhu, X.; Wang, N.; Zhang, X.; Yang, D.; Nie, J.; Ma, G. Biodegradable core-shell electrospun nanofibers based on PLA and γ-PGA for wound healing. *Eur. Polym. J.* **2019**, *116*, 30–37. [CrossRef]

3. Khan, N. Applications of electrospun nanofibers in the biomedical field. *SURG J.* **2012**, *5*, 63–73. [CrossRef]
4. Miguel, S.P.; Sequeira, R.S.; Moreira, A.F.; Cabral, C.S.; Mendonça, A.G.; Ferreira, P.; Correia, I.J. An overview of electrospun membranes loaded with bioactive molecules for improving the wound healing process. *Eur. J. Pharm. Biopharm.* **2019**, *139*, 1–22. [CrossRef] [PubMed]
5. Dhivya, S.; Padma, V.V.; Santhini, E. Wound dressings—A review. *BioMedicine* **2015**, *5*, 22. [CrossRef] [PubMed]
6. Gong, W.; Li, J.; Ren, G.; Lv, L. Wound healing and inflammation characteristics of the submicrometric mats prepared from electrospinning. *J. Bioact. Compat. Polym.* **2019**, *34*, 83–96. [CrossRef]
7. Zahedi, E.; Esmaeili, A.; Eslahi, N.; Shokrgozar, M.A.; Simchi, A. Fabrication and characterization of core-shell electrospun fibrous mats containing medicinal herbs for wound healing and skin tissue engineering. *Mar. Drugs* **2019**, *17*, 27. [CrossRef]
8. Karimi, K.; Odhav, A.; Kollipara, R.; Fike, J.; Stanford, C.; Hall, J.C. Acute cutaneous necrosis: A guide to early diagnosis and treatment. *J. Cutan. Med. Surg.* **2017**, *21*, 425–437. [CrossRef]
9. Lazarus, G.S.; Cooper, D.M.; Knighton, D.R.; Margolis, D.J.; Percoraro, R.E.; Rodeheaver, G.; Robson, M.C. Definitions and guidelines for assessment of wounds and evaluation of healing. *Wound Repair Regen.* **1994**, *2*, 165–170. [CrossRef]
10. Guo, S.a.; DiPietro, L.A. Factors affecting wound healing. *J. Dent. Res.* **2010**, *89*, 219–229. [CrossRef]
11. Ward, J.; Holden, J.; Grob, M.; Soldin, M. Management of wounds in the community: Five principles. *Br. J. Community Nurs.* **2019**, *24* (Suppl. S6), S20–S23. [CrossRef] [PubMed]
12. Zindle, J.K.; Wolinsky, E.; Bogie, K.M. A review of animal models from 2015 to 2020 for preclinical chronic wounds relevant to human health. *J. Tissue Viability* **2021**, *30*, 291–300. [CrossRef] [PubMed]
13. Lindholm, C.; Searle, R. Wound management for the 21st century: Combining effectiveness and efficiency. *Int. Wound J.* **2016**, *13*, 5–15. [CrossRef] [PubMed]
14. Mustoe, T. Understanding chronic wounds: A unifying hypothesis on their pathogenesis and implications for therapy. *Am. J. Surg.* **2004**, *187*, S65–S70. [CrossRef] [PubMed]
15. Zhao, G.; Usui, M.L.; Lippman, S.I.; James, G.A.; Stewart, P.S.; Fleckman, P.; Olerud, J.E. Biofilms and inflammation in chronic wounds. *Adv. Wound Care* **2013**, *2*, 389–399. [CrossRef] [PubMed]
16. McCarty, S.M.; Percival, S.L. Proteases and delayed wound healing. *Adv. Wound Care* **2013**, *2*, 438–447. [CrossRef]
17. Ben-Porath, I.; Weinberg, R.A. The signals and pathways activating cellular senescence. *Int. J. Biochem. Cell Biol.* **2005**, *37*, 961–976. [CrossRef]
18. Humphrey, P.R.; Maureen, M.D.; Ritter, J.M. *Rang & Dale's Pharmacology*; Elsevier: Amsterdam, The Netherlands, 2012.
19. Hoffman, M. Remodeling the blood coagulation cascade. *J. Thromb. Thrombolysis* **2003**, *16*, 17–20. [CrossRef]
20. Rivera-Caravaca, J.M.; Camelo-Castillo, A.; Ramírez-Macías, I.; Gil-Pérez, P.; López-García, C.; Esteve-Pastor, M.A.; Orenes-Piñero, E.; Tello-Montoliu, A.; Marín, F. Antithrombotic therapy in patients with peripheral artery disease: A focused review on oral anticoagulation. *Int. J. Mol. Sci.* **2021**, *22*, 7113. [CrossRef]
21. Schultz, G.; Chin, G.; Moldawer, L.; Diegelmann, R. *Ch23 Mechanisms of Vascular Disease*; University of Adelaide Press: Adelaide, Australia, 2011.
22. Akombaetwa, N.; Bwanga, A.; Makoni, P.A.; Witika, B.A. Applications of electrospun drug-eluting nanofibers in wound healing: Current and future perspectives. *Polymers* **2022**, *14*, 2931. [CrossRef]
23. Marshall, C.D.; Hu, M.S.; Leavitt, T.; Barnes, L.A.; Lorenz, H.P.; Longaker, M.T. Cutaneous scarring: Basic science, current treatments, and future directions. *Adv. Wound Care* **2018**, *7*, 29–45. [CrossRef]
24. George Broughton, I.; Janis, J.E.; Attinger, C.E. Wound healing: An overview. *Plast. Reconstr. Surg.* **2006**, *117*, 1e-S–32e-S. [CrossRef]
25. Ben Amar, M.; Wu, M. Re-epithelialization: Advancing epithelium frontier during wound healing. *J. R. Soc. Interface* **2014**, *11*, 20131038. [CrossRef]
26. de Oliveira Gonzalez, A.C.; Costa, T.F.; de Araújo Andrade, Z.; Medrado, A.R.A.P. Wound healing-A literature review. *An. Bras. Dermatol.* **2016**, *91*, 614–620. [CrossRef]
27. Azimi, B.; Milazzo, M.; Lazzeri, A.; Berrettini, S.; Uddin, M.J.; Qin, Z.; Buehler, M.J.; Danti, S. Electrospinning piezoelectric fibers for biocompatible devices. *Adv. Healthc. Mater.* **2020**, *9*, 1901287. [CrossRef] [PubMed]
28. Guenday, C.; Anand, S.; Gencer, H.B.; Munafo, S.; Moroni, L.; Fusco, A.; Donnarumma, G.; Ricci, C.; Hatir, P.C.; Tuereli, N.G. Ciprofloxacin-loaded polymeric nanoparticles incorporated electrospun fibers for drug delivery in tissue engineering applications. *Drug Deliv. Transl. Res.* **2020**, *10*, 706–720. [CrossRef] [PubMed]
29. Laudenslager, M.J.; Sigmund, W.M. Electrospinning. In *Encyclopedia of Nanotechnology*; Bhushan, B., Ed.; Springer: Dordrecht, The Netherlands, 2012; pp. 769–775.
30. Sill, T.J.; Von Recum, H.A. Electrospinning: Applications in drug delivery and tissue engineering. *Biomaterials* **2008**, *29*, 1989–2006. [CrossRef]
31. Deitzel, J.M.; Kleinmeyer, J.; Harris, D.; Tan, N.B. The effect of processing variables on the morphology of electrospun nanofibers and textiles. *Polymer* **2001**, *42*, 261–272. [CrossRef]
32. Baumgarten, P.K. Electrostatic spinning of acrylic microfibers. *J. Colloid Interface Sci.* **1971**, *36*, 71–79. [CrossRef]
33. Megelski, S.; Stephens, J.S.; Chase, D.B.; Rabolt, J.F. Micro-and nanostructured surface morphology on electrospun polymer fibers. *Macromolecules* **2002**, *35*, 8456–8466. [CrossRef]

34. Theron, S.; Zussman, E.; Yarin, A. Experimental investigation of the governing parameters in the electrospinning of polymer solutions. *Polymer* **2004**, *45*, 2017–2030. [CrossRef]
35. Matabola, K.; Moutloali, R. The influence of electrospinning parameters on the morphology and diameter of poly (vinyledene fluoride) nanofibers-effect of sodium chloride. *J. Mater. Sci.* **2013**, *48*, 5475–5482. [CrossRef]
36. Bhardwaj, N.; Kundu, S.C. Electrospinning: A fascinating fiber fabrication technique. *Biotechnol. Adv.* **2010**, *28*, 325–347. [CrossRef] [PubMed]
37. Pillay, V.; Dott, C.; Choonara, Y.E.; Tyagi, C.; Tomar, L.; Kumar, P.; du Toit, L.C.; Ndesendo, V.M. A review of the effect of processing variables on the fabrication of electrospun nanofibers for drug delivery applications. *J. Nanomater.* **2013**, *2013*, 789289. [CrossRef]
38. Zong, X.; Kim, K.; Fang, D.; Ran, S.; Hsiao, B.S.; Chu, B. Structure and process relationship of electrospun bioabsorbable nanofiber membranes. *Polymer* **2002**, *43*, 4403–4412. [CrossRef]
39. Doshi, J.; Reneker, D.H. Electrospinning process and applications of electrospun fibers. *J. Electrost.* **1995**, *35*, 151–160. [CrossRef]
40. Sun, B.; Long, Y.; Zhang, H.; Li, M.; Duvail, J.; Jiang, X.; Yin, H. Advances in three-dimensional nanofibrous macrostructures via electrospinning. *Prog. Polym. Sci.* **2014**, *39*, 862–890. [CrossRef]
41. Kanani, A.G.; Bahrami, S.H. Effect of changing solvents on poly (ε-caprolactone) nanofibrous webs morphology. *J. Nanomater.* **2011**, *2011*, 724153.
42. Fong, H.; Chun, I.; Reneker, D.H. Beaded nanofibers formed during electrospinning. *Polymer* **1999**, *40*, 4585–4592. [CrossRef]
43. Zhang, Y.; Feng, Y.; Huang, Z.; Ramakrishna, S.; Lim, C. Fabrication of porous electrospun nanofibres. *Nanotechnology* **2006**, *17*, 901. [CrossRef]
44. Jarusuwannapoom, T.; Hongrojjanawiwat, W.; Jitjaicham, S.; Wannatong, L.; Nithitanakul, M.; Pattamaprom, C.; Koombhongse, P.; Rangkupan, R.; Supaphol, P. Effect of solvents on electro-spinnability of polystyrene solutions and morphological appearance of resulting electrospun polystyrene fibers. *Eur. Polym. J.* **2005**, *41*, 409–421. [CrossRef]
45. Pelipenko, J.; Kristl, J.; Janković, B.; Baumgartner, S.; Kocbek, P. The impact of relative humidity during electrospinning on the morphology and mechanical properties of nanofibers. *Int. J. Pharm.* **2013**, *456*, 125–134. [CrossRef]
46. De Vrieze, S.; Van Camp, T.; Nelvig, A.; Hagström, B.; Westbroek, P.; De Clerck, K. The effect of temperature and humidity on electrospinning. *J. Mater. Sci.* **2009**, *44*, 1357–1362. [CrossRef]
47. Dodero, A.; Brunengo, E.; Alloisio, M.; Sionkowska, A.; Vicini, S.; Castellano, M. Chitosan-based electrospun membranes: Effects of solution viscosity, coagulant and crosslinker. *Carbohydr. Polym.* **2020**, *235*, 115976. [CrossRef]
48. Zeng, J.; Haoqing, H.; Schaper, A.; Wendorff, J.H.; Greiner, A. Poly-L-lactide nanofibers by electrospinning–Influence of solution viscosity and electrical conductivity on fiber diameter and fiber morphology. *e-Polymers* **2003**, *3*, 9. [CrossRef]
49. Gupta, P.; Elkins, C.; Long, T.E.; Wilkes, G.L. Electrospinning of linear homopolymers of poly (methyl methacrylate): Exploring relationships between fiber formation, viscosity, molecular weight and concentration in a good solvent. *Polymer* **2005**, *46*, 4799–4810. [CrossRef]
50. Koski, A.; Yim, K.; Shivkumar, S. Effect of molecular weight on fibrous PVA produced by electrospinning. *Mater. Lett.* **2004**, *58*, 493–497. [CrossRef]
51. Demir, M.M.; Yilgor, I.; Yilgor, E.; Erman, B. Electrospinning of polyurethane fibers. *Polymer* **2002**, *43*, 3303–3309. [CrossRef]
52. Geng, X.; Kwon, O.-H.; Jang, J. Electrospinning of chitosan dissolved in concentrated acetic acid solution. *Biomaterials* **2005**, *26*, 5427–5432. [CrossRef]
53. Zuo, W.; Zhu, M.; Yang, W.; Yu, H.; Chen, Y.; Zhang, Y. Experimental study on relationship between jet instability and formation of beaded fibers during electrospinning. *Polym. Eng. Sci.* **2005**, *45*, 704–709. [CrossRef]
54. Casper, C.L.; Stephens, J.S.; Tassi, N.G.; Chase, D.B.; Rabolt, J.F. Controlling surface morphology of electrospun polystyrene fibers: Effect of humidity and molecular weight in the electrospinning process. *Macromolecules* **2004**, *37*, 573–578. [CrossRef]
55. Kumar, P.; Lakshmanan, V.-K.; Biswas, R.; Nair, S.V.; Jayakumar, R. Synthesis and biological evaluation of chitin hydrogel/nano ZnO composite bandage as antibacterial wound dressing. *J. Biomed. Nanotechnol.* **2012**, *8*, 891–900. [CrossRef]
56. Stoica, A.E.; Chircov, C.; Grumezescu, A.M. Nanomaterials for wound dressings: An up-to-date overview. *Molecules* **2020**, *25*, 2699. [CrossRef]
57. Chen, K.; Wang, F.; Liu, S.; Wu, X.; Xu, L.; Zhang, D. In situ reduction of silver nanoparticles by sodium alginate to obtain silver-loaded composite wound dressing with enhanced mechanical and antimicrobial property. *Int. J. Biol. Macromol.* **2020**, *148*, 501–509. [CrossRef] [PubMed]
58. Fouda, M.M.; El-Aassar, M.; Al-Deyab, S.S. Antimicrobial activity of carboxymethyl chitosan/polyethylene oxide nanofibers embedded silver nanoparticles. *Carbohydr. Polym.* **2013**, *92*, 1012–1017. [CrossRef] [PubMed]
59. Rajendran, N.K.; Kumar, S.S.D.; Houreld, N.N.; Abrahamse, H. A review on nanoparticle based treatment for wound healing. *J. Drug Deliv. Sci. Technol.* **2018**, *44*, 421–430. [CrossRef]
60. Dastidar, D.G.; Ghosh, D. Silver nanoparticle decorated chitosan scaffold for wound healing and tissue regeneration. *Macromolecules* **2018**, *105 Pt 1*, 1241–1249.
61. Ganesh, M.; Aziz, A.S.; Ubaidulla, U.; Hemalatha, P.; Saravanakumar, A.; Ravikumar, R.; Peng, M.M.; Choi, E.Y.; Jang, H.T. Sulfanilamide and silver nanoparticles-loaded polyvinyl alcohol-chitosan composite electrospun nanofibers: Synthesis and evaluation on synergism in wound healing. *J. Ind. Eng. Chem.* **2016**, *39*, 127–135. [CrossRef]

62. Lee, S.J.; Heo, D.N.; Moon, J.-H.; Ko, W.-K.; Lee, J.B.; Bae, M.S.; Park, S.W.; Kim, J.E.; Lee, D.H.; Kim, E.-C. Electrospun chitosan nanofibers with controlled levels of silver nanoparticles. Preparation, characterization and antibacterial activity. *Carbohydr. Polym.* **2014**, *111*, 530–537. [CrossRef]
63. Bharathi, B.S.; Stalin, T. Cerium oxide and peppermint oil loaded polyethylene oxide/graphene oxide electrospun nanofibrous mats as antibacterial wound dressings. *Mater. Today Commun.* **2019**, *21*, 100664. [CrossRef]
64. Eghbalifam, N.; Shojaosadati, S.A.; Hashemi-Najafabadi, S.; Khorasani, A.C. Synthesis and characterization of antimicrobial wound dressing material based on silver nanoparticles loaded gum Arabic nanofibers. *Int. J. Biol. Macromol.* **2020**, *155*, 119–130. [CrossRef] [PubMed]
65. Cai, N.; Li, C.; Han, C.; Luo, X.; Shen, L.; Xue, Y.; Yu, F. Tailoring mechanical and antibacterial properties of chitosan/gelatin nanofiber membranes with Fe3O4 nanoparticles for potential wound dressing application. *Appl. Surf. Sci.* **2016**, *369*, 492–500. [CrossRef]
66. Son, W.K.; Youk, J.H.; Lee, T.S.; Park, W.H. Preparation of antimicrobial ultrafine cellulose acetate fibers with silver nanoparticles. *Macromol. Rapid Commun.* **2004**, *25*, 1632–1637. [CrossRef]
67. Yan, J.; Wang, D.; Bai, T.; Cheng, W.; Han, G.; Ni, X.; Shi, Q.S. Electrospun PVA Nanofibrous Membranes Reinforced with Silver Nanoparticles Impregnated Cellulosic Fibers: Morphology and Antibacterial Property. *Chem. Res. Chin. Univ.* **2021**, *37*, 505–511. [CrossRef]
68. Lee, E.J.; Huh, B.K.; Kim, S.N.; Lee, J.Y.; Park, C.G.; Mikos, A.G.; Choy, Y.B. Application of materials as medical devices with localized drug delivery capabilities for enhanced wound repair. *Prog. Mater. Sci.* **2017**, *89*, 392–410. [CrossRef]
69. Schneider, A.; Wang, X.; Kaplan, D.; Garlick, J.; Egles, C. Biofunctionalized electrospun silk mats as a topical bioactive dressing for accelerated wound healing. *Acta Biomater.* **2009**, *5*, 2570–2578. [CrossRef]
70. Chen, S.; Liu, B.; Carlson, M.A.; Gombart, A.F.; Reilly, D.A.; Xie, J. Recent advances in electrospun nanofibers for wound healing. *Nanomedicine* **2017**, *12*, 1335–1352. [CrossRef]
71. Li, J.; Zhang, Y.P.; Kirsner, R.S. Angiogenesis in wound repair: Angiogenic growth factors and the extracellular matrix. *Microsc. Res. Tech.* **2003**, *60*, 107–114. [CrossRef]
72. Değer, S. Preparation and Characterization of Herbal Extract Loaded Bilayer Sponges for Wound Dressing Applications. Ph.D. Thesis, Izmir Institute of Technology, Urla, Turkey, 2019.
73. Norouzi, M.; Shabani, I.; Ahvaz, H.H.; Soleimani, M. PLGA/gelatin hybrid nanofibrous scaffolds encapsulating EGF for skin regeneration. *J. Biomed. Mater. Res. Part A* **2015**, *103*, 2225–2235. [CrossRef]
74. Jin, G.; Prabhakaran, M.P.; Kai, D.; Ramakrishna, S. Controlled release of multiple epidermal induction factors through core–shell nanofibers for skin regeneration. *Eur. J. Pharm. Biopharm.* **2013**, *85*, 689–698. [CrossRef]
75. Kumar, S.A. Wound healing: Current understanding and future prospect. *Int. J. Drug Discov. ISSN* **2017**, 0975–4423.
76. Stechmiller, J.K. Understanding the role of nutrition and wound healing. *Nutr. Clin. Pract.* **2010**, *25*, 61–68. [CrossRef] [PubMed]
77. Velnar, T.; Bailey, T.; Smrkolj, V. The wound healing process: An overview of the cellular and molecular mechanisms. *J. Int. Med. Res.* **2009**, *37*, 1528–1542. [CrossRef] [PubMed]
78. Sheng, X.; Fan, L.; He, C.; Zhang, K.; Mo, X.; Wang, H. Vitamin E-loaded silk fibroin nanofibrous mats fabricated by green process for skin care application. *Int. J. Biol. Macromol.* **2013**, *56*, 49–56. [CrossRef]
79. Kheradvar, S.A.; Nourmohammadi, J.; Tabesh, H.; Bagheri, B. Starch nanoparticle as a vitamin E-TPGS carrier loaded in silk fibroin-poly (vinyl alcohol)-Aloe vera nanofibrous dressing. *Colloids Surf. B Biointerfaces* **2018**, *166*, 9–16. [CrossRef]
80. Fan, L.; Wang, H.; Zhang, K.; Cai, Z.; He, C.; Sheng, X.; Mo, X. Vitamin C-reinforcing silk fibroin nanofibrous matrices for skin care application. *RSC Adv.* **2012**, *2*, 4110–4119. [CrossRef]
81. Ammon, H.P.; Wahl, M.A. Pharmacology of Curcuma longa. *Planta Med.* **1991**, *57*, 1–7. [CrossRef]
82. Abe, Y.; Hashimoto, S.; Horie, T. Curcumin inhibition of inflammatory cytokine production by human peripheral blood monocytes and alveolar macrophages. *Pharmacol. Res.* **1999**, *39*, 41–47. [CrossRef]
83. Merrell, J.G.; McLaughlin, S.W.; Tie, L.; Laurencin, C.T.; Chen, A.F.; Nair, L.S. Curcumin loaded poly (ε-caprolactone) nanofibers: Diabetic wound dressing with antioxidant and anti-inflammatory properties. *Clin. Exp. Pharmacol. Physiol.* **2009**, *36*, 1149. [CrossRef]
84. Cho, H.; Yun, C.-W.; Park, W.-K.; Kong, J.-Y.; Kim, K.S.; Park, Y.; Lee, S.; Kim, B.-K. Modulation of the activity of pro-inflammatory enzymes, COX-2 and iNOS, by chrysin derivatives. *Pharmacol. Res.* **2004**, *49*, 37–43. [CrossRef]
85. Deldar, Y.; Pilehvar-Soltanahmadi, Y.; Dadashpour, M.; Montazer Saheb, S.; Rahmati-Yamchi, M.; Zarghami, N. An in vitro examination of the antioxidant, cytoprotective and anti-inflammatory properties of chrysin-loaded nanofibrous mats for potential wound healing applications. *Artif. Cells Nanomed. Biotechnol.* **2018**, *46*, 706–716. [CrossRef] [PubMed]
86. Mohiti-Asli, M.; Saha, S.; Murphy, S.; Gracz, H.; Pourdeyhimi, B.; Atala, A.; Loboa, E. Ibuprofen loaded PLA nanofibrous scaffolds increase proliferation of human skin cells in vitro and promote healing of full thickness incision wounds in vivo. *J. Biomed. Mater. Res. Part B Appl. Biomater.* **2017**, *105*, 327–339. [CrossRef] [PubMed]
87. Santoro, M.; Shah, S.R.; Walker, J.L.; Mikos, A.G. Poly (lactic acid) nanofibrous scaffolds for tissue engineering. *Adv. Drug Deliv. Rev.* **2016**, *107*, 206–212. [CrossRef] [PubMed]
88. Dart, A.; Bhave, M.; Kingshott, P. Antimicrobial peptide-based electrospun fibers for wound healing applications. *Macromol. Biosci.* **2019**, *19*, 1800488. [CrossRef]

89. Li, W.; Cicek, N.; Levin, D.B.; Logsetty, S.; Liu, S. Bacteria-triggered release of a potent biocide from core-shell polyhydroxyalkanoate (PHA)-based nanofibers for wound dressing applications. *J. Biomater. Sci. Polym. Ed.* **2020**, *31*, 394–406. [CrossRef]
90. Zhao, J.; Han, F.; Zhang, W.; Yang, Y.; You, D.; Li, L. Toward improved wound dressings: Effects of polydopamine-decorated poly (lactic-co-glycolic acid) electrospinning incorporating basic fibroblast growth factor and ponericin G1. *RSC Adv.* **2019**, *9*, 33038–33051. [CrossRef]
91. Chen, Q.; Wu, J.; Liu, Y.; Li, Y.; Zhang, C.; Qi, W.; Yeung, K.W.; Wong, T.M.; Zhao, X.; Pan, H. Electrospun chitosan/PVA/bioglass Nanofibrous membrane with spatially designed structure for accelerating chronic wound healing. *Mater. Sci. Eng. C* **2019**, *105*, 110083. [CrossRef]
92. Cui, S.; Sun, X.; Li, K.; Gou, D.; Zhou, Y.; Hu, J.; Liu, Y. Polylactide nanofibers delivering doxycycline for chronic wound treatment. *Mater. Sci. Eng. C* **2019**, *104*, 109745. [CrossRef]
93. Abdalkarim, S.Y.H.; Yu, H.-Y.; Wang, D.; Yao, J. Electrospun poly (3-hydroxybutyrate-co-3-hydroxy-valerate)/cellulose reinforced nanofibrous membranes with ZnO nanocrystals for antibacterial wound dressings. *Cellulose* **2017**, *24*, 2925–2938. [CrossRef]
94. Pankongadisak, P.; Sangklin, S.; Chuysinuan, P.; Suwantong, O.; Supaphol, P. The use of electrospun curcumin-loaded poly (L-lactic acid) fiber mats as wound dressing materials. *J. Drug Deliv. Sci. Technol.* **2019**, *53*, 101121. [CrossRef]
95. Liu, X.; Lin, T.; Gao, Y.; Xu, Z.; Huang, C.; Yao, G.; Jiang, L.; Tang, Y.; Wang, X. Antimicrobial electrospun nanofibers of cellulose acetate and polyester urethane composite for wound dressing. *J. Biomed. Mater. Res. Part B Appl. Biomater.* **2012**, *100*, 1556–1565. [CrossRef] [PubMed]
96. Thakur, V.K.; Thakur, M.K.; Kessler, M.R. *Handbook of Composites from Renewable Materials, Biodegradable Materials*; John Wiley & Sons: Hoboken, NJ, USA, 2017; Volume 5.
97. Czaja, W.; Krystynowicz, A.; Bielecki, S.; Brown Jr, R.M. Microbial cellulose—The natural power to heal wounds. *Biomaterials* **2006**, *27*, 145–151. [CrossRef] [PubMed]
98. Sahana, T.; Rekha, P. Biopolymers: Applications in wound healing and skin tissue engineering. *Mol. Biol. Rep.* **2018**, *45*, 2857–2867. [CrossRef] [PubMed]
99. Vatankhah, E.; Prabhakaran, M.P.; Jin, G.; Mobarakeh, L.G.; Ramakrishna, S. Development of nanofibrous cellulose acetate/gelatin skin substitutes for variety wound treatment applications. *J. Biomater. Appl.* **2014**, *28*, 909–921. [CrossRef]
100. He, X.; Cheng, L.; Zhang, X.; Xiao, Q.; Zhang, W.; Lu, C. Tissue engineering scaffolds electrospun from cotton cellulose. *Carbohydr. Polym.* **2015**, *115*, 485–493. [CrossRef]
101. Rao, S.S.; Jeyapal, S.G.; Rajiv, S. Biodegradable electrospun nanocomposite fibers based on Poly (2-hydroxy ethyl methacrylate) and bamboo cellulose. *Compos. Part B Eng.* **2014**, *60*, 43–48. [CrossRef]
102. Song, J.; Birbach, N.L.; Hinestroza, J.P. Deposition of silver nanoparticles on cellulosic fibers via stabilization of carboxymethyl groups. *Cellulose* **2012**, *19*, 411–424. [CrossRef]
103. Min, B.-M.; Lee, S.W.; Lim, J.N.; You, Y.; Lee, T.S.; Kang, P.H.; Park, W.H. Chitin and chitosan nanofibers: Electrospinning of chitin and deacetylation of chitin nanofibers. *Polymer* **2004**, *45*, 7137–7142. [CrossRef]
104. Jayakumar, R.; Prabaharan, M.; Kumar, P.S.; Nair, S.; Tamura, H. Biomaterials based on chitin and chitosan in wound dressing applications. *Biotechnol. Adv.* **2011**, *29*, 322–337. [CrossRef]
105. Milazzo, M.; Gallone, G.; Marcello, E.; Mariniello, M.D.; Bruschini, L.; Roy, I.; Danti, S. Biodegradable polymeric micro/nanostructures with intrinsic antifouling/antimicrobial properties: Relevance in damaged skin and other biomedical applications. *J. Funct. Biomater.* **2020**, *11*, 60. [CrossRef]
106. Zarghami, A.; Irani, M.; Mostafazadeh, A.; Golpour, M.; Heidarinasab, A.; Haririan, I. Fabrication of PEO/chitosan/PCL/olive oil nanofibrous scaffolds for wound dressing applications. *Fibers Polym.* **2015**, *16*, 1201–1212. [CrossRef]
107. Yang, X.; Li, L.; Yang, D.; Nie, J.; Ma, G. Electrospun core–shell fibrous 2D scaffold with biocompatible poly (glycerol sebacate) and poly-l-lactic acid for wound healing. *Adv. Fiber Mater.* **2020**, *2*, 105–117. [CrossRef]
108. Alves, P.E.; Soares, B.G.; Lins, L.C.; Livi, S.; Santos, E.P. Controlled delivery of dexamethasone and betamethasone from PLA electrospun fibers: A comparative study. *Eur. Polym. J.* **2019**, *117*, 1–9. [CrossRef]
109. Moradkhannejhad, L.; Abdouss, M.; Nikfarjam, N.; Shahriari, M.H.; Heidary, V. The effect of molecular weight and content of PEG on in vitro drug release of electrospun curcumin loaded PLA/PEG nanofibers. *J. Drug Deliv. Sci. Technol.* **2020**, *56*, 101554. [CrossRef]
110. Yang, C.; Yan, Z.; Lian, Y.; Wang, J.; Zhang, K. Graphene oxide coated shell-core structured chitosan/PLLA nanofibrous scaffolds for wound dressing. *J. Biomater. Sci. Polym. Ed.* **2020**, *31*, 622–641. [CrossRef]
111. Augustine, R.; Zahid, A.A.; Hasan, A.; Wang, M.; Webster, T.J. CTGF loaded electrospun dual porous core-shell membrane for diabetic wound healing. *Int. J. Nanomed.* **2019**, 8573–8588. [CrossRef]
112. Patel, S.K.; Sandeep, K.; Singh, M.; Singh, G.P.; Lee, J.-K.; Bhatia, S.K.; Kalia, V.C. Biotechnological application of polyhydroxyalkanoates and their composites as anti-microbials agents. In *Biotechnological Applications of Polyhydroxyalkanoates*; Springer: Singapore, 2019; pp. 207–225.
113. Shishatskaya, E.I.; Nikolaeva, E.D.; Vinogradova, O.N.; Volova, T.G. Experimental wound dressings of degradable PHA for skin defect repair. *J. Mater. Sci. Mater. Med.* **2016**, *27*, 165. [CrossRef]
114. Wu, Q.; Wang, Y.; Chen, G.-Q. Medical application of microbial biopolyesters polyhydroxyalkanoates. *Artif. Cells Blood Substit. Biotechnol.* **2009**, *37*, 1–12. [CrossRef]

115. Yang, X.-D.; Zou, X.-H.; Dai, Z.-W.; Luo, R.-C.; Wei, C.-J.; Chen, G.-Q. Effects of oligo (3-hydroxyalkanoates) on the viability and insulin secretion of murine beta cells. *J. Biomater. Sci. Polym. Ed.* **2009**, *20*, 1729–1746. [CrossRef]
116. Yuan, J.; Geng, J.; Xing, Z.; Shim, K.J.; Han, I.; Kim, J.C.; Kang, I.K.; Shen, J. Novel wound dressing based on nanofibrous PHBV–keratin mats. *J. Tissue Eng. Regen. Med.* **2015**, *9*, 1027–1035. [CrossRef]
117. Azimi, B.; Thomas, L.; Fusco, A.; Kalaoglu-Altan, O.I.; Basnett, P.; Cinelli, P.; De Clerck, K.; Roy, I.; Donnarumma, G.; Coltelli, M.-B. Electrosprayed chitin nanofibril/electrospun polyhydroxyalkanoate fiber mesh as functional nonwoven for skin application. *J. Funct. Biomater.* **2020**, *11*, 62. [CrossRef]
118. Danti, S.; Trombi, L.; Fusco, A.; Azimi, B.; Lazzeri, A.; Morganti, P.; Coltelli, M.-B.; Donnarumma, G. Chitin nanofibrils and nanolignin as functional agents in skin regeneration. *Int. J. Mol. Sci.* **2019**, *20*, 2669. [CrossRef] [PubMed]
119. Kandhasamy, S.; Perumal, S.; Madhan, B.; Umamaheswari, N.; Banday, J.A.; Perumal, P.T.; Santhanakrishnan, V.P. Synthesis and fabrication of collagen-coated ostholamide electrospun nanofiber scaffold for wound healing. *ACS Appl. Mater. Interfaces* **2017**, *9*, 8556–8568. [CrossRef] [PubMed]
120. Ali Akbari Ghavimi, S.; Ebrahimzadeh, M.H.; Solati-Hashjin, M.; Abu Osman, N.A. Polycaprolactone/starch composite: Fabrication, structure, properties, and applications. *J. Biomed. Mater. Res. Part A* **2015**, *103*, 2482–2498. [CrossRef] [PubMed]
121. Dias, J.; Baptista-Silva, S.; Sousa, A.; Oliveira, A.; Bártolo, P.; Granja, P. Biomechanical performance of hybrid electrospun structures for skin regeneration. *Mater. Sci. Eng. C* **2018**, *93*, 816–827. [CrossRef] [PubMed]
122. Mirzaei-Parsa, M.J.; Ghanbari, H.; Alipoor, B.; Tavakoli, A.; Najafabadi, M.R.H.; Faridi-Majidi, R. Nanofiber-acellular dermal matrix as a bilayer scaffold containing mesenchymal stem cell for healing of full-thickness skin wounds. *Cell Tissue Res.* **2019**, *375*, 709–721. [CrossRef] [PubMed]
123. Rad, Z.P.; Mokhtari, J.; Abbasi, M. Calendula officinalis extract/PCL/Zein/Gum arabic nanofibrous bio-composite scaffolds via suspension, two-nozzle and multilayer electrospinning for skin tissue engineering. *Int. J. Biol. Macromol.* **2019**, *135*, 530–543.
124. Tığlı, R.S.; Kazaroğlu, N.M.; Mavış, B.; Gümüşderelioğlu, M. Cellular behavior on epidermal growth factor (EGF)-immobilized PCL/gelatin nanofibrous scaffolds. *J. Biomater. Sci. Polym. Ed.* **2011**, *22*, 207–223. [CrossRef]
125. Kasafírek, E.; Rybák, M.; Krejčí, I.; Šturc, A.; Křepela, E.; Šedo, A. Two-step generation of spirocyclic dipeptides from linear peptide ethyl ester precursors. *Life Sci.* **1992**, *50*, 187–193. [CrossRef]
126. Pokorna, A.; Bobal, P.; Oravec, M.; Rarova, L.; Bobalova, J.; Jampilek, J. Investigation of permeation of theophylline through skin using selected piperazine-2, 5-diones. *Molecules* **2019**, *24*, 566. [CrossRef]
127. Kocic, H.; Arsic, I.; Stankovic, M.; Tiodorovic, D.; Ciric, V.; Kocic, G. Proliferative, anti-apoptotic and immune-enhancing effects of L-arginine in culture of skin fibroblasts. *J. Biol. Regul. Homeost. Agents* **2017**, *31*, 667–672. [PubMed]
128. Kanji, S.; Das, M.; Aggarwal, R.; Lu, J.; Joseph, M.; Basu, S.; Pompili, V.J.; Das, H. Nanofiber-expanded human umbilical cord blood-derived CD34+ cell therapy accelerates murine cutaneous wound closure by attenuating pro-inflammatory factors and secreting IL-10. *Stem Cell Res.* **2014**, *12*, 275–288. [CrossRef] [PubMed]
129. Motealleh, B.; Zahedi, P.; Rezaeian, I.; Moghimi, M.; Abdolghaffari, A.H.; Zarandi, M.A. Morphology, drug release, antibacterial, cell proliferation, and histology studies of chamomile-loaded wound dressing mats based on electrospun nanofibrous poly (ε-caprolactone)/polystyrene blends. *J. Biomed. Mater. Res. Part B Appl. Biomater.* **2014**, *102*, 977–987. [CrossRef] [PubMed]
130. Sun, T.; Mai, S.; Norton, D.; Haycock, J.W.; Ryan, A.J.; Macneil, S. Self-organization of skin cells in three-dimensional electrospun polystyrene scaffolds. *Tissue Eng.* **2005**, *11*, 1023–1033. [CrossRef] [PubMed]
131. Altinbasak, I.; Jijie, R.; Barras, A.; Golba, B.; Sanyal, R.; Bouckaert, J.; Drider, D.; Bilyy, R.; Dumych, T.; Paryzhak, S. Reduced graphene-oxide-embedded polymeric nanofiber mats: An "on-demand" photothermally triggered antibiotic release platform. *ACS Appl. Mater. Interfaces* **2018**, *10*, 41098–41106. [CrossRef]
132. Johnson, C.D.; D'Amato, A.R.; Puhl, D.L.; Wich, D.M.; Vesperman, A.; Gilbert, R.J. Electrospun fiber surface nanotopography influences astrocyte-mediated neurite outgrowth. *Biomed. Mater.* **2018**, *13*, 054101. [CrossRef]
133. Calori, I.R.; Braga, G.; de Jesus, P.d.C.C.; Bi, H.; Tedesco, A.C. Polymer scaffolds as drug delivery systems. *Eur. Polym. J.* **2020**, *129*, 109621. [CrossRef]
134. Karthikeyan, A.; Senthil, N.; Min, T. Nanocurcumin: A promising candidate for therapeutic applications. *Front. Pharmacol.* **2020**, *11*, 487. [CrossRef]
135. Lee, C.-H.; Hung, K.-C.; Hsieh, M.-J.; Chang, S.-H.; Juang, J.-H.; Hsieh, I.-C.; Wen, M.-S.; Liu, S.-J. Core-shell insulin-loaded nanofibrous scaffolds for repairing diabetic wounds. *Nanomed. Nanotechnol. Biol. Med.* **2020**, *24*, 102123. [CrossRef]
136. Teng, S.-H.; Wang, P.; Kim, H.-E. Blend fibers of chitosan–agarose by electrospinning. *Mater. Lett.* **2009**, *63*, 2510–2512. [CrossRef]
137. Ajmal, G.; Bonde, G.V.; Mittal, P.; Khan, G.; Pandey, V.K.; Bakade, B.V.; Mishra, B. Biomimetic PCL-gelatin based nanofibers loaded with ciprofloxacin hydrochloride and quercetin: A potential antibacterial and anti-oxidant dressing material for accelerated healing of a full thickness wound. *Int. J. Pharm.* **2019**, *567*, 118480. [CrossRef]
138. Parai, D.; Dey, P.; Mukherjee, S.K. Biofilm: A Challenge to Overcome in Wound Healing. In *Wound Healing Research: Current Trends and Future Directions*; Springer: Singapore, 2021; pp. 661–677.
139. Hosseini, M.; Shafiee, A. Engineering bioactive scaffolds for skin regeneration. *Small* **2021**, *17*, 2101384. [CrossRef]
140. Silva, S.Y.; Rueda, L.C.; Márquez, G.A.; López, M.; Smith, D.J.; Calderón, C.A.; Castillo, J.C.; Matute, J.; Rueda-Clausen, C.F.; Orduz, A. Double blind, randomized, placebo controlled clinical trial for the treatment of diabetic foot ulcers, using a nitric oxide releasing patch: PATHON. *Trials* **2007**, *8*, 26. [CrossRef]

141. Floyd, C.T.; Rothwell, S.W.; Risdahl, J.; Martin, R.; Olson, C.; Rose, N. Salmon thrombin-fibrinogen dressing allows greater survival and preserves distal blood flow compared to standard kaolin gauze in coagulopathic Swine with a standardized lethal femoral artery injury. *J. Spec. Oper. Med. A Peer Rev. J. SOF Med. Prof.* **2012**, *12*, 16–26. [CrossRef]
142. Azimi, B.; Maleki, H.; Zavagna, L.; De la Ossa, J.G.; Linari, S.; Lazzeri, A.; Danti, S. Bio-based electrospun fibers for wound healing. *J. Funct. Biomater.* **2020**, *11*, 67. [CrossRef]
143. Arenbergerova, M.; Arenberger, P.; Bednar, M.; Kubat, P.; Mosinger, J. Light-activated nanofibre textiles exert antibacterial effects in the setting of chronic wound healing. *Exp. Dermatol.* **2012**, *21*, 619–624. [CrossRef]
144. Augustine, R.; Hasan, A.; Patan, N.K.; Dalvi, Y.B.; Varghese, R.; Antony, A.; Unni, R.N.; Sandhyarani, N.; Moustafa, A.-E.A. Cerium oxide nanoparticle incorporated electrospun poly (3-hydroxybutyrate-co-3-hydroxyvalerate) membranes for diabetic wound healing applications. *ACS Biomater. Sci. Eng.* **2019**, *6*, 58–70. [CrossRef]
145. Lee, C.-H.; Chang, S.-H.; Chen, W.-J.; Hung, K.-C.; Lin, Y.-H.; Liu, S.-J.; Hsieh, M.-J.; Pang, J.-H.S.; Juang, J.-H. Augmentation of diabetic wound healing and enhancement of collagen content using nanofibrous glucophage-loaded collagen/PLGA scaffold membranes. *J. Colloid Interface Sci.* **2015**, *439*, 88–97. [CrossRef]
146. Yu, J.-W.; Deng, Y.-P.; Han, X.; Ren, G.-F.; Cai, J.; Jiang, G.-J. Metformin improves the angiogenic functions of endothelial progenitor cells via activating AMPK/eNOS pathway in diabetic mice. *Cardiovasc. Diabetol.* **2016**, *15*, 88. [CrossRef]
147. Mohammadi, M.R.; Kargozar, S.; Bahrami, S.; Rabbani, S. An excellent nanofibrous matrix based on gum tragacanth-poly (ϵ-caprolactone)-poly (vinyl alcohol) for application in diabetic wound healing. *Polym. Degrad. Stab.* **2020**, *174*, 109105. [CrossRef]

pharmaceuticals

MDPI

Review

Silk Fibroin Nanofibers: Advancements in Bioactive Dressings through Electrospinning Technology for Diabetic Wound Healing

Afaf Aldahish [1], Nirenjen Shanmugasundaram [2], Rajalakshimi Vasudevan [1], Taha Alqahtani [1], Saud Alqahtani [1], Ahmad Mohammad Asiri [3], Praveen Devanandan [4], Tamilanban Thamaraikani [2], Chitra Vellapandian [2] and Narayanan Jayasankar [2,*]

1 Department of Pharmacology, College of Pharmacy, King Khalid University, Abha, Saudi Arabia
2 Department of Pharmacology, SRM College of Pharmacy, SRM Institute of Science and Technology, Kattankulathur, Chengalpattu 603203, India
3 Khamis Mushayt General Hospital, Aseer Health Cluster, Ministry of Health, Khamis Mushait 62433, Saudi Arabia
4 Department of Pharmacy Practice, St. Peter's Institute of Pharmaceutical Sciences, Vidya Nagar, Hanamkonda 506001, India
* Correspondence: narayanj@srmist.edu.in

Abstract: Background: Non-healing diabetic wounds represent a significant clinical challenge globally, necessitating innovative approaches in drug delivery to enhance wound healing. Understanding the pathogenesis of these wounds is crucial for developing effective treatments. Bioactive dressings and polymeric nanofibers have emerged as promising modalities, with silk biomaterials gaining attention for their unique properties in diabetic wound healing. Purpose of Review: The purpose of this review is to examine the challenges and innovations in treating non-healing diabetic wounds, emphasizing the global burden and the need for effective solutions. This review explores the complex mechanisms of wound healing in diabetes and evaluates the therapeutic potential of bioactive dressings and polymeric nanofibers. Special focus is given to the application of silk biomaterials, particularly silk fibroin, for wound healing, detailing their properties, mechanisms, and clinical translation. This review also describes various nanofiber fabrication methods, especially electrospinning technology, and presents existing evidence on the effectiveness of electrospun silk fibroin formulations. Recent Findings: Recent advancements highlight the potential of silk biomaterials in diabetic wound healing, owing to their biocompatibility, mechanical strength, and controlled drug release properties. Electrospun silk fibroin-based formulations have shown promising results in preclinical and clinical studies, demonstrating accelerated wound closure and tissue regeneration. Summary: Non-healing diabetic wounds present a significant healthcare burden globally, necessitating innovative therapeutic strategies. Bioactive dressings and polymeric nanofibers, particularly silk-based formulations fabricated through electrospinning, offer promising avenues for enhancing diabetic wound healing. Further research is warranted to optimize formulation parameters and validate efficacy in larger clinical trials.

Keywords: diabetic wounds; wound healing; bioactive dressings; polymeric nanofibers; silk biomaterials; electrospinning; silk fibroin; drug delivery

1. Introduction

Diabetes mellitus (DM) is a widespread and impactful metabolic disorder marked by chronic hyperglycemia due to defects in insulin secretion or action [1]. This persistent elevation of blood glucose levels leads to a spectrum of complications, one of the most problematic being non-healing diabetic wounds [2]. These chronic wounds, particularly those occurring in the lower extremities, pose substantial challenges in patient care due to their tendency to develop infections, delay in healing, and risk of progression to severe outcomes such as amputation. Understanding the pathophysiological mechanisms behind these non-healing wounds is crucial for developing effective therapeutic strategies [3]. The healing of diabetic wounds is hindered by a range of factors related to the underlying pathophysiology of diabetes. Persistent inflammation is another critical factor that obstructs the healing process. Chronic inflammation in diabetic wounds is driven by sustained high levels of pro-inflammatory cytokines and oxidative stress. This constant inflammatory state can lead to further tissue damage and delays in the resolution of the inflammatory phase, thereby prolonging the healing process [4].

The global burden of non-healing diabetic wounds is substantial and growing. As of 2019, approximately 463 million people worldwide were diagnosed with diabetes. With the global prevalence of diabetes expected to rise to 700 million by 2040, the incidence of diabetic wounds is also projected to increase significantly [5]. This rise in diabetic cases is accompanied by an increased prevalence of chronic wounds, which impose a considerable economic burden on healthcare systems and adversely affect patients' quality of life. The economic impact of diabetic wounds extends beyond direct medical costs, such as expenses for hospitalizations, treatments, and medications. It also includes indirect costs related to loss of productivity, long-term care needs, and diminished quality of life for patients [6]. Non-healing wounds often lead to frequent hospital visits, prolonged treatment durations, and higher rates of morbidity and mortality. Consequently, addressing this health crisis requires innovative and effective solutions to improve wound management and patient outcomes [7].

Traditional wound care methods often fall short when dealing with the complexities of diabetic wound healing. Common dressings such as gauze, semi-permeable films, foam, and hydrogel dressings have various limitations. For instance, gauze dressings may not adequately absorb wound exudate or maintain a moist environment, which is critical for promoting healing. Semi-permeable films and foam dressings can sometimes cause discomfort or lead to infection if not properly managed. Hydrogel dressings, while beneficial in maintaining moisture, may not always provide the sustained release of therapeutic agents needed for effective wound management [8]. To address these shortcomings, there is a growing need for advanced wound dressings that offer controlled and sustained release of therapeutic agents while creating an optimal environment for healing. Recent advancements in wound care technology have focused on developing bioactive dressings and polymeric nanofibers, which have shown promising results in enhancing drug delivery and supporting wound healing processes. Among the innovative approaches, Electrospun nanofibers, particularly those derived from silk fibroin, have emerged as a highly promising solution for diabetic wound care. Electrospinning technology allows for the precise fabrication of nanofibers with customizable properties, such as fiber diameter, porosity, and surface chemistry. These nanofibers exhibit a high surface area-to-volume ratio, which enhances their ability to deliver therapeutic agents effectively [9].

Silk fibroin, in particular, is known for its biocompatibility, biodegradability, and excellent mechanical properties. When used in electrospun nanofibers, silk fibroin provides a supportive scaffold that mimics the extracellular matrix, facilitating cell attachment, proliferation, and migration. This scaffold structure also allows for the continuous release of drugs and bioactive factors, thereby addressing the limitations of traditional dressings. The unique properties of electrospun nanofibers enable them to create a conducive microenvironment for wound healing. They support essential processes such as tissue regeneration, angiogenesis, and exudate absorption [10]. Furthermore, the ability to load nanofibers with various therapeutic agents, including growth factors, anti-inflammatory agents, and antimicrobial agents, enhances their effectiveness in managing diabetic wounds. The challenge of non-healing diabetic wounds highlights the need for advanced therapeutic strategies and innovative wound care technologies [11]. The limitations of traditional wound care methods necessitate the development of more effective solutions. Electrospun nanofibers, especially those made from silk fibroin, offer a promising advancement in wound care technology. Their ability to provide controlled drug release, support tissue regeneration, and enhance the healing environment positions them as a valuable tool in addressing the global burden of diabetic wounds.

The purpose of this Comprehensive review is to examine the challenges and innovations in treating non-healing diabetic wounds, emphasizing the global burden and the need for effective solutions. This review explores the complex mechanisms of wound healing in diabetes and evaluates the therapeutic potential of bioactive dressings and polymeric nanofibers. Special focus is given to the application of silk biomaterials, particularly silk fibroin, for wound healing, detailing their properties, mechanisms, and clinical translation. This review also describes fabrication methods, especially electrospinning technology, and presents existing evidence on the effectiveness of electrospun silk fibroin formulations.

2. Pathogenesis and Intricate Mechanisms of Non-Healing Diabetic Wounds

Wound healing is a complex, highly intricate biological process, activated in response to compromise of the integrity of tissue, which leads the series of cellular and molecular events through a well-coordinated sequence aimed at restitution of the structure and function of damaged tissue back to normal. This is typically divided into four different stages: Hemostasis, inflammation, proliferation, and remodeling. First, there is the stage of hemostasis mediated by platelets. These, upon contact with the exposed collagen of the injured tissue, are activated, aggregate, and adhere to the distorted endothelium, thereby triggering the coagulation cascade. This leads to the conversion of fibrinogen to fibrin and, hence, the formation of a thrombus that provides a provisional extracellular matrix. At the same time, activated platelets express proteins that promote migration and adhesion of neutrophils and monocytes to the site of injury. In addition, these platelets produce growth factors, including TGF-β (transforming growth factor -β) and PDGF (platelet-derived growth factor), required in the healing process [12] and the role of the various growth factors in wound healing is given in Table 1.

Table 1. Role of various growth factors in the wound healing process.

S.No.	Growth Factors	Sources of Growth Factors	Function
1.	EGF	Platelets and macrophages	Re-epithelialization; granulation tissue formation
2.	PDGF	Platelets; keratinocytes; macrophages; endothelial cells; fibroblasts	Inflammation; granulation tissue formation/angiogenesis; re-epithelialization; matrix formation and remodeling
3.	TGF-β	Platelets; keratinocytes; macrophages; lymphocytes; fibroblasts	Inflammation; granulation tissue formation; re-epithelialization; matrix formation and remodeling
4.	TNF-α	Neutrophils; macrophages	collagen expression; re-epithelialization
5.	VEGF	Platelets; neutrophils; macrophages; endothelial cells; smooth muscle cells; fibroblasts	granulation tissue formation/angiogenesis/neo-vascularization
6.	FGF	Macrophages, fibroblasts, endothelial cells	Angiogenesis, granulation tissue formation, re-epithelialization, collagen synthesis
7.	IGF	Platelets, macrophages, fibroblasts	Re-epithelialization, matrix formation and remodeling, cell migration
8.	KGF	Fibroblasts	Stimulates keratinocyte proliferation and migration, re-epithelialization
9.	HGF	Mesenchymal cells, fibroblasts	Promotes epithelial and endothelial cell proliferation, re-epithelialization, angiogenesis

The table outlines the key growth factors involved in the wound healing process, highlighting their primary sources and functions. Epidermal growth factor (EGF), platelet-derived growth factor (PDGF), transforming growth factor-beta (TGF-β), tumor necrosis factor alpha (TNF-α), vascular endothelial growth factor (VEGF), fibroblast growth factor (FGF), insulin-like growth factor (IGF), keratinocyte growth factor (KGF), and hepatocyte growth factor (HGF).

Following hemostasis, there is the inflammatory phase characterized by infiltration of cells of inflammation to the wound site. Neutrophils, as the first responders, assume the role for tissue debridement and control of infection. The process entered into by these cells is: cells adhere to the endothelium near the area of wounding and then cross damaged capillaries or move across intercellular gaps of endothelial cells in a process called diapedesis. They also secrete growth factors, which stimulate cell growth and proteases, which digest extracellular matrix components, thereby further promoting wound healing. As the inflammatory process chronicles, circulating monocytes infiltrate into the tissue and mature into macrophages. These macrophages are polarized first into a pro-inflammatory M1 phenotype and participate in the phagocytosis of the wound, clearing it of pathogens, foreign bodies, apoptotic neutrophils, and damaged tissue. They also aid in the production of cytokines and other mediators that sustain the inflammatory response. Soon after tissue injury, the resident mast cells respond by liberating proteases that hydrolyze the matrix and cytokines involved in recruiting neutrophils. Later on, this is coordinated by T-lymphocytes that come later to coordinate tissue remodeling. As inflammation declines, the healing process enters into its proliferative phase, characterized by a change in macrophage phenotype from M1 to M2. In essence, the underlying process is determined by the interplay of complex molecular and cellular mechanisms where the macrophage changes from a pro-inflammatory to anti-inflammatory role. During this phase, M2 macrophages release growth factors such as VEGF and TGF-β, which are involved in the cell proliferation and protein synthesis. They also secrete protease inhibitors, proteases, and anti-inflammatory mediators that promote the formation of granulation tissue. Further subtypes of the M2 macrophages include M2a, M2b, and M2c subtypes, all of which have their role distinct in this proliferative phase. M2a macrophages, polarized by IL-4 and IL-13, produce fibroblasts and extracellular matrix components. In contrast, M2b macrophages produce IL-10, TNF, and IL-6, which have an anti-inflammatory effect. It is polarized by M2c macrophages that secrete vascular structure and extracellular matrix remodeling in this phase, thanks to IL-10 and TGF-β. This process is accompanied by a characteristic process called angiogenesis or the formation of new blood vessels, which is driven by proangiogenic factors of which FGF-2 and VEGF are examples. This newly formed capillary network provides oxygen and nutrition for the rapidly growing cells of healing wound. Meanwhile, proliferating capillaries account for the granular nature of granulation tissue in appearance, which acts as a scaffolding for keratinocyte migration to re-epithelialize the wound [13,14].

The final stage is the remodeling phase, after the initial injury in between two to three weeks, when granulation tissue is gradually replaced by scar tissue. The blood vessels become less dense in number and collagen fibers are arranged and altered. There is continuous synthesis and breakdown of collagen and that is in turn controlled by matrix metalloproteinases. Through cross-linking and alignment of collagen fibers along lines of tension, tensile strength of the wound is achieved. Wound contraction also takes place where myofibroblasts draw the edges of the wound closer thereby decreasing the size of the wound [15,16]. Ultimately, it is the highly coordinated and dynamic process involving multiple cellular and molecular mechanisms which goes into the restoration of tissue integrity and function as clearly depicted in Figure 1. While the general process of wound healing is a well-coordinated sequence of events, the presence of certain pathological conditions can significantly alter this process. One such condition is diabetes, which profoundly impacts wound healing dynamics. Diabetic wounds, particularly in the context of chronic hyperglycemia, present a unique set of challenges that disrupt the normal wound healing cascade. Understanding the specific pathogenesis of diabetic wound healing is crucial, as it sheds light on the mechanisms that lead to delayed wound closure and chronic wound formation in diabetic patients as shown in Figure 2. Diabetic wounds face numerous challenges that significantly impede the healing process. A key issue is vasculopathy, where macrovascular complications in diabetes hinder the delivery of oxygen and essential nutrients to the wound site [17,18]. This is compounded by microcirculatory deficiencies, such as basement membrane thickening and reduced capillary size, which restrict physiological exchanges and impair blood flow. The situation is further exacerbated by endothelial dysfunction, which limits the production of nitric oxide, leading to suboptimal blood flow and delayed healing [19]. Another critical factor is neuropathy, where disruptions in motor, autonomic, and sensory nerve fibers diminish the ability to sense external stimuli, such as heat and pressure, delaying the healing process [20]. This sensory loss, coupled with motor fiber defects, increases physical stress on the wound, making it more prone to bacterial infections. Infections are a major concern in diabetic wounds, often leading to severe complications like abscesses, osteomyelitis, and cellulitis. These infections can rapidly develop in the hypoxic environment of a diabetic wound, further delaying the healing process [21–23]. The immune system also plays a role in delayed healing, as diabetes weakens immune cells, reducing their ability to combat infections. High blood sugar levels further inhibit immune function, increasing the risk of complications like sepsis or gangrene [24]. Additionally, interrupted growth factor activity is a significant contributor to delayed healing in diabetic wounds. Growth factors such as FGF, TGF-β and VEGF are critical for wound healing, but their levels are markedly reduced in diabetic patients, leading to prolonged inflammation and delayed tissue development [25]. Cellular dysfunction in key skin cells, including keratinocytes and fibroblasts, further hinders the healing process. The presence of specific microRNAs in diabetic foot ulcer fibroblasts has been shown to impair cellular functions, making wound recovery even more challenging [26]. Understanding the pathology of wound healing and the specific challenges presented by diabetic wound healing provides a foundational context for exploring the critical role of wound dressings. These dressings are not merely supplementary but play a pivotal role in managing wound healing by addressing the unique needs and complexities associated with different types of wounds, particularly those complicated by diabetes.

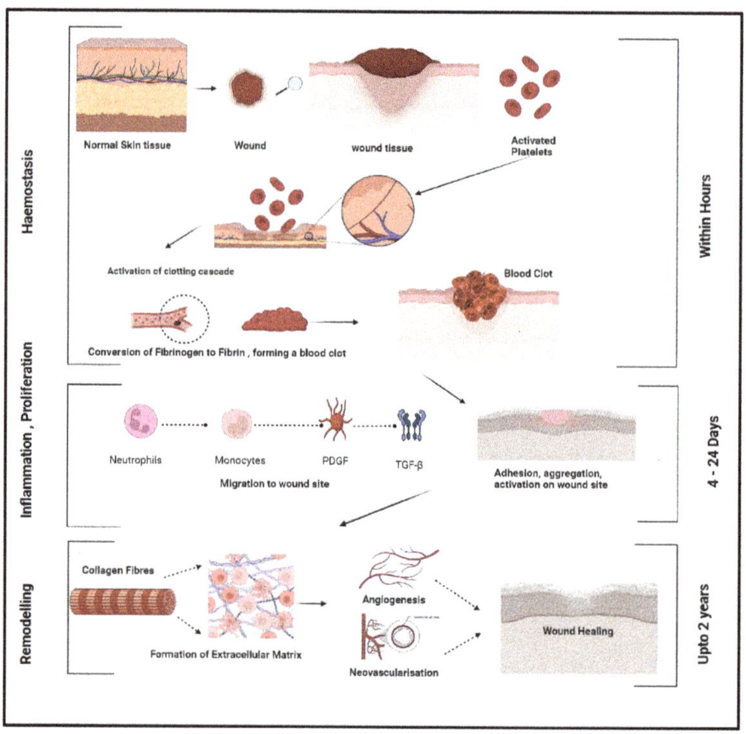

Figure 1. General Mechanisms of Wound Healing [26]—Wound healing progresses through three phases. The inflammatory phase starts with clot formation and immune response to prevent infection.

During the proliferative phase, new tissue and blood vessels develop to restore the wound. The remodeling phase then involves the strengthening and reorganization of the new tissue for final repair and recovery.

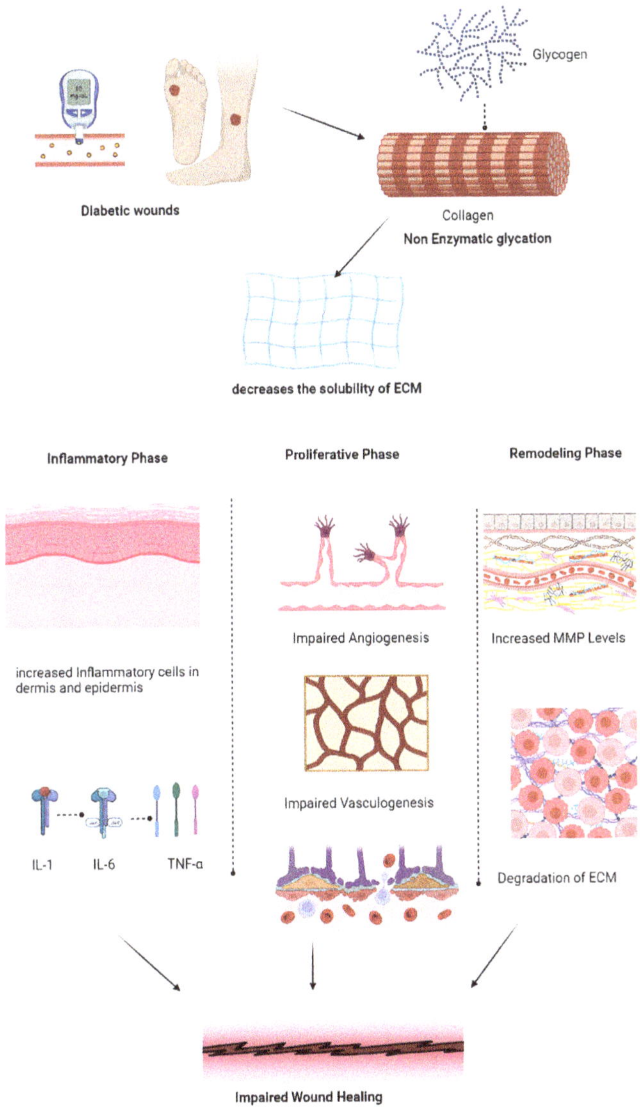

Figure 2. In diabetic wounds, impaired wound healing is primarily due to decreased collagen synthesis, which reduces the solubility of the extracellular matrix (ECM) and triggers an enhanced inflammatory response [26]. During the inflammatory phase, pro-inflammatory cytokines such as IL-1, IL-6, and TNF-α are released. The proliferative phase is characterized by impaired angiogenesis and vasculogenesis, while in the remodeling phase, increased levels of matrix metalloproteinases (MMPs) lead to further degradation of the ECM, ultimately contributing to impaired wound healing. (IL—interleukin, TNF—tumor necrosis factor, MMP—matrix metalloproteinase, and ECM—extracellular matrix).

3. Role of Bioactive Wound Dressings and Its Types

Wound dressings are integral to the effective management of various injuries, primarily by shielding wounds from bacterial invasion and expediting the process of wound healing [27]. Despite the availability of numerous wound dressings, some currently used materials exhibit limitations such as delayed healing, inadequate gaseous permeability, insufficient moisture retention, and the potential to trigger allergic reactions [28]. These shortcomings underscore the urgent need for the development of more effective wound dressing materials. Wound dressings are broadly categorized into four types: traditional/passive dressings, interactive materials, skin substitutes, and bioactive dressings as shown in Figure 3 [29]. Traditional dressings, such as wool dressings, plasters, gauze, and bandages, primarily function to protect the injury from foreign contaminants, control bleeding, cushion the wound, and absorb exudate. However, these dressings have limitations, including the risk of wound exudate leakage, which can lead to bacterial infections, and the potential for skin damage during removal.

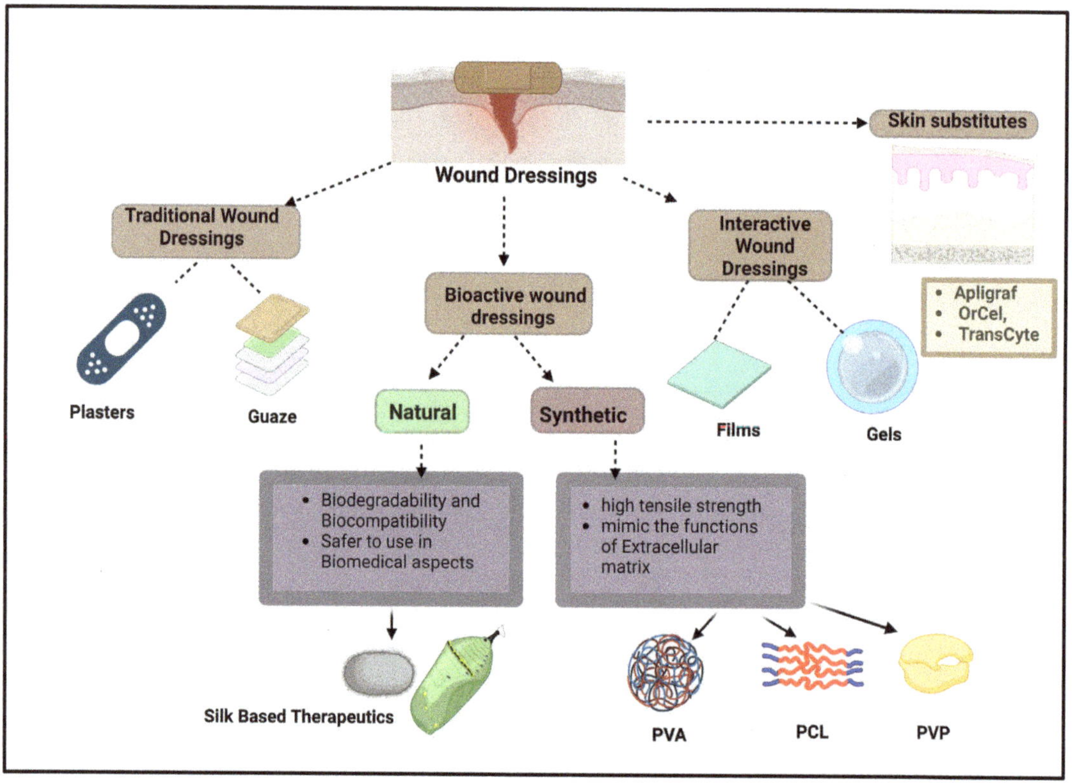

Figure 3. Overview of Wound Dressing Types and Their Characteristics: This figure categorizes wound dressings into traditional, interactive, and bioactive types. Traditional dressings, like plasters and gauze, offer basic protection. Interactive dressings (films, gels) and bioactive dressings (natural and synthetic) enhance healing. Natural materials, such as silk-based therapeutics, provide biodegradability and biocompatibility, while synthetic materials like PVA, PCL, and PVP offer high tensile strength. Skin substitutes like Apligraf, OrCel, and TransCyte represent advanced wound care options.

Interactive dressings, which include composites, films, gels, foams, and sprays, offer a more advanced approach to wound care by providing a moist environment conducive to healing enhancing re-epithelialization and granulation and promoting water transmission. These dressings can also be infused with bioactive agents to further accelerate the healing process. Skin substitutes, such as OrCel, Apligraf, and TransCyte, are sophisticated tissue-engineered structures typically developed from cell co-cultures or cell-seeded scaffolds. These substitutes are particularly effective in skin regeneration. However, they come with challenges, such as the risk of wound infections, disease transmission, potential rejection by the body, high costs, and limited shelf life [30]. Dermal grafts, including acellular xenografts, autografts, and allografts, are essential in dermatology and plastic surgery for treating traumatic wounds, burn reconstruction, post-oncologic resection defects, vitiligo, scar contracture release, hair restoration, and congenital skin deficiencies. Despite their utility, these materials are not suitable for managing complex injuries, particularly those involving exposed bones or deep tissue spaces [31]. Bioactive dressings, such as hydrocolloids, sponges, wafers, foams, nanofibers, hydrogels, and collagen-based materials, represent a significant advancement in wound care. These dressings are biodegradable, biocompatible, and can serve as drug delivery systems for therapeutic agents, including nanoparticles, growth factors, vitamins, and antibiotics, all of which contribute to improved wound healing [32]. Nanofibers [33] and hydrogels [34], in particular, stand out for their ability to be loaded with drugs and provide controlled delivery of bioactive agents, thus categorizing them as bioactive wound dressings.

While these wound dressings have played a significant role in wound management, the advent of advanced materials has led to the development of more sophisticated options. Among these, polymeric nanofibers have emerged as a promising class of wound dressings, offering unique properties that enhance healing outcomes. These nanofibers not only provide a physical barrier but also deliver therapeutic agents in a controlled manner, making them particularly suitable for addressing the complex needs of modern wound care [35]. Building on the foundation of bioactive wound dressings, the incorporation of polymeric nanofibers offers a promising approach to further enhance the therapeutic potential of these dressings, particularly by enabling controlled drug delivery, improved mechanical properties, and better integration with the wound microenvironment.

4. Mechanical Properties and Biocompatibility in Wound Dressings

As wound dressing technologies continue to evolve, the integration of advanced materials, particularly polymeric nanofibers, has opened new avenues for enhancing wound care. However, to fully realize the therapeutic potential of these innovations, it is essential to consider not only their ability to deliver bioactive agents but also their inherent mechanical properties and biocompatibility. The mechanical properties of wound dressing materials play a pivotal role in their effectiveness in promoting wound healing. Tensile strength, elasticity, porosity, permeability, flexibility, and adhesion are key factors that determine the material's performance. Tensile strength ensures the material can withstand mechanical stress without breaking, contributing to the durability of the dressing during wound care. Elasticity is critical for the material to conform to the wound bed and accommodate movement, especially in dynamic areas. Adequate porosity and permeability allow for oxygen exchange and moisture management while preventing bacterial invasion, maintaining an optimal healing environment. Flexibility is essential to ensure patient comfort and to avoid causing additional trauma to the wound during movement. Adhesion properties should enable the dressing to adhere securely to the wound bed without causing excessive pain or damage during dressing changes. In addition to mechanical properties, several parameters influence the wound healing process. Biocompatibility is a crucial consideration, as the material must not elicit an immune response or cause cytotoxicity. The degradation rate of biodegradable materials should be in harmony with tissue regeneration, as rapid degradation can result in premature loss of material, while slow degradation may cause irritation. Moisture retention capabilities are vital for maintaining the appropriate hydration levels in the wound, fostering cellular migration and proliferation. Materials designed for drug delivery can incorporate therapeutic agents such as antimicrobial peptides or growth factors, which directly address infection and promote tissue regeneration. Furthermore, material-cell interactions, influenced by surface properties such as roughness and charge, can enhance cell attachment, migration, and proliferation, contributing to effective wound closure. Some advanced materials may even provide mechanical stimulation to the wound, which can enhance cellular activity and collagen deposition, further accelerating the healing process. Considering both mechanical properties and these influential parameters allows for the design of wound dressings that not only protect but actively promote healing [36].

5. Polymeric Nanofibers Used in Wound Dressings

Polymeric nanofibers have emerged as a promising tool in the treatment of diabetic wounds due to their unique properties and potential to enhance wound healing. Among the various materials explored, silk fibroin stands out due to its exceptional biocompatibility and mechanical strength. Understanding the broader landscape of polymeric nanofibers, including both synthetic and natural variants, is crucial to appreciating the specific advantages silk fibroin offers in wound healing applications. These nanofibers, typically fabricated using both synthetic polymers such as polylactic acid (PLA), polycaprolactone (PCL), and polyvinyl alcohol (PVA), as well as natural polymers like chitosan, collagen, and gelatin, are characterized by their high surface area-to-volume ratio, porosity, and ability to mimic the extracellular matrix (ECM) [37]. Natural polymers offer additional benefits such as biocompatibility and bioactivity, which are particularly advantageous in promoting cell adhesion, proliferation and Natural polymers typically exhibit minimal immune response, while synthetic polymers are often preferred for their ease of electrospinning and excellent mechanical properties, including flexibility and stiffness The combination of these materials in nanofiber form supports cellular attachment, proliferation, and migration- key processes in wound healing [38,39]. Moreover, polymeric nanofibers can be engineered to incorporate and gradually release therapeutic agents directly at the wound site, ensuring sustained delivery of active ingredients, improving the healing process, and reducing infection risks [40]. The structure of these nanofibers closely resembles the ECM, providing a scaffold for tissue regeneration and enhancing natural healing processes, which are often impaired in diabetic patients. Additionally, polymeric nanofibers can promote angiogenesis by delivering factors such as VEGF, improve moisture retention, and can be functionalized with antimicrobial agents to prevent bacterial colonization. Despite the promising potential, challenges remain, including issues of biocompatibility, biodegradability, and large-scale production, which future research will need to address to realize the full potential of nanofiber-based therapies in clinical settings [39,41,42]. The selection of polymers for nanofiber-based wound dressings is not governed by a universal standard but is rather dictated by the specific functions desired from the nanofibers. The choice of polymers significantly influences properties such as the viscosity of the spinning solution, morphology of the nanofibers, mechanical strength, biocompatibility, and physicochemical characteristics [43]. Polymers used in this context are generally categorized into synthetic and natural types, each offering distinct advantages. To delve into the synthetic polymers utilized in wound dressings, The following are the synthetic polymers used in Bioactive wound dressings intended for Diabetic wound healing and Table 2 summarizes the various synthetic polymer formulations and their experimental applications in wound healing studies. By highlighting the strengths of synthetic polymers, we can better understand the context in which silk fibroin can be integrated as a viable alternative or complement to these materials.

Table 2. Synthetic polymer formulations and their effects on wound healing in experimental animals.

S.No.	Synthetic Polymers	Formulation	Experimental Animals	Highlights
1.	Polyethylene Glycol (PEG)	Chitosan crosslinked PEG Hydrogels loaded with silver nanoparticles	Rabbits	High porosity and improved antioxidant property and antimicrobial property. Boosted wound healing in experimental animals [44]
		Quaternized chitosan Combined PEG-CHO hydrogels	Rats	Good mechanical properties and Biocompatibilty, and improved angiogenesis and accelerated the process of wound healing in experimental animals [45]
		PEG-PDLLA Hydrogels	Mice	Enhanced angiogenesis and decreases the ROS, IL-6 and TNF. Promotes the healing of wounds [46]
2.	Polycaprolactone (PCL)	Composite PCL/electrospun nanocoated scaffolds with ACP and Si	Diabetic mice	Better mechanical stability, enhanced wound healing of full thickness wound by stimulating angiogenesis, collagen deposition and re-epithelialization [47]
		Composite nanofibrous scaffolds made of chitosan, gelatin, PCL, PVP	Diabetic rats	Cytocompatibility with respect to L929 cells. Accelerated the wound healing process by improving the collagen synthesis, lowering the inflammatory cytokines TNF, IL-6, IL-1 and NFkB [48]
3.	Polylactic acid (PLA)	Multilayered nanofibrous PLA patches	Diabetic rats	Better wound healing activity by adequate fibroblasts proliferation, angiogenesis and resulting in a healing of full thickness wound [49]
		Electrospun fibers made of PLA and PVP	Diabetic mice	Possesses anti-inflammatory and antibacterial activity prompting wound healing process [50]
4.	Poly(lactic-co-glycolic acid) (PLGA)	Composite PLGA/CNC nanofiber	Diabetic mice	Better cytocompatibility by fibroblast adhesion and accelerated full thickness wound healing decreasing the expression of IL-6 and IL-1B [51]
		PLGA incorporated nanoparticles	Diabetic mice	Very beneficial against MRSA diabetic wounds possess better wound healing efficiency [52]
5.	Polyvinyl alcohol (PVA)	PVA incorporated nanofibers	Diabetic mice	Accelerated closure of full-thickness • Wounds in diabetic mice, with • Enhanced revascularization and • re-epithelialization, increased • collagen deposition and remodeling, • and improved hair follicle • regeneration [53]
		PVA/GO hydrogels	Fibroblast cell lines	Good cytocompatibility and antibacterial activity and promote better wound healing activity [54]

Table 2. *Cont.*

S.No.	Synthetic Polymers	Formulation	Experimental Animals	Highlights
6.	Polyvinyl pyrrolidone (PVP)	Composite nanofibrous scaffolds made of chitosan, gelatin and PVP	Diabetic rats	High tensile strength, accelerated wound healing by improving the collagen remodelling by decreasing the levels of TNF, IL-6 and NFKB [55]
		PVP-grafted microspheres	Diabetic mice	Antibacterial and accelerated wound healing activity in experimental animal [55]

This table summarizes the various synthetic polymer formulations and their experimental applications in wound healing studies. The abbreviations used represent key compounds and biological markers relevant to the study, including polyethylene glycol (PEG), aldehyde group (CHO), poly(D,L-lactic acid) (PDLLA), polycaprolactone (PCL), amorphous calcium phosphate (ACP), silicon (Si), polyvinyl pyrrolidone (PVP), polylactic acid (PLA), Poly(lactic-co-glycolic acid) (PLGA), cellulose nanocrystals (CNC), methicillin-resistant *Staphylococcus aureus* (MRSA), polyvinyl alcohol (PVA), graphene oxide (GO), tumor necrosis factor, interleukin 6 (IL-6), interleukin 1 (IL-1), and nuclear factor kappa B (NF-κB).

Poly(lactic-co-glycolic acid) (PLGA) is a biocompatible and biodegradable polymer synthesized from lactic acid and glycolic acid. It is widely recognized for its excellent mechanical strength and flexibility, making it suitable for nanofibrous wound dressing applications. The degradation rate of PLGA can be adjusted by modifying the ratio of lactic acid to glycolic acid, molecular weight, and crystallinity [56]. However, PLGA's poor water solubility often necessitates the use of organic solvents, which can introduce cytotoxicity and hinder diabetic wound healing. To address this, modifications such as the synthesis of N-carboxyethyl PLGA have been explored to enhance water solubility. Additionally, the inclusion of chitosan and recombinant human platelet-derived growth factor in PLGA-based nanofibers has been shown to increase hydrophilicity, promoting wound healing in diabetic models [57]. The study by Castro et al. focuses on creating electrospun fibrous membranes made from β-tricalcium phosphate (β-TCP) and Poly(lactic-co-glycolic acid) (PLGA) for guided bone regeneration. The research demonstrates that combining the biodegradable nature of PLGA with the osteoconductive properties of β-TCP results in membranes that effectively support bone tissue regeneration [58]. Poly(lactic acid) (PLA) is a thermoplastic aliphatic polyester derived from renewable resources. Widely used in pharmaceuticals and medical devices, PLA offers biocompatibility and mechanical strength [59,60]. However, PLA may exhibit poor compatibility with blood, a limitation that can be mitigated by blending it with other polymers like chitosan derivatives. This blending enhances its blood compatibility, making PLA a valuable component in wound healing platforms that support cell attachment and proliferation. The work carried out by Chengyi Liu and colleagues details the development of a polylactic acid (PLA) electrospun wound dressing, modified with polyethylene glycol (PEG), rosmarinic acid, and graphite oxide. These modifications were aimed at enhancing the dressing's properties—PLA improved its flexibility and biocompatibility, rosmarinic acid contributed antioxidant properties, and graphite oxide increased mechanical strength. Through careful fabrication and characterization, the study demonstrates that this multifunctional wound dressing shows significant potential for promoting wound healing, making it a promising option for advanced wound care [61]. Poly(ε-caprolactone) (PCL) is another biocompatible and biodegradable polymer known for its functional ester bonds, which allow degradation into non-toxic byproducts in physiological conditions [62]. Despite its ability to mimic the extracellular matrix (ECM), PCL's hydrophobicity can limit cell attachment and proliferation [63]. To overcome this, PCL is often combined with hydrophilic polymers such as collagen, gelatin and chitosan. The research conducted by Deiviga Murugan et al. presents an innovative approach to wound healing with poly(ε-caprolactone) (PCL) nanofibrous scaffolds infused with the homeopathic mother tincture of *Syzygium cumini*. The study emphasizes PCL's pivotal role in providing structural stability and mechanical strength to the scaffolds. Its biocompatibility and controlled degradation characteristics complement the healing properties of *Syzygium cumini*, creating a synergistic effect that enhances wound healing outcomes [64]. Polyvinyl alcohol (PVA) is a water-soluble, non-toxic polymer with excellent mechanical properties and chemical resistance [65]. Its flexibility and swelling capacity make it a strong candidate for wound dressings. However, PVA tends to be unstable in aqueous environments, leading researchers to explore crosslinking, grafting and copolymerization with other polymers like polyvinyl pyrrolidone (PVP) and sterculia to enhance stability [66]. PVA-based nanofibers have also been incorporated with silver nanoparticles to provide antibacterial properties, which are critical for wound healing [67]. The study by Fatahian et al. explores the fabrication of electrospun polyvinyl alcohol (PVA) nanofibers with antibacterial and hemostatic properties for wound healing applications. The researchers developed a novel PVA-based nanofiber scaffold designed to offer both antimicrobial protection and promote blood clotting. This dual-functionality aims to enhance wound management by providing a protective barrier against infections while facilitating rapid Hemostasis [68].

Natural polymers are biopolymers derived from living organisms and have been widely used in various biomedical applications due to their inherent biocompatibility and biodegradability [69]. These polymers, which include chitosan, alginate, collagen, and silk fibroin, offer unique advantages in tissue engineering and wound care [70]. They are often favored for their ability to interact favorably with biological tissues, support cell growth, and promote healing processes. However, each natural polymer has its limitations, such as varying mechanical properties, degradation rates, and ease of processing. Among natural polymers, silk is distinguished by its exceptional biocompatibility, biodegradability, and mechanical strength. Its unique porous structure enhances cellular infiltration and tissue regeneration, addressing many of the limitations associated with other natural polymers and making it a valuable material for advanced wound care applications [71].

6. Silk Biomaterials and Silk Based Therapeutics in Diabetic Wound Healing

Silks are polymer derived proteins produced by various insects, including silkworms, spiders, bees, and others. Among these, silkworm silk, particularly from the domesticated species *Bombyx mori* (*B. mori*), is the most extensively studied and commercially utilized due to its favorable properties and availability [72]. Silks can be broadly categorized into mulberry and non-mulberry types, with mulberry silk being derived from the domesticated *Bombyx mori* silkworms. Non-mulberry silks, also known as wild silks, are produced by various species within the Saturniidae family, such as *Antheraea mylitta* (Tasar), *Antheraea assama* (Muga), and *Samia ricini* (Eri) [73,74]. These wild varieties differ in fibroin sequences and structural properties, leading to variations in mechanical strength, bioactivity, and degradation behavior. Spider silk, produced by species such as *Nephila clavipes* and *Araneus diadematus*, is renowned for its exceptional mechanical strength, surpassing that of silkworm silk. However, the production of spider silk on a commercial scale is challenging due to its heterogeneous nature and the difficulty in obtaining sufficient quantities [75–77]. As a result, *Bombyx mori silk* remains the primary source for silk-based biomaterials.

6.1. *Silk Fibroin's Structure and Properties*

Silk from the *Bombyx mori* silkworm comprises two primary proteins: fibroin and sericin. Fibroin, a core protein surrounded by sericin proteins [78]. The repetitive hydrophobic sequences within fibroin, mainly composed of glycine and alanine, contribute to its high strength and durability, making it a desirable biomaterial [79]. Fibroin, which constitutes approximately 70% of the silk's weight, forms the inner core of the silk thread, providing mechanical strength. The remaining 30% is composed of sericin, a protein that surrounds the fibroin core in a thin layer and also contains fat/wax (0.8–1%) and color/ash (1–1.4%) [80]. Silk, a natural protein polymer, is recognized by the U.S. Food and Drug Administration (FDA) for medical applications due to its biocompatibility and unique properties [81]. Silk fibroin is derived from mulberry silk after the removal of the outer sericin layer, which is known to trigger an immune response when combined with fibroin.

During the spinning process, the silkworm larvae extrude two fine fibroin filaments (approximately 10 μm in diameter) through their spinnerets, which are simultaneously coated with sericin from the silk glands. Upon exposure to air, these protein fibers become stronger and tougher [82,83].

The major structural component of silk, fibroin, contributes to its mechanical strength, while sericin acts as a glue-like coating that holds the fibroin filaments together. Each silk Fiber consists of two fibroin filaments encased in sericin [84]. These nanofibrils are the fundamental building blocks of silk and are tightly intertwined to form larger fibril units known as microfibrils, which range from 20 to 200 nm in diameter. Both microfibrils and nanofibrils are aligned parallel to the silk fibroin filaments, contributing to the silk's robust fibrous properties [85,86]. Silk fibroin's molecular structure consists of polypeptide chains with molecular weights ranging from 200 to 350 kDa. The primary structure of fibroin is an H-L complex, which includes a heavy (H) chain polypeptide and a light (L) chain polypeptide connected by a single disulfide bond at the C-terminus of the H-chain. Additionally, a glycoprotein called P25 is noncovalently bound to the H-L chains, playing a crucial role in maintaining the overall structural integrity of silk fibroin. The H-chain is largely responsible for the fibrous properties of silk, with glycine (46%), serine (12%), and alanine (30%) being the most prevalent amino acids in this chain. In contrast, the non-fibrous L-chains contain amino acids such as isoleucine, leucine, valine, and other acidic amino acids [87]. Owing to its biocompatibility, gradual degradation, low immunogenicity, versatility, and excellent mechanical properties, silk fibroin is increasingly being explored for various biomedical applications. Its ability to adapt to biological environments suggests that it may integrate better into the body with potentially reduced material-associated thrombosis [88–90]. This potential pave the way for developing biomaterials with tailored properties based on silk motifs. Historically, specific amino acid patterns have been linked to functional properties, and these patterns can be genetically or chemically modified to create recombinant silk polymers that control chemical reactivity, polymer size, and bulk material characteristics while preserving essential secondary structural features [91].

6.2. *Wound Healing Mechanism of Silk Fibroin*

Silk fibroin (SF) plays a pivotal role in various stages of the wound healing process, demonstrating its effectiveness across multiple mechanisms as clearly described in Figure 4. One of the key contributions of SF is in promoting hemostasis, the initial and crucial step in healing. The structure of SF provides an ideal environment for the rapid adsorption of platelets, leading to the activation of the coagulation cascade and subsequent clot formation. This is facilitated by the porous nature of SF matrices, which efficiently trap blood cells and platelets, thereby accelerating the process of hemostasis. By minimizing blood loss and creating a stable environment at the wound site, SF sets the stage for the healing process to proceed smoothly [92–94]. As healing progresses, SF continues to support critical cellular behaviors such as attachment, migration, and proliferation. Its biochemical and physical properties mimic the extracellular matrix, promoting integrin-mediated cell adhesion. This encourages the attachment of various cell types, including keratinocytes and fibroblasts, to the wound bed, while also guiding cell migration—a process essential for wound closure. Additionally, SF modulates the release of growth factors and cytokines, enhancing cellular proliferation and ensuring effective tissue regeneration. The impact of SF extends further as it supports neovascularization and angiogenesis, processes vital for supplying nutrients and oxygen to the healing tissue. SF matrices, with their porous structure and biodegradability, provide a conducive environment for endothelial cell infiltration and new blood vessel formation [95–97]. By facilitating the release of angiogenic factors like VEGF in a controlled manner, SF enhances the formation of a capillary network, ensuring the regenerating tissue receives an adequate blood supply. This vascular support is crucial for effective healing, preventing tissue necrosis and promoting overall tissue health [98]. SF plays an instrumental role in re-epithelialization, the phase of wound healing that restores the epidermal barrier. The biocompatibility and structural mimicry of natural ECM by SF enable keratinocytes to adhere, spread, and form a new epithelial layer over the wound. By maintaining an optimal moisture balance and protecting the wound from external contaminants, SF creates an ideal microenvironment for re-epithelialization, speeding up wound closure and improving the quality of the regenerated skin [99].

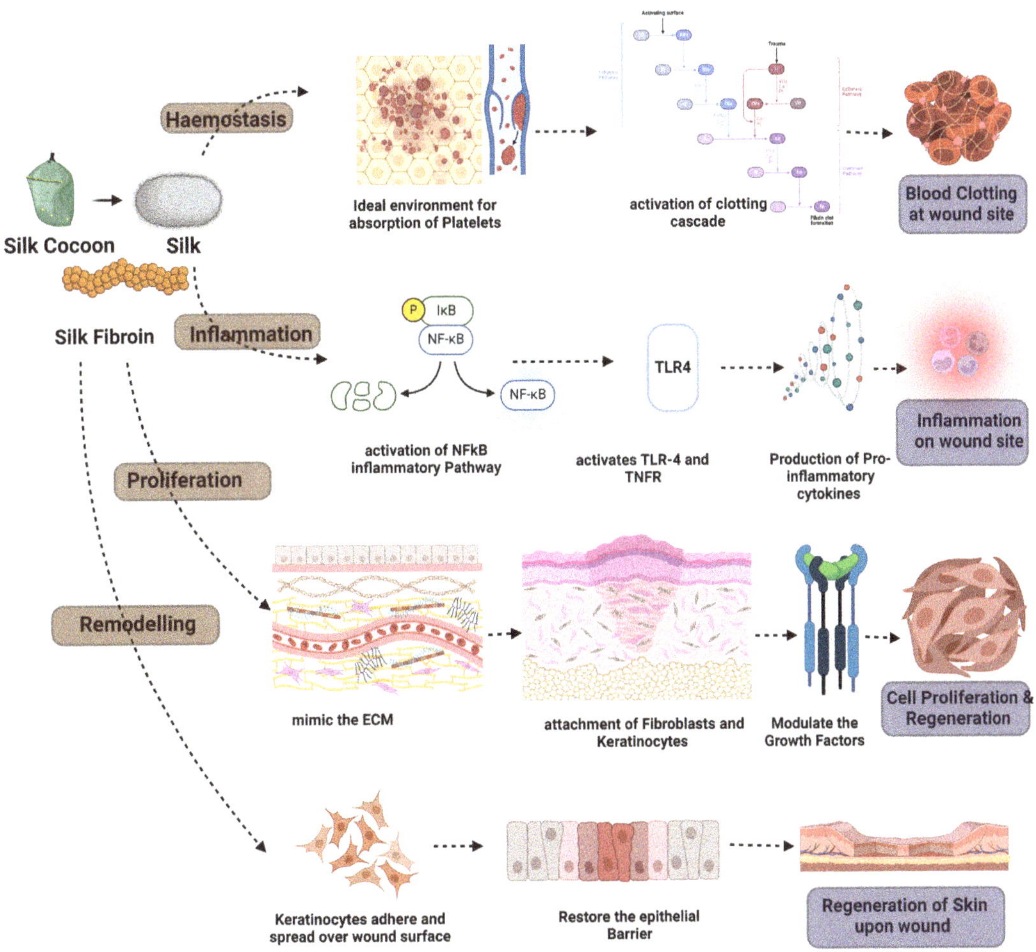

Figure 4. Silk fibroin aids wound healing by modulating inflammation, supporting angiogenesis, and enhancing ECM remodeling. It reduces inflammatory cytokines, promotes cell growth and migration, and improves ECM organization throughout the healing phases.

The mechanisms by which silk fibroin enhances wound healing involve several intricate cellular signaling pathways. Silk fibroin accelerates wound healing primarily by modulating the NF-κB signaling pathway, a critical regulator of numerous cellular processes essential for tissue repair. NF-κB, or nuclear factor kappa light-chain-enhancer of activated B cells, is a transcription factor that controls the expression of genes involved in various cellular behaviors such as proliferation, adhesion, the clearance of reactive oxygen species (ROS), and inflammation. When silk fibroin interacts with cells, it stimulates the NF-κB signaling pathway by increasing the expression of receptors such as tumor necrosis factor receptor (TNFR) and Toll-like receptors (TLRs). These receptors, upon activation, initiate a cascade of intracellular events that lead to the activation of NF-κB. Once activated, NF-κB translocates into the cell nucleus, where it binds to specific DNA sequences to regulate the transcription of a broad array of genes. These genes encode proteins that play vital roles in the wound healing process [100]. For instance, NF-κB upregulates the production of cytokines and growth factors such as EGF and VEGF, which are essential for promoting cell proliferation and new blood vessel formation. Additionally, NF-κB enhances the expression of adhesion molecules like fibronectin, which are crucial for cell attachment and migration, facilitating the re-epithelialization of the wound. Moreover, NF-κB's role in controlling the inflammatory response is particularly significant in wound healing. By regulating the production of pro-inflammatory cytokines like interleukin-1 beta (IL-1β) and anti-inflammatory cytokines like interleukin-10 (IL-10), NF-κB helps balance the inflammation process, ensuring that it is sufficient to combat infection without causing excessive tissue damage. This balance is vital for clearing the wound of pathogens and debris while allowing tissue regeneration to proceed efficiently. Furthermore, NF-κB influences the production of proteins such as vimentin, which is involved in cell shape and movement, and transforming growth factor-beta (TGF-β), which is key in tissue remodeling and scar formation [101]. By orchestrating these complex cellular responses, NF-κB, activated by silk fibroin, plays an integral role in advancing the wound healing process from the initial inflammatory phase through to the proliferation and remodeling stages. These processes are vital for effective wound healing, particularly in diverse types of wounds such as corneal epithelial wounds. In silk fibroin-induced cells, there is an upregulation of key mediators of NF-κB, including tumor necrosis factor receptor (TNFR) and Toll-like receptors (TLRs). By influencing the expression of these proteins, silk fibroin plays a critical role in the remodeling and proliferation phases of wound healing [102].

Moreover, silk fibroin has been shown to have protective effects in various models of injury. For example, in a rat model of burn injury, silk fibroin was found to inactivate the apoptotic pathway, thereby protecting cells from programmed cell death. This protective effect is likely mediated through the regulation of several complex cellular signaling pathways, including Wnt and Notch signaling, TGF-β signaling, mitogen-activated protein kinase (MAPK) signaling, and AKT/mTOR signaling [103]. Both MAPK and AKT/mTOR pathways are well-known for their roles in wound healing, where they contribute to cell proliferation, migration, and survival [104]. The ability of silk fibroin to modulate critical signaling pathways, particularly NF-κB, along with its biocompatibility, user-friendly nature, and minimal immune response, positions it as a highly promising material for wound healing applications.

Silk fibroin can be utilized in various forms, including solutions, films, electrospun nanofiber mats, hydrogels, hydrocolloid dressings, and sponges, to enhance wound healing. Among these various forms, electrospun nanofiber mats stand out as the most promising option due to their unique properties and superior performance in enhancing wound healing. This brings us to a closer examination of the electrospinning technique and its advantages in the development of silk fibroin-based wound dressings. However, silk fibroin can be formed using several other methods, each with its own set of advantages and limitations. To provide a comprehensive overview, the following Table 3 outlines the benefits and drawbacks of various methods for forming silk fibroin. Additionally, 3D printing is emerging as an innovative technique that holds great potential for creating wound-healing materials. 3D Printing provides superior control over scaffold architecture, enabling precise customization in terms of pore size, shape, and spatial distribution, which can enhance the material's interaction with cells and improve wound healing. Electrospinning and freeze drying, while established methods, lack the same level of control over scaffold structure. Additionally, 3D printing eliminates the need for potentially harmful solvents, making it a more biocompatible option for some applications. However, 3D printing can struggle with mechanical strength, similar to hydrogel methods, and its use in processing silk fibroin still requires further optimization to match the efficiency of established methods like electrospinning [105].

Table 3. Comparison of various methods for forming silk fibroin and their application in wound healing [105].

S.No.	Methods	Advantages	Disadvantages
1.	Electrospinning	• Produces nanofibers with high surface area • Mimics extracellular matrix (ECM) • Easy functionalization	• Requires volatile solvents • Limited fiber control and alignment
2.	Freeze Drying	• Creates porous structures • Good for tissue scaffolds • Retains bioactivity	• Fragile structures • Time-consuming process
3.	Solvent Casting	• Simple and inexpensive • Suitable for film production • Good control over film thickness	• Limited pore structure • Residual solvent toxicity issues
4.	Hydrogel Formation	• Excellent moisture retention • Mimics ECM • Ideal for drug delivery systems	• Poor mechanical strength • Limited scalability
5.	Lyophilization	• Suitable for highly porous scaffolds • No need for organic solvents	• Slow process • High cost • Can cause structural collapse
6.	3D Printing	• Precise control over geometry and pore size • Customizable designs • No need for toxic solvents	• Limited mechanical strength in some cases • Requires optimization for silk fibroin processing

This table compares methods for forming silk fibroin in wound healing. Each method has strengths, like the high surface area of electrospun nanofibers and the precision of 3D printing, but also limitations such as solvent use and scalability.

7. Electrospinning—Fabrication Method of Silk Fibroin

7.1. Electrospinning

Electrospinning has emerged as a prominent technique for the fabrication of nanofibers, especially in the field of biomedical applications such as wound healing. Among the various methods available for nanofiber preparation such as drawing, phase separation, template synthesis, extraction, and self-assembly [106]. Electrospinning is considered the most feasible and straightforward. The primary advantages of electrospinning over other methods include its ability to produce nanofibers at a large scale, the use of a wide range of polymers, and the elimination of the need for post-synthetic processing, which are often required in other techniques [107]. This method has seen significant advancements in recent years, particularly for applications in diabetic wounds (DWs) [108]. Electrospinning operates on a simple yet highly effective principle. A polymer solution or melt is placed within a syringe equipped with a needle, which serves as the spinneret. An electric potential is then applied to this polymer solution, resulting in the formation of fibers with diameters ranging from 50 to 1000 nm or even greater. The process begins with the polymer solution being extruded through the needle, forming a droplet at the tip. Under the influence of the applied electric field, this droplet elongates, creating a cone shape known as the Taylor cone. As the electric potential increases, it reaches a critical point where the electrostatic forces overcome the surface tension of the polymer solution, leading to the ejection of a fine jet of the solution. This jet undergoes rapid stretching and thinning due to solvent evaporation and electrostatic forces, ultimately forming nanofibers that are collected on a stationary or rotating metal collector [109,110]. The electrospinning setup is relatively simple and typically consists of three main components: a high-voltage power supply, a syringe with a needle, and a conductive collector. The high-voltage supply provides the necessary driving force to generate an electric field between the spinneret and the collector. The polymer solution, housed within the syringe, is fed at a controlled rate toward the needle tip, where it is subjected to the electric field. As the polymeric jet is ejected from the Taylor cone, it travels towards the collector, where the solvent evaporates, leaving behind solid nanofibers [111]. Several key parameters influence the electrospinning process and the resulting nanofiber morphology. They are 1. Applied Voltage: The strength of the electric field directly affects the formation of the Taylor cone and the ejection of the polymer jet. Higher voltages can increase the rate of fiber production but may also lead to defects such as beading if not carefully controlled [112]. 2. Solution Flow Rate: The rate at which the polymer solution is fed through the needle influences the thickness and uniformity of the fibers. A higher flow rate can result in thicker fibers, while a lower flow rate produces finer fibers. 3. Needle Diameter: The internal diameter of the needle determines the initial diameter of the polymer jet and, consequently, the final Fiber diameter. A smaller needle diameter generally leads to finer Fibers. 4. Tip-to-Collector Distance: The distance between the needle tip and the collector affects the time available for the jet to stretch and the solvent to evaporate. A longer distance allows for more thinning of the fibers, while a shorter distance may lead to incomplete solvent evaporation and thicker fibers. 5. Ambient Conditions: Temperature, humidity, air velocity, and pressure within the electrospinning chamber play significant roles in the process [113,114]. For example, higher humidity can cause the fibers to retain moisture, leading to defects, while temperature fluctuations can affect the viscosity of the polymer solution and the rate of solvent evaporation.

Electrospinning has a rich history, dating back to its first patent in 1934 by Anton Formhals, who originally intended it for textile production. The technique was initially used to produce threads, which were collected and converted into fabric using a ground collector. Over time, electrospinning has evolved into a powerful method for producing nanoscale fibers, particularly for biomedical applications. The technique gained prominence in the late 20th and early 21st centuries as researchers recognized its potential for creating nanofibers that closely mimic the extracellular matrix, an essential component in tissue engineering and wound healing [115,116], Table 4 compared and contrasted the role of ECM and electrospun mats in the process of wound Healing. In the context of wound healing, especially for diabetic wounds, electrospun nanofibers offer several advantages. These fibers have a high surface-to-volume ratio, which enhances cell attachment and proliferation, crucial for tissue regeneration. The porosity of the nanofibrous scaffolds allows for adequate nutrient and oxygen exchange while providing a barrier against bacterial invasion. Furthermore, the chemical versatility of electrospun fibers enables the incorporation of bioactive molecules, such as growth factors or antimicrobial agents, to promote faster and more effective wound healing. The recent advancements in electrospinning have enabled the production of nanofibers with diverse structural and morphological organizations, tailored to meet specific biomedical applications. For example, researchers have developed core-shell nanofibers for controlled drug release, aligned nanofibers to guide cell growth, and multilayered scaffolds that mimic the complex structure of natural tissues. These innovations highlight the potential of electrospinning as a standard method for fabricating nanofibers in regenerative medicine. Electrospinning is a highly adaptable and efficient technique for producing nanofibers with a wide range of applications, particularly in wound healing. Its ability to control fibers morphology and tailor the properties of nanofibers to specific needs has made it a cornerstone in the development of advanced biomaterials [117,118]. As research in this area continues to progress, electrospinning is likely to play an increasingly important role in creating innovative solutions for medical challenges, such as the treatment of diabetic wounds.

Table 4. Comparison of electrospun nanofiber scaffolds and extracellular matrix.

Comparison	Extracellular Matrix (ECM)	Electrospun Scaffolds
Components	Comprised of a dynamic 3D network of polysaccharides and natural polymers (collagen, elastin, fibrinogen, etc.)	Primarily made from synthetic and natural polymers
Structure	Consists mainly of fibers with diameters between 50 and 500 nm	Nanofibers typically range from 10 μm to 500 nm in diameter, produced via electrospinning
Role in Wound Healing	• Facilitates pattern formation, morphogenesis, and phenotype maintenance during development • Mediates clot formation, wound healing, inflammation, granulation tissue formation, and tissue remodeling • Supports cell adhesion, migration, growth, differentiation, and apoptosis	• Offers suitable porosity for cell migration and penetration • Provides ample surface area and chemistry for cell adhesion, growth, migration, and differentiation • Degrades at a rate that aligns with tissue regeneration, supporting proper tissue integration

The table provides a comparative overview of electrospun nanofiber scaffolds and the extracellular matrix (ECM) with respect to their components, structure, and roles in wound healing.

7.2. Types of Electrospinning

As a "top-down" fiber-production technique, electrospinning offers several advantages, including simplicity in operation, low production costs, and minimal energy consumption. This method effectively combines polymer materials with inorganic nanoparticles to produce fibers with diameters in the nano- to micrometer range relatively quickly. The earliest and most commonly used electrospinning system is the single-spinneret system. Over time, advancements in technology have led to the development of more complex systems, such as double- and multineedle configurations. Researchers have also tailored nanofibers with specific shapes and structures by varying parameters such as polymer type, molecular weight, solution conductivity, voltage, flow rate, temperature, and humidity. These adjustments can produce a range of fiber structures, including porous, pleated, hollow, beaded, and reticulated forms, making electrospinning a prominent research area in various fields [119]. Uniaxial electrospinning, also known as single-fluid or traditional electrospinning, is one of the most widely utilized techniques for fabricating nanofibers. This process involves using a single polymer solution or melt, which is extruded through a spinneret under the influence of a high electric field [120]. Due to the limitations of single-fluid electrospinning, multifluid electrospinning techniques have been developed. These methods involve two or more working fluids, allowing for the creation of more complex nanofiber structures. Multifluid electrospinning includes coaxial electrospinning, side-by-side electrospinning, triaxial electrospinning [121–124].

7.3. Mechanism of Wound Healing by Electrospun Fibers in the Various Phases of Wound Healing

Electrospun fibers are proving to be transformative in wound healing due to their versatile and beneficial properties across various phases of the healing process. In the initial Hemostasis phase, which is crucial for stopping bleeding and forming a stable clot, electrospun fibers provide essential mechanical support [125]. Their highly porous structure aids in trapping blood cells and platelets, thereby facilitating effective clot formation. This early intervention helps stabilize the wound environment, minimizing excessive bleeding and creating a foundation for the subsequent phases of healing. During the inflammation phase, which focuses on cleaning the wound and initiating repair processes, electrospun fibers play a significant role in modulating the inflammatory response [126]. Many of these fibers are designed to incorporate anti-inflammatory agents or possess intrinsic properties that help mitigate excessive inflammation, which is critical as prolonged inflammation can delay healing. The fibrous network also supports the migration of inflammatory cells, such as macrophages and neutrophils, to the wound site. This migration is essential for clearing out cellular debris and pathogens. Additionally, the fibers can be engineered to release growth factors gradually, which aids in controlling inflammation and preparing the wound bed for the next phase of healing. As the wound transitions into the proliferation phase, electrospun fibers provide a scaffold that is pivotal for cellular activities such as fibroblast and keratinocyte proliferation and migration. The fibers micro and nanostructures closely mimic the extracellular matrix (ECM), offering a supportive environment that guides the orientation and growth of these cells. This mimicry is crucial as it helps in forming new tissue layers [126]. Furthermore, electrospun fibers enhance angiogenesis—the formation of new blood vessels—by providing a conducive environment for vascular growth. This process is vital for supplying the growing tissue with necessary nutrients and oxygen. In addition, the fibers can be tailored to support collagen deposition, which is key for reinforcing tissue strength and integrity. In the final remodeling phase, which involves the maturation and reorganization of the newly formed tissue, electrospun fibers contribute significantly to tissue development [127]. By replicating the ECM, these fibers help in the proper alignment and maturation of collagen fibers, which is crucial for enhancing tissue strength and elasticity. Biodegradable electrospun fibers are particularly advantageous as they degrade in a controlled manner, aligning with the natural timeline of ECM replacement. This controlled degradation helps in minimizing scar formation and ensuring the stability of the newly formed tissue [128].

7.4. Electrospun Silk Based Scaffolds from Bench to Bed Side

The evolution of wound care and tissue engineering has brought forth numerous innovations, among which electrospun silk-based scaffolds stand as a significant milestone. These scaffolds have garnered widespread attention due to their unique combination of biocompatibility, biodegradability, and mechanical strength, which closely mimics the extracellular matrix (ECM) of human tissues. The electrospinning process, a versatile technique capable of producing nanofibers with high surface area-to-volume ratios, plays a crucial role in enhancing the functional properties of silk fibroin. This has led to the development of advanced wound dressings and tissue scaffolds that support cellular adhesion, proliferation, and differentiation. Despite these challenges, the potential benefits of electrospun silk-based scaffolds are immense. Their ability to deliver bioactive agents, such as growth factors and antimicrobial peptides, in a controlled and sustained manner is particularly advantageous for treating chronic wounds, such as those associated with diabetes.

The synthesis of silk-based dressings and the application of electrospinning techniques converge to form a powerful strategy in wound management. By harnessing the natural biocompatibility and structural integrity of silk fibroin and combining it with the versatility of electrospinning, researchers have developed electrospun silk-based scaffolds that offer a unique blend of properties ideal for wound healing. These advanced dressings not only capitalize on the inherent advantages of silk fibers but also leverage the fine-tuned control over fiber morphology, porosity, and surface functionality provided by electrospinning. The resulting electrospun silk-based dressings represent a sophisticated integration of material science and bioengineering, designed to meet the complex demands of wound repair and tissue regeneration. In the study conducted by K. Karthikeyan et al. [129] novel biofibers were fabricated by coating silk fibroin with chitosan impregnated with silver nanoparticles, resulting in scaffolds that exhibited potent antibacterial properties and enhanced wound healing potential. Similarly, Salvador Aznar-Cervantes et al. [130] developed electrospun silk fibroin scaffolds coated with graphene oxide and reduced graphene, which demonstrated improved electrical conductivity, mechanical strength, and biocompatibility, crucial for promoting cell adhesion and proliferation in wound healing. Sónia P. Miguel et al. [131] produced and characterized electrospun silk fibroin-based asymmetric membranes, which featured a porous top layer for moisture management and a denser bottom layer for structural support, thus creating an ideal wound environment that promotes healing while preventing infection. Additionally, M. Rama and U. Vijayalakshmi [132] investigated the influence of silk fibroin in nanofibrous scaffolds designed for osteoregenerative applications, revealing enhanced osteoconductive properties that could be particularly beneficial in cases where bone exposure is involved in deep wound healing. Win chun Juo et.al [133,134] focused on the fabrication and characterization of electrospun silk fibroin/TiO_2 nanofibrous mats, where the inclusion of TiO_2 was shown to improve mechanical properties, enhance cell proliferation, and provide antibacterial activity, making these mats promising candidates for wound dressings. Kuberasampathkumar Shanmugam and Subramanian Sundaramoorthy [135] explored the development of electrospun mats from Eri silk fibroin and PLA blends, highlighting their balanced mechanical strength, biodegradability, and biocompatibility, which support cell proliferation and effective wound healing as shown in Figure 5. These studies collectively underscore the versatility and effectiveness of electrospun silk fibroin-based scaffolds in various wound healing applications, from antibacterial treatments to supporting tissue regeneration.

In recent years, the integration of electrospun silk-based scaffolds into clinical practice is a rapidly advancing field. Ongoing research aims to optimize their properties, explore their multifunctional capabilities, and establish standardized protocols for their use in various medical applications. As these scaffolds continue to move through the pipeline from experimental models to clinical trials, they represent a beacon of hope for patients suffering from non-healing wounds and other tissue defects. The application of biomaterials as wound dressings for diabetic wounds has been extensively studied in Clinical research settings. However, only a limited number of these have progressed to clinical testing, and even fewer have received approval and have become commercially available for diabetic wound management in the past five years. Several barriers hinder the clinical translation of these wound dressings from research to market. One significant challenge is the necessity for additional validation by regulatory bodies such as the U.S. Food and Drug Administration (FDA) or the European Union Medical Device Regulation when chemical modifications are made to biomaterials to enhance their inherent properties. This requirement introduces an extra step in the process of material safety and quality assessment, which must be completed before the already time-intensive technology validation can begin. Moreover, the standard methods used to characterize traditional wound dressings may not be sufficient to demonstrate the advanced capabilities of innovative wound dressings in enhancing wound healing. More sophisticated models of diabetic wound conditions and more comprehensive techniques are often needed to simultaneously assess tissue regeneration rates, drug release efficiency, and stimuli-responsive mechanisms. In addition, the complexity of these advanced wound dressings, often featuring multicomponent and multifunctional cores, complicates the processes of device classification and validation. It can be challenging to determine the primary mode of action of a wound dressing, given that many exhibits combined mechanisms.

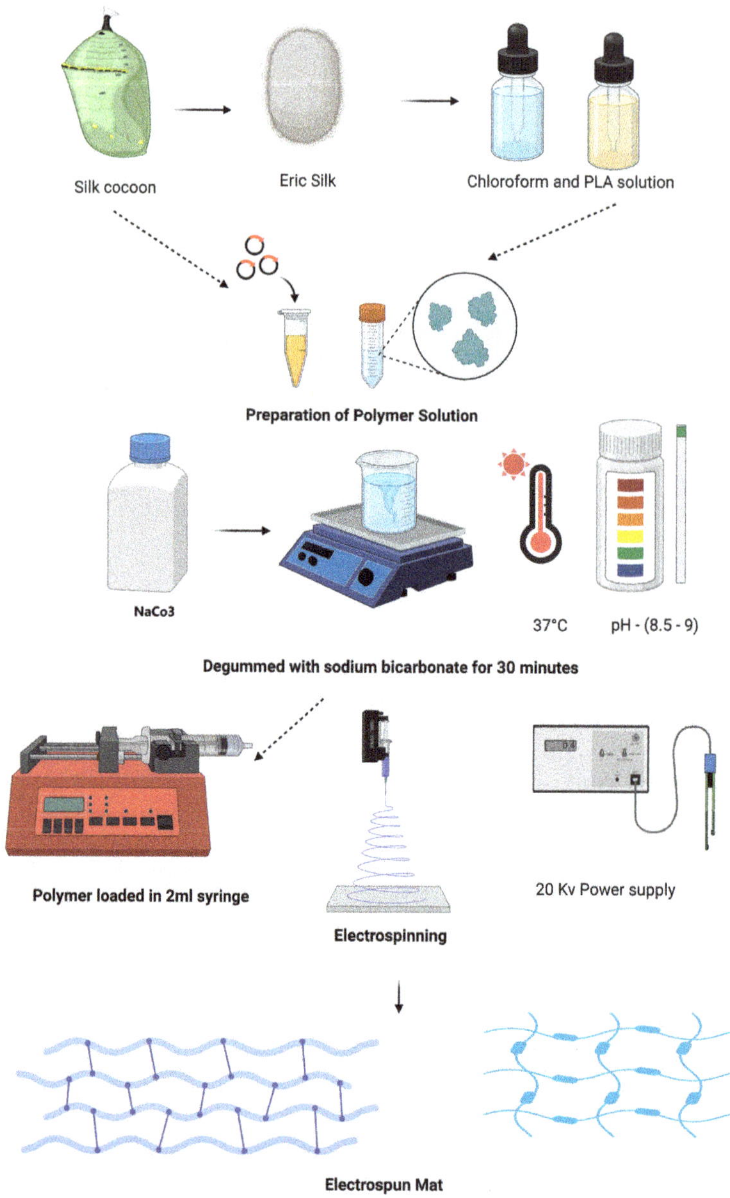

Figure 5. The electrospun mat formulation by Kuberasampathkumar Shanmugam and Subramanian Sundaramoorthy involves dissolving Eri silk fibroin and PLA in suitable solvents, blending the solutions, and electrospinning the blend into nanofibers. The resulting mat is dried and characterized for its properties using techniques such as SEM and tensile testing to ensure its suitability for wound dressing applications [135].

8. Conclusions and Future Perspectives

The clinical translation of electrospun silk fibroin-based formulations holds great promise but faces significant challenges, including the scalability of production, regulatory hurdles, and the need for thorough safety and efficacy evaluations. Overcoming these obstacles will require collaborative efforts and rigorous testing to ensure these innovative biomaterials can be effectively and safely integrated into medical practice. Looking ahead, the future of electrospun silk fibroin-based formulations appears bright. Ongoing advancements in biofabrication techniques, along with a deeper understanding of silk fibroin's interactions within biological systems, are expected to drive the development of next-generation biomaterials. These innovations have the potential to revolutionize medical treatments, offering personalized and highly effective therapeutic solutions that could significantly impact the field of regenerative medicine.

Funding: The authors extend their appreciation to the Deanship of Scientific Research and Graduate Studies at King Khalid University for funding this work through Large Research Project under grant number "RGP2/402/45".

Acknowledgments: The authors would like to thank the Deanship of Scientific Research and Graduate Studies at King Khalid University, by supporting the Research (RGP2/402/45). The authors would like to thank the Management of SRM Institute of Science and Technology and St. Peters Institute of Pharmaceutical Sciences for their support towards the work.

Conflicts of Interest: The authors declare no conflict of interest.

Abbreviations

DM	Diabetes Mellitus
VEGF	Vascular Endothelial Growth Factor
TGF	Transforming Growth Factor
IL-4	Interleukin-4
IL-13	Interleukin-13
TNF	Tumor Necrosis Factor
FGF	Fibroblast Growth Factor
PLA	Polylactic Acid
PCL	Polycaprolactone
PLGA	Poly(lactic-co-glycolic acid)
PVA	Polyvinyl Alcohol
ECM	Extracellular Matrix
SF	Silk Fibroin
NFkB	Nuclear Factor-kappa B
ROS	Reactive Oxygen Species
TLR	Toll-Like Receptor
TNFR	Tumor Necrosis Factor Receptor
MAPK	Mitogen-Activated Protein Kinase
AKT	Protein Kinase B
IL-10	Interleukin-10
FGF	Fibroblast Growth Factor
IGF	Insulin Like Growth Factor
KGF	Keratinocyte Growth Factor
HGF	Hepatocyte Growth Factor

References

1. American Diabetes Association. Diagnosis and Classification of Diabetes Mellitus. *Diabetes Care* **2009**, *32*, S62–S67. [CrossRef] [PubMed]
2. Burgess, J.L.; Wyant, W.A.; Abdo Abujamra, B.; Kirsner, R.S.; Jozic, I. Diabetic Wound-Healing Science. *Medicina* **2021**, *57*, 1072. [CrossRef]
3. Frykberg, R.G.; Banks, J. Challenges in the Treatment of Chronic Wounds. *Adv. Wound Care* **2015**, *4*, 560–582. [CrossRef]

4. Dasari, N.; Jiang, A.; Skochdopole, A.; Chung, J.; Reece, E.M.; Vorstenbosch, J.; Winocour, S. Updates in Diabetic Wound Healing, Inflammation, and Scarring. *Semin. Plast. Surg.* **2021**, *35*, 153–158. [CrossRef] [PubMed]
5. Saeedi, P.; Petersohn, I.; Salpea, P.; Malanda, B.; Karuranga, S.; Unwin, N.; Colagiuri, S.; Guariguata, L.; Motala, A.A.; Ogurtsova, K.; et al. Global and Regional Diabetes Prevalence Estimates for 2019 and Projections for 2030 and 2045: Results from the International Diabetes Federation Diabetes Atlas, 9th Edition. *Diabetes Res. Clin. Pract.* **2019**, *157*, 107843. [CrossRef] [PubMed]
6. Järbrink, K.; Ni, G.; Sönnergren, H.; Schmidtchen, A.; Pang, C.; Bajpai, R.; Car, J. The Humanistic and Economic Burden of Chronic Wounds: A Protocol for a Systematic Review. *Syst. Rev.* **2017**, *6*, 15. [CrossRef] [PubMed]
7. Sharma, A.; Shankar, R.; Yadav, A.K.; Pratap, A.; Ansari, M.A.; Srivastava, V. Burden of Chronic Nonhealing Wounds: An Overview of the Worldwide Humanistic and Economic Burden to the Healthcare System. *Int. J. Low Extrem. Wounds* **2024**. [CrossRef] [PubMed]
8. Shi, C.; Wang, C.; Liu, H.; Li, Q.; Li, R.; Zhang, Y.; Liu, Y.; Shao, Y.; Wang, J. Selection of Appropriate Wound Dressing for Various Wounds. *Front. Bioeng. Biotechnol.* **2020**, *8*, 182. [CrossRef]
9. Al-Abduljabbar, A.; Farooq, I. Electrospun Polymer Nanofibers: Processing, Properties, and Applications. *Polymers* **2022**, *15*, 65. [CrossRef]
10. Yang, L.; Wang, X.; Xiong, M.; Liu, X.; Luo, S.; Luo, J.; Wang, Y. Electrospun Silk Fibroin/Fibrin Vascular Scaffold with Superior Mechanical Properties and Biocompatibility for Applications in Tissue Engineering. *Sci. Rep.* **2024**, *14*, 3942. [CrossRef] [PubMed]
11. Moazzami Goudarzi, Z.; Zaszczyńska, A.; Kowalczyk, T.; Sajkiewicz, P. Electrospun Antimicrobial Drug Delivery Systems and Hydrogels Used for Wound Dressings. *Pharmaceutics* **2024**, *16*, 93. [CrossRef]
12. Wilkinson, H.N.; Hardman, M.J. Wound Healing: Cellular Mechanisms and Pathological Outcomes. *Open Biol.* **2020**, *10*, 200223. [CrossRef] [PubMed]
13. Choudhary, V.; Choudhary, M.; Bollag, W.B. Exploring Skin Wound Healing Models and the Impact of Natural Lipids on the Healing Process. *Int. J. Mol. Sci.* **2024**, *25*, 3790. [CrossRef] [PubMed]
14. Gonzalez, A.C.D.O.; Costa, T.F.; de Araújo Andrade, Z.; Medrado, A.R.A.P. Wound Healing—A Literature Review. *Bras. Dermatol.* **2016**, *91*, 614–620. [CrossRef] [PubMed]
15. Tamilarasi, G.P.; Krishnan, M.; Sabarees, G.; Gouthaman, S.; Alagarsamy, V.; Solomon, V.R. Emerging Trends in Curcumin Embedded Electrospun Nanofibers for Impaired Diabetic Wound Healing. *Appl. Nano* **2022**, *3*, 202–232. [CrossRef]
16. Fernández-Guarino, M.; Hernández-Bule, M.L.; Bacci, S. Cellular and Molecular Processes in Wound Healing. *Biomedicines* **2023**, *11*, 2526. [CrossRef]
17. Cade, W.T. Diabetes-Related Microvascular and Macrovascular Diseases in the Physical Therapy Setting. *Phys. Ther.* **2008**, *88*, 1322–1335. [CrossRef]
18. Mieczkowski, M.; Mrozikiewicz-Rakowska, B.; Kowara, M.; Kleibert, M.; Czupryniak, L. The Problem of Wound Healing in Diabetes—From Molecular Pathways to the Design of an Animal Model. *Int. J. Mol. Sci.* **2022**, *23*, 7930. [CrossRef] [PubMed]
19. Maheshwari, P.; Nirenjen, S.; Bergin, R.V.B.; Pavithradevi, M.; Arun, S.; Shanmugasundaram, P. Improvement of Patient Compliance through Patient Counselling in Patients with Diabetic Foot Ulcer. *Res. J. Pharm. Technol.* **2018**, *11*, 2248. [CrossRef]
20. Mansour, A.; Mousa, M.; Abdelmannan, D.; Tay, G.; Hassoun, A.; Alsafar, H. Microvascular and Macrovascular Complications of Type 2 Diabetes Mellitus: Exome Wide Association Analyses. *Front. Endocrinol.* **2023**, *14*, 1143067. [CrossRef] [PubMed]
21. Lauri, C.; Leone, A.; Cavallini, M.; Signore, A.; Giurato, L.; Uccioli, L. Diabetic Foot Infections: The Diagnostic Challenges. *J. Clin. Med.* **2020**, *9*, 1779. [CrossRef]
22. Eisenbud, D.E. Oxygen in Wound Healing. *Clin. Plast. Surg.* **2012**, *39*, 293–310. [CrossRef] [PubMed]
23. Guan, Y.; Niu, H.; Liu, Z.; Dang, Y.; Shen, J.; Zayed, M.; Ma, L.; Guan, J. Sustained Oxygenation Accelerates Diabetic Wound Healing by Promoting Epithelialization and Angiogenesis and Decreasing Inflammation. *Sci. Adv.* **2021**, *7*, abj0153. [CrossRef] [PubMed]
24. Berbudi, A.; Rahmadika, N.; Tjahjadi, A.I.; Ruslami, R. Type 2 Diabetes and Its Impact on the Immune System. *Curr. Diabetes Rev.* **2020**, *16*, 442–449. [CrossRef] [PubMed]
25. Zheng, S.-Y.; Wan, X.-X.; Kambey, P.A.; Luo, Y.; Hu, X.-M.; Liu, Y.-F.; Shan, J.-Q.; Chen, Y.-W.; Xiong, K. Therapeutic Role of Growth Factors in Treating Diabetic Wound. *World J. Diabetes* **2023**, *14*, 364–395. [CrossRef]
26. Nirenjen, S.; Narayanan, J.; Tamilanban, T.; Subramaniyan, V.; Chitra, V.; Fuloria, N.K.; Wong, L.S.; Ramachawolran, G.; Sekar, M.; Gupta, G.; et al. Exploring the Contribution of Pro-Inflammatory Cytokines to Impaired Wound Healing in Diabetes. *Front. Immunol.* **2023**, *14*, 1216321. [CrossRef]
27. Sood, A.; Granick, M.S.; Tomaselli, N.L. Wound Dressings and Comparative Effectiveness Data. *Adv. Wound Care* **2014**, *3*, 511–529. [CrossRef] [PubMed]
28. Su, L.; Jia, Y.; Fu, L.; Guo, K.; Xie, S. The Emerging Progress on Wound Dressings and Their Application in Clinic Wound Management. *Heliyon* **2023**, *9*, e22520. [CrossRef] [PubMed]
29. Alven, S.; Peter, S.; Mbese, Z.; Aderibigbe, B.A. Polymer-Based Wound Dressing Materials Loaded with Bioactive Agents: Potential Materials for the Treatment of Diabetic Wounds. *Polymers* **2022**, *14*, 724. [CrossRef]
30. Urciuolo, F.; Casale, C.; Imparato, G.; Netti, P.A. Bioengineered Skin Substitutes: The Role of Extracellular Matrix and Vascularization in the Healing of Deep Wounds. *J. Clin. Med.* **2019**, *8*, 2083. [CrossRef] [PubMed]
31. Oualla-Bachiri, W.; Fernández-González, A.; Quiñones-Vico, M.I.; Arias-Santiago, S. From Grafts to Human Bioengineered Vascularized Skin Substitutes. *Int. J. Mol. Sci.* **2020**, *21*, 8197. [CrossRef] [PubMed]

32. Polverino, G.; Russo, F.; D'Andrea, F. Bioactive Dressing: A New Algorithm in Wound Healing. *J. Clin. Med.* **2024**, *13*, 2488. [CrossRef]
33. Jiang, Z.; Zheng, Z.; Yu, S.; Gao, Y.; Ma, J.; Huang, L.; Yang, L. Nanofiber Scaffolds as Drug Delivery Systems Promoting Wound Healing. *Pharmaceutics* **2023**, *15*, 1829. [CrossRef]
34. Yasin, S.N.N.; Said, Z.; Halib, N.; Rahman, Z.A.; Mokhzani, N.I. Polymer-Based Hydrogel Loaded with Honey in Drug Delivery System for Wound Healing Applications. *Polymers* **2023**, *15*, 3085. [CrossRef] [PubMed]
35. Sethuram, L.; Thomas, J. Therapeutic Applications of Electrospun Nanofibers Impregnated with Various Biological Macromolecules for Effective Wound Healing Strategy—A Review. *Biomed. Pharmacother.* **2023**, *157*, 113996. [CrossRef]
36. Liu, Y.; Li, C.; Feng, Z.; Han, B.; Yu, D.-G.; Wang, K. Advances in the Preparation of Nanofiber Dressings by Electrospinning for Promoting Diabetic Wound Healing. *Biomolecules* **2022**, *12*, 1727. [CrossRef] [PubMed]
37. Shalaby, M.A.; Anwar, M.M.; Saeed, H. Nanomaterials for Application in Wound Healing: Current State-of-the-Art and Future Perspectives. *J. Polym. Res.* **2022**, *29*, 91. [CrossRef]
38. Zhang, H.; Lin, X.; Cao, X.; Wang, Y.; Wang, J.; Zhao, Y. Developing Natural Polymers for Skin Wound Healing. *Bioact. Mater.* **2024**, *33*, 355–376. [CrossRef] [PubMed]
39. Sell, S.A.; Wolfe, P.S.; Garg, K.; McCool, J.M.; Rodriguez, I.A.; Bowlin, G.L. The Use of Natural Polymers in Tissue Engineering: A Focus on Electrospun Extracellular Matrix Analogues. *Polymers* **2010**, *2*, 522–553. [CrossRef]
40. Oliveira, C.; Sousa, D.; Teixeira, J.A.; Ferreira-Santos, P.; Botelho, C.M. Polymeric Biomaterials for Wound Healing. *Front. Bioeng. Biotechnol.* **2023**, *11*, 1136077. [CrossRef] [PubMed]
41. Zhao, Y.; Qiu, Y.; Wang, H.; Chen, Y.; Jin, S.; Chen, S. Preparation of Nanofibers with Renewable Polymers and Their Application in Wound Dressing. *Int. J. Polym. Sci.* **2016**, *2016*, 4672839. [CrossRef]
42. Satchanska, G.; Davidova, S.; Petrov, P.D. Natural and Synthetic Polymers for Biomedical and Environmental Applications. *Polymers* **2024**, *16*, 1159. [CrossRef] [PubMed]
43. Liu, X.; Xu, H.; Zhang, M.; Yu, D.-G. Electrospun Medicated Nanofibers for Wound Healing: Review. *Membranes* **2021**, *11*, 770. [CrossRef] [PubMed]
44. Masood, N.; Ahmed, R.; Tariq, M.; Ahmed, Z.; Masoud, M.S.; Ali, I.; Asghar, R.; Andleeb, A.; Hasan, A. Silver Nanoparticle Impregnated Chitosan-PEG Hydrogel Enhances Wound Healing in Diabetes Induced Rabbits. *Int. J. Pharm.* **2019**, *559*, 23–36. [CrossRef] [PubMed]
45. Wu, C.; Long, L.; Zhang, Y.; Xu, Y.; Lu, Y.; Yang, Z.; Guo, Y.; Zhang, J.; Hu, X.; Wang, Y. Injectable Conductive and Angiogenic Hydrogels for Chronic Diabetic Wound Treatment. *J. Control. Release* **2022**, *344*, 249–260. [CrossRef] [PubMed]
46. Xu, Z.; Liu, Y.; Ma, R.; Chen, J.; Qiu, J.; Du, S.; Li, C.; Wu, Z.; Yang, X.; Chen, Z.; et al. Thermosensitive Hydrogel Incorporating Prussian Blue Nanoparticles Promotes Diabetic Wound Healing via ROS Scavenging and Mitochondrial Function Restoration. *ACS Appl. Mater. Interfaces* **2022**, *14*, 14059–14071. [CrossRef] [PubMed]
47. Jiang, Y.; Han, Y.; Wang, J.; Lv, F.; Yi, Z.; Ke, Q.; Xu, H. Space-Oriented Nanofibrous Scaffold with Silicon-Doped Amorphous Calcium Phosphate Nanocoating for Diabetic Wound Healing. *ACS Appl. Bio Mater.* **2019**, *2*, 787–795. [CrossRef] [PubMed]
48. Cam, M.E.; Ertas, B.; Alenezi, H.; Hazar-Yavuz, A.N.; Cesur, S.; Ozcan, G.S.; Ekentok, C.; Guler, E.; Katsakouli, C.; Demirbas, Z.; et al. Accelerated Diabetic Wound Healing by Topical Application of Combination Oral Antidiabetic Agents-Loaded Nanofibrous Scaffolds: An in Vitro and in Vivo Evaluation Study. *Mater. Sci. Eng. C* **2021**, *119*, 111586. [CrossRef]
49. Ali, I.H.; Khalil, I.A.; El-Sherbiny, I.M. Design, Development, in-Vitro and in-Vivo Evaluation of Polylactic Acid-Based Multifunctional Nanofibrous Patches for Efficient Healing of Diabetic Wounds. *Sci. Rep.* **2023**, *13*, 3215. [CrossRef]
50. Di Cristo, F.; Valentino, A.; De Luca, I.; Peluso, G.; Bonadies, I.; Di Salle, A.; Calarco, A. Polylactic Acid/Poly(Vinylpyrrolidone) Co-Electrospun Fibrous Membrane as a Tunable Quercetin Delivery Platform for Diabetic Wounds. *Pharmaceutics* **2023**, *15*, 805. [CrossRef]
51. Zheng, Z.; Liu, Y.; Huang, W.; Mo, Y.; Lan, Y.; Guo, R.; Cheng, B. Neurotensin-Loaded PLGA/CNC Composite Nanofiber Membranes Accelerate Diabetic Wound Healing. *Artif. Cells Nanomed. Biotechnol.* **2018**, *46*, 493–501. [CrossRef]
52. Hasan, N.; Cao, J.; Lee, J.; Naeem, M.; Hlaing, S.P.; Kim, J.; Jung, Y.; Lee, B.-L.; Yoo, J.-W. PEI/NONOates-Doped PLGA Nanoparticles for Eradicating Methicillin-Resistant *Staphylococcus aureus* Biofilm in Diabetic Wounds via Binding to the Biofilm Matrix. *Mater. Sci. Eng. C* **2019**, *103*, 109741. [CrossRef]
53. Lv, H.; Zhao, M.; Li, Y.; Li, K.; Chen, S.; Zhao, W.; Wu, S.; Han, Y. Electrospun Chitosan–Polyvinyl Alcohol Nanofiber Dressings Loaded with Bioactive Ursolic Acid Promoting Diabetic Wound Healing. *Nanomaterials* **2022**, *12*, 2933. [CrossRef]
54. Ningrum, D.R.; Hanif, W.; Mardhian, D.F.; Asri, L.A.T.W. In Vitro Biocompatibility of Hydrogel Polyvinyl Alcohol/Moringa Oleifera Leaf Extract/Graphene Oxide for Wound Dressing. *Polymers* **2023**, *15*, 468. [CrossRef] [PubMed]
55. Yu, J.; Wang, P.; Yin, M.; Zhang, K.; Wang, X.; Han, B. Carboxymethyl Chitosan-Grafted Polyvinylpyrrolidone-Iodine Microspheres for Promoting the Healing of Chronic Wounds. *Bioengineered* **2022**, *13*, 8735–8746. [CrossRef] [PubMed]
56. Makadia, H.K.; Siegel, S.J. Poly Lactic-Co-Glycolic Acid (PLGA) as Biodegradable Controlled Drug Delivery Carrier. *Polymers* **2011**, *3*, 1377–1397. [CrossRef]
57. Liu, Y.; Zhou, S.; Gao, Y.; Zhai, Y. Electrospun Nanofibers as a Wound Dressing for Treating Diabetic Foot Ulcer. *Asian J. Pharm. Sci.* **2019**, *14*, 130–143. [CrossRef]

58. Castro, V.O.; Fredel, M.C.; Aragones, Á.; de Oliveira Barra, G.M.; Cesca, K.; Merlini, C. Electrospun Fibrous Membranes of Poly (Lactic-Co-Glycolic Acid) with β-Tricalcium Phosphate for Guided Bone Regeneration Application. *Polym. Test.* **2020**, *86*, 106489. [CrossRef]
59. Nofar, M.; Sacligil, D.; Carreau, P.J.; Kamal, M.R.; Heuzey, M.-C. Poly (Lactic Acid) Blends: Processing, Properties and Applications. *Int. J. Biol. Macromol.* **2019**, *125*, 307–360. [CrossRef] [PubMed]
60. Capuana, E.; Lopresti, F.; Ceraulo, M.; La Carrubba, V. Poly-l-Lactic Acid (PLLA)-Based Biomaterials for Regenerative Medicine: A Review on Processing and Applications. *Polymers* **2022**, *14*, 1153. [CrossRef]
61. Liu, C.; Du, G.; Guo, Q.; Li, R.; Li, C.; He, H. Fabrication and Characterization of Polylactic Acid Electrospun Wound Dressing Modified with Polyethylene Glycol, Rosmarinic Acid and Graphite Oxide. *Nanomaterials* **2023**, *13*, 2000. [CrossRef] [PubMed]
62. Raina, N.; Pahwa, R.; Khosla, J.K.; Gupta, P.N.; Gupta, M. Polycaprolactone-Based Materials in Wound Healing Applications. *Polym. Bull.* **2022**, *79*, 7041–7063. [CrossRef]
63. Song, R.; Murphy, M.; Li, C.; Ting, K.; Soo, C.; Zheng, Z. Current Development of Biodegradable Polymeric Materials for Biomedical Applications. *Drug Des. Dev. Ther.* **2018**, *12*, 3117–3145. [CrossRef]
64. Murugan, D.; Suresh, A.; Thakur, G.; Singh, B.N. Fabrication and Evaluation of Poly(ε-Caprolactone) Based Nanofibrous Scaffolds Loaded with Homoeopathic Mother Tincture of Syzygium Cumini for Wound Healing Applications. *OpenNano* **2023**, *14*, 100189. [CrossRef]
65. Zhong, Y.; Lin, Q.; Yu, H.; Shao, L.; Cui, X.; Pang, Q.; Zhu, Y.; Hou, R. Construction Methods and Biomedical Applications of PVA-Based Hydrogels. *Front. Chem.* **2024**, *12*, 1376799. [CrossRef]
66. Costa-Júnior, E.S.; Barbosa-Stancioli, E.F.; Mansur, A.A.P.; Vasconcelos, W.L.; Mansur, H.S. Preparation and Characterization of Chitosan/Poly(Vinyl Alcohol) Chemically Crosslinked Blends for Biomedical Applications. *Carbohydr. Polym.* **2009**, *76*, 472–481. [CrossRef]
67. Sabarees, G.; Velmurugan, V.; Tamilarasi, G.P.; Alagarsamy, V.; Raja Solomon, V. Recent Advances in Silver Nanoparticles Containing Nanofibers for Chronic Wound Management. *Polymers* **2022**, *14*, 3994. [CrossRef]
68. Fatahian, R.; Mirjalili, M.; Khajavi, R.; Rahimi, M.K.; Nasirizadeh, N. Fabrication of Antibacterial and Hemostatic Electrospun PVA Nanofibers for Wound Healing. *SN Appl. Sci.* **2020**, *2*, 1288. [CrossRef]
69. Baranwal, J.; Barse, B.; Fais, A.; Delogu, G.L.; Kumar, A. Biopolymer: A Sustainable Material for Food and Medical Applications. *Polymers* **2022**, *14*, 983. [CrossRef] [PubMed]
70. Tuwalska, A.; Grabska-Zielińska, S.; Sionkowska, A. Chitosan/Silk Fibroin Materials for Biomedical Applications—A Review. *Polymers* **2022**, *14*, 1343. [CrossRef] [PubMed]
71. Radulescu, D.-M.; Andronescu, E.; Vasile, O.R.; Ficai, A.; Vasile, B.S. Silk Fibroin-Based Scaffolds for Wound Healing Applications with Metal Oxide Nanoparticles. *J. Drug Deliv. Sci. Technol.* **2024**, *96*, 105689. [CrossRef]
72. Vepari, C.; Kaplan, D.L. Silk as a Biomaterial. *Prog. Polym. Sci.* **2007**, *32*, 991–1007. [CrossRef] [PubMed]
73. Fang, G.; Sapru, S.; Behera, S.; Yao, J.; Shao, Z.; Kundu, S.C.; Chen, X. Exploration of the Tight Structural–Mechanical Relationship in Mulberry and Non-Mulberry Silkworm Silks. *J. Mater. Chem. B* **2016**, *4*, 4337–4347. [CrossRef] [PubMed]
74. Schmidt, T.; Puchalla, N.; Schendzielorz, M.; Kramell, A.E. Degumming and Characterization of Bombyx Mori and Non-Mulberry Silks from Saturniidae Silkworms. *Sci. Rep.* **2023**, *13*, 19504. [CrossRef]
75. Lewis, R.V. Spider Silk: Ancient Ideas for New Biomaterials. *Chem. Rev.* **2006**, *106*, 3762–3774. [CrossRef]
76. Murugesh Babu, K. Silk from Silkworms and Spiders as High-Performance Fibers. In *Structure and Properties of High-Performance Fibers*; Elsevier: Amsterdam, The Netherlands, 2017; pp. 327–366.
77. Römer, L.; Scheibel, T. The Elaborate Structure of Spider Silk: Structure and Function of a Natural High Performance Fiber. *Prion* **2008**, *2*, 154–161. [CrossRef] [PubMed]
78. Kunz, R.I.; Brancalhão, R.M.C.; Ribeiro, L.d.F.C.; Natali, M.R.M. Silkworm Sericin: Properties and Biomedical Applications. *BioMed Res. Int.* **2016**, *2016*, 8175701. [CrossRef]
79. Reizabal, A.; Costa, C.M.; Pérez-Álvarez, L.; Vilas-Vilela, J.L.; Lanceros-Méndez, S. Silk Fibroin as Sustainable Advanced Material: Material Properties and Characteristics, Processing, and Applications. *Adv. Funct. Mater.* **2023**, *33*, 202210764. [CrossRef]
80. Vidya, M.; Rajagopal, S. Silk Fibroin: A Promising Tool for Wound Healing and Skin Regeneration. *Int. J. Polym. Sci.* **2021**, *2021*, 9069924. [CrossRef]
81. Nguyen, T.P.; Nguyen, Q.V.; Nguyen, V.-H.; Le, T.-H.; Huynh, V.Q.N.; Vo, D.-V.N.; Trinh, Q.T.; Kim, S.Y.; Le, Q. Van Silk Fibroin-Based Biomaterials for Biomedical Applications: A Review. *Polymers* **2019**, *11*, 1933. [CrossRef] [PubMed]
82. Yonesi, M.; Garcia-Nieto, M.; Guinea, G.V.; Panetsos, F.; Pérez-Rigueiro, J.; González-Nieto, D. Silk Fibroin: An Ancient Material for Repairing the Injured Nervous System. *Pharmaceutics* **2021**, *13*, 429. [CrossRef]
83. Yao, X.; Zou, S.; Fan, S.; Niu, Q.; Zhang, Y. Bioinspired Silk Fibroin Materials: From Silk Building Blocks Extraction and Reconstruction to Advanced Biomedical Applications. *Mater. Today Bio* **2022**, *16*, 100381. [CrossRef] [PubMed]
84. Qi, Y.; Wang, H.; Wei, K.; Yang, Y.; Zheng, R.-Y.; Kim, I.; Zhang, K.-Q. A Review of Structure Construction of Silk Fibroin Biomaterials from Single Structures to Multi-Level Structures. *Int. J. Mol. Sci.* **2017**, *18*, 237. [CrossRef] [PubMed]
85. Wang, Q.; Schniepp, H.C. Nanofibrils as Building Blocks of Silk Fibers: Critical Review of the Experimental Evidence. *JOM* **2019**, *71*, 1248–1263. [CrossRef]
86. Ling, S.; Chen, W.; Fan, Y.; Zheng, K.; Jin, K.; Yu, H.; Buehler, M.J.; Kaplan, D.L. Biopolymer Nanofibrils: Structure, Modeling, Preparation, and Applications. *Prog. Polym. Sci.* **2018**, *85*, 1–56. [CrossRef] [PubMed]

87. Sashina, E.S.; Bochek, A.M.; Novoselov, N.P.; Kirichenko, D.A. Structure and Solubility of Natural Silk Fibroin. *Russ. J. Appl. Chem.* **2006**, *79*, 869–876. [CrossRef]
88. Bandyopadhyay, A.; Chowdhury, S.K.; Dey, S.; Moses, J.C.; Mandal, B.B. Silk: A Promising Biomaterial Opening New Vistas Towards Affordable Healthcare Solutions. *J. Indian Inst. Sci.* **2019**, *99*, 445–487. [CrossRef]
89. De Giorgio, G.; Matera, B.; Vurro, D.; Manfredi, E.; Galstyan, V.; Tarabella, G.; Ghezzi, B.; D'Angelo, P. Silk Fibroin Materials: Biomedical Applications and Perspectives. *Bioengineering* **2024**, *11*, 167. [CrossRef] [PubMed]
90. Sun, W.; Gregory, D.A.; Tomeh, M.A.; Zhao, X. Silk Fibroin as a Functional Biomaterial for Tissue Engineering. *Int. J. Mol. Sci.* **2021**, *22*, 1499. [CrossRef]
91. Deptuch, T.; Dams-Kozlowska, H. Silk Materials Functionalized via Genetic Engineering for Biomedical Applications. *Materials* **2017**, *10*, 1417. [CrossRef]
92. Mazurek, Ł.; Szudzik, M.; Rybka, M.; Konop, M. Silk Fibroin Biomaterials and Their Beneficial Role in Skin Wound Healing. *Biomolecules* **2022**, *12*, 1852. [CrossRef] [PubMed]
93. Wang, S.-L.; Li, X.-W.; Xu, W.; Yu, Q.-Y.; Fang, S.-M. Advances of Regenerated and Functionalized Silk Biomaterials and Application in Skin Wound Healing. *Int. J. Biol. Macromol.* **2024**, *254*, 128024. [CrossRef]
94. Lehmann, T.; Vaughn, A.E.; Seal, S.; Liechty, K.W.; Zgheib, C. Silk Fibroin-Based Therapeutics for Impaired Wound Healing. *Pharmaceutics* **2022**, *14*, 651. [CrossRef]
95. Li, Y.-Y.; Ji, S.-F.; Fu, X.-B.; Jiang, Y.-F.; Sun, X.-Y. Biomaterial-Based Mechanical Regulation Facilitates Scarless Wound Healing with Functional Skin Appendage Regeneration. *Mil. Med. Res.* **2024**, *11*, 13. [CrossRef] [PubMed]
96. Muncie, J.M.; Weaver, V.M. The Physical and Biochemical Properties of the Extracellular Matrix Regulate Cell Fate. *Curr. Top. Dev. Biol.* **2018**, *130*, 1–37. [PubMed]
97. Chen, Z.; Du, C.; Liu, S.; Liu, J.; Yang, Y.; Dong, L.; Zhao, W.; Huang, W.; Lei, Y. Progress in Biomaterials Inspired by the Extracellular Matrix. *Giant* **2024**, *19*, 100323. [CrossRef]
98. Kolimi, P.; Narala, S.; Nyavanandi, D.; Youssef, A.A.A.; Dudhipala, N. Innovative Treatment Strategies to Accelerate Wound Healing: Trajectory and Recent Advancements. *Cells* **2022**, *11*, 2439. [CrossRef] [PubMed]
99. Zhang, J.; Wang, L.; Xu, C.; Cao, Y.; Liu, S.; Reis, R.L.; Kundu, S.C.; Yang, X.; Xiao, B.; Duan, L. Transparent Silk Fibroin Film-Facilitated Infected-Wound Healing through Antibacterial, Improved Fibroblast Adhesion and Immune Modulation. *J. Mater. Chem. B* **2024**, *12*, 475–488. [CrossRef] [PubMed]
100. Park, Y.R.; Sultan, M.T.; Park, H.J.; Lee, J.M.; Ju, H.W.; Lee, O.J.; Lee, D.J.; Kaplan, D.L.; Park, C.H. NF-KB Signaling Is Key in the Wound Healing Processes of Silk Fibroin. *Acta Biomater.* **2018**, *67*, 183–195. [CrossRef] [PubMed]
101. Barrientos, S.; Stojadinovic, O.; Golinko, M.S.; Brem, H.; Tomic-Canic, M. Growth Factors and Cytokines in Wound Healing. *Wound Repair Regen.* **2008**, *16*, 585–601. [CrossRef]
102. Bao, P.; Kodra, A.; Tomic-Canic, M.; Golinko, M.S.; Ehrlich, H.P.; Brem, H. The Role of Vascular Endothelial Growth Factor in Wound Healing. *J. Surg. Res.* **2009**, *153*, 347–358. [CrossRef]
103. Aykac, A.; Karanlik, B.; Sehirli, A.O. Protective Effect of Silk Fibroin in Burn Injury in Rat Model. *Gene* **2018**, *641*, 287–291. [CrossRef]
104. Indrakumar, S.; Dash, T.K.; Mishra, V.; Tandon, B.; Chatterjee, K. Silk Fibroin and Its Nanocomposites for Wound Care: A Comprehensive Review. *ACS Polym. Au* **2024**, *4*, 168–188. [CrossRef]
105. Sta Agueda, J.R.H.; Chen, Q.; Maalihan, R.D.; Ren, J.; da Silva, Í.G.M.; Dugos, N.P.; Caldona, E.B.; Advincula, R.C. 3D Printing of Biomedically Relevant Polymer Materials and Biocompatibility. *MRS Commun.* **2021**, *11*, 197–212. [CrossRef]
106. Anusiya, G.; Jaiganesh, R. A Review on Fabrication Methods of Nanofibers and a Special Focus on Application of Cellulose Nanofibers. *Carbohydr. Polym. Technol. Appl.* **2022**, *4*, 100262. [CrossRef]
107. Abdulhussain, R.; Adebisi, A.; Conway, B.R.; Asare-Addo, K. Electrospun Nanofibers: Exploring Process Parameters, Polymer Selection, and Recent Applications in Pharmaceuticals and Drug Delivery. *J. Drug Deliv. Sci. Technol.* **2023**, *90*, 105156. [CrossRef]
108. Jiang, X.; Zeng, Y.-E.; Li, C.; Wang, K.; Yu, D.-G. Enhancing Diabetic Wound Healing: Advances in Electrospun Scaffolds from Pathogenesis to Therapeutic Applications. *Front. Bioeng. Biotechnol.* **2024**, *12*, 1354286. [CrossRef] [PubMed]
109. Reneker, D.H.; Yarin, A.L.; Zussman, E.; Xu, H. Electrospinning of Nanofibers from Polymer Solutions and Melts. *Adv. Appl. Mech.* **2007**, *41*, 43–346.
110. Nadaf, A.; Gupta, A.; Hasan, N.; Fauziya; Ahmad, S.; Kesharwani, P.; Ahmad, F.J. Recent Update on Electrospinning and Electrospun Nanofibers: Current Trends and Their Applications. *RSC Adv.* **2022**, *12*, 23808–23828. [CrossRef] [PubMed]
111. Ahmadi Bonakdar, M.; Rodrigue, D. Electrospinning: Processes, Structures, and Materials. *Macromol* **2024**, *4*, 58–103. [CrossRef]
112. Şener, A.G.; Altay, A.S.; Altay, F. Effect of Voltage on Morphology of Electrospun Nanofibers. In Proceedings of the 2011 7th International Conference on Electrical and Electronics Engineering (ELECO), Bursa, Turkey, 1–4 December 2011; pp. 324–328.
113. Xue, J.; Wu, T.; Dai, Y.; Xia, Y. Electrospinning and Electrospun Nanofibers: Methods, Materials, and Applications. *Chem. Rev.* **2019**, *119*, 5298–5415. [CrossRef] [PubMed]
114. Deitzel, J.M.; Kleinmeyer, J.; Harris, D.; Beck Tan, N.C. The Effect of Processing Variables on the Morphology of Electrospun Nanofibers and Textiles. *Polymer* **2001**, *42*, 261–272. [CrossRef]
115. Keirouz, A.; Wang, Z.; Reddy, V.S.; Nagy, Z.K.; Vass, P.; Buzgo, M.; Ramakrishna, S.; Radacsi, N. The History of Electrospinning: Past, Present, and Future Developments. *Adv. Mater. Technol.* **2023**, *8*, 202201723. [CrossRef]

116. Tucker, N.; Stanger, J.J.; Staiger, M.P.; Razzaq, H.; Hofman, K. The History of the Science and Technology of Electrospinning from 1600 to 1995. *J. Eng. Fiber. Fabr.* **2012**, *7*, 155892501200702. [CrossRef]
117. Ghajarieh, A.; Habibi, S.; Talebian, A. Biomedical Applications of Nanofibers. *Russ. J. Appl. Chem.* **2021**, *94*, 847–872. [CrossRef]
118. Azimi, B.; Maleki, H.; Zavagna, L.; De la Ossa, J.G.; Linari, S.; Lazzeri, A.; Danti, S. Bio-Based Electrospun Fibers for Wound Healing. *J. Funct. Biomater.* **2020**, *11*, 67. [CrossRef] [PubMed]
119. Venmathi Maran, B.A.; Jeyachandran, S.; Kimura, M. A Review on the Electrospinning of Polymer Nanofibers and Its Biomedical Applications. *J. Compos. Sci.* **2024**, *8*, 32. [CrossRef]
120. Muthukrishnan, L. An Overview on Electrospinning and Its Advancement toward Hard and Soft Tissue Engineering Applications. *Colloid Polym. Sci.* **2022**, *300*, 875–901. [CrossRef] [PubMed]
121. Buzgo, M.; Mickova, A.; Rampichova, M.; Doupnik, M. Blend Electrospinning, Coaxial Electrospinning, and Emulsion Electrospinning Techniques. In *Core-Shell Nanostructures for Drug Delivery and Theranostics*; Elsevier: Amsterdam, The Netherlands, 2018; pp. 325–347.
122. Qin, X. Coaxial Electrospinning of Nanofibers. In *Electrospun Nanofibers*; Elsevier: Amsterdam, The Netherlands, 2017; pp. 41–71.
123. Abadi, B.; Goshtasbi, N.; Bolourian, S.; Tahsili, J.; Adeli-Sardou, M.; Forootanfar, H. Electrospun Hybrid Nanofibers: Fabrication, Characterization, and Biomedical Applications. *Front. Bioeng. Biotechnol.* **2022**, *10*, 986975. [CrossRef] [PubMed]
124. Gupta, P.; Wilkes, G.L. Some Investigations on the Fiber Formation by Utilizing a Side-by-Side Bicomponent Electrospinning Approach. *Polymer* **2003**, *44*, 6353–6359. [CrossRef]
125. Zhang, X.; Wang, Y.; Gao, Z.; Mao, X.; Cheng, J.; Huang, L.; Tang, J. Advances in Wound Dressing Based on Electrospinning Nanofibers. *J. Appl. Polym. Sci.* **2024**, *141*, 54746. [CrossRef]
126. Opneja, A.; Kapoor, S.; Stavrou, E.X. Contribution of Platelets, the Coagulation and Fibrinolytic Systems to Cutaneous Wound Healing. *Thromb. Res.* **2019**, *179*, 56–63. [CrossRef] [PubMed]
127. Rickel, A.P.; Deng, X.; Engebretson, D.; Hong, Z. Electrospun Nanofiber Scaffold for Vascular Tissue Engineering. *Mater. Sci. Eng. C Mater. Biol. Appl.* **2021**, *129*, 112373. [CrossRef]
128. Nazarnezhad, S.; Baino, F.; Kim, H.-W.; Webster, T.J.; Kargozar, S. Electrospun Nanofibers for Improved Angiogenesis: Promises for Tissue Engineering Applications. *Nanomaterials* **2020**, *10*, 1609. [CrossRef]
129. Karthikeyan, K.; Sekar, S.; Pandima Devi, M.; Inbasekaran, S.; Lakshminarasaiah, C.H.; Sastry, T.P. Fabrication of Novel Biofibers by Coating Silk Fibroin with Chitosan Impregnated with Silver Nanoparticles. *J. Mater. Sci. Mater. Med.* **2011**, *22*, 2721–2726. [CrossRef] [PubMed]
130. Aznar-Cervantes, S.; Martínez, J.G.; Bernabeu-Esclapez, A.; Lozano-Pérez, A.A.; Meseguer-Olmo, L.; Otero, T.F.; Cenis, J.L. Fabrication of Electrospun Silk Fibroin Scaffolds Coated with Graphene Oxide and Reduced Graphene for Applications in Biomedicine. *Bioelectrochemistry* **2016**, *108*, 36–45. [CrossRef]
131. Miguel, S.P.; Simões, D.; Moreira, A.F.; Sequeira, R.S.; Correia, I.J. Production and Characterization of Electrospun Silk Fibroin Based Asymmetric Membranes for Wound Dressing Applications. *Int. J. Biol. Macromol.* **2019**, *121*, 524–535. [CrossRef] [PubMed]
132. Rama, M.; Vijayalakshmi, U. Influence of Silk Fibroin on the Preparation of Nanofibrous Scaffolds for the Effective Use in Osteoregenerative Applications. *J. Drug Deliv. Sci. Technol.* **2021**, *61*, 102182. [CrossRef]
133. Jao, W.; Yang, M.; Lin, C.; Hsu, C. Fabrication and Characterization of Electrospun Silk Fibroin/TiO_2 Nanofibrous Mats for Wound Dressings. *Polym. Adv. Technol.* **2012**, *23*, 1066–1076. [CrossRef]
134. Khan, A.U.R.; Morsi, Y.; Zhu, T.; Ahmad, A.; Xie, X.; Yu, F.; Mo, X. Electrospinning: An Emerging Technology to Construct Polymer-Based Nanofibrous Scaffolds for Diabetic Wound Healing. *Front. Mater. Sci.* **2021**, *15*, 10–35. [CrossRef]
135. Kubera Sampath Kumar, S.; Prakash, C.; Vaidheeswaran, S.; Karthic Kumar, B.; Subramanian, S. Design and Characterization of Secondary and Tertiary Layers of a Multilayer Wound Dressing System. *J. Test. Eval.* **2020**, *48*, 2683–2698. [CrossRef]

pharmaceuticals

MDPI

Article

Supporting the Wound Healing Process—Curcumin, Resveratrol and Baicalin in In Vitro Wound Healing Studies

Kacper Jagiełło [1,*], Oliwia Uchańska [2], Konrad Matyja [3], Mateusz Jackowski [3], Benita Wiatrak [4], Paweł Kubasiewicz-Ross [5] and Ewa Karuga-Kuźniewska [6]

1 Department of Process Engineering and Technology of Polymer and Carbon Materials, Faculty of Chemistry, Wroclaw University of Science and Technology, ul. Gdańska 7/9, 50-344 Wrocław, Poland
2 Department of Reproduction and Clinic of Farm Animals, Faculty of Veterinary Medicine, Wrocław University of Environmental and Life Sciences, pl. Grunwaldzki 49, 50-366 Wrocław, Poland
3 Department of Micro, Nano, and Bioprocess Engineering, Faculty of Chemistry, Wroclaw University of Science and Technology, ul. Norwida 4/6, 50-373 Wrocław, Poland
4 Department of Pharmacology, Wroclaw Medical University, ul. Jana Mikulicza-Radeckiego 2, 50-345 Wrocław, Poland
5 Department and Clinic of Dental Surgery, Wroclaw Medical University, ul. Krakowska 26, 50-425 Wrocław, Poland
6 Department of Epizootiology with Exotic Animal and Bird Clinic, Faculty of Veterinary Medicine, Wrocław University of Environmental and Life Sciences, pl. Grunwaldzki 45, 50-366 Wrocław, Poland
* Correspondence: kacper.jagiello@pwr.edu.pl

Abstract: The purpose of the investigation was to evaluate the effect of the selected bioflavonoids curcumin, resveratrol and baicalin on the wound healing process in an in vitro model. In the study, Balb3t3 and L929 cell lines were used. The first step was the evaluation of the cytotoxicity of the substances tested (MTT assay). Then, using the scratch test (ST), the influence of bioflavonoids on the healing process was evaluated in an in vitro model. The second stage of the work was a mathematical analysis of the results obtained. On the basis of experimental data, the parameters of the Brian and Cousens model were determined in order to determine the maximum value of the cellular and metabolic response that occurs for the examined range of concentrations of selected bioflavonoids. In the MTT assays, no cytotoxic effect of curcumin, resveratrol and baicalin was observed in selected concentrations, while in the ST tests for selected substances, a stimulatory effect was observed on the cell division rate regardless of the cell lines tested. The results obtained encourage further research on the use of substances of natural origin to support the wound healing process.

Keywords: bioflavonoids; difficult-to-heal wounds; Brian and Cousens model; scratch assay; MTT assay

1. Introduction

Difficult-to-heal wounds are one of the most serious problems in the daily practice of veterinarians. Healing processes are generally effective in healthy animals. The organism reacts to skin damage by initiating numerous complex repair processes. Depending on the scale and type of defect, the healing process takes between a few days and several weeks. The effect of healing is to close the skin loss by filling it with scar tissue. Then, the scar rebuilds, which can take weeks, months, or even years [1–4].

The wound becomes clinically difficult in the event of a problem related to the defect itself, such as infection, damage to deep tissue structures or the nature of the damage (e.g., mechanical, chemical, radiation) [1]. The mentioned conditions have a significant influence on the speed and quality of the healing process. Geriatric patients, who suffer from chronic diseases and metabolic disorders, experience a much more difficult wound healing process [2]. The time it takes to close the wound can take months or even years, and the wound often renews itself [3,4].

The basis for the treatment of chronic skin defects is a holistic approach, i.e., the treatment of the general condition of the patient and local wound therapy [2,5]. Local wound treatment consists of selecting the appropriate dressing material. The dressing is not only to protect the wound surface but also to actively support the healing process [6]. A suitable moist environment is ensured by the use of hydrogel dressings that support cell proliferation and debridement of non-viable tissue. Most wound dressings work by providing moisture to the wound or keeping the moisture in the wound bed for a longer period of time. For example, dressings that use hydrofiber technology such as AQUACEL, which further supports debridement, provides a moist environment and absorbs excessive exudate [7]. There are various medical dressings available on the market for wound treatment. Their healing activity often depends on the additives used, e.g., different kinds of dressings containing silver ions, which strongly support the antibacterial effect. Research has shown that nanocomposite hydrogels used for wound treatment exhibited significant inhibition against Gram-positive and Gram-negative bacteria due to Ag^+ ions released from silver nitrate [8–10]. Another readily used wound healing material is, for example, honey extract, which improves wound removal and cell proliferation, leading to faster closure of wound edges [11–15]. It is also beneficial due to its high sugar content, which creates a higher osmotic gradient that pulls fluid through the subdermal tissue and provides an additional source of glucose for the growth of cellular components in the wounded area [11]. The use of growth factors is also observed in dressings due to their ability to activate fibroblasts, increase their proliferation and, as in the case of the aforementioned substances, accelerate the healing of skin loss [16–18]. For years, scientists have focused their attention on the potential of substances of plant origin [19–21]. Among this group, flavonoids deserve special attention, of which the following substances caught our attention: curcumin, resveratrol and baicalin.

Curcumin is a substance extracted from the *Curcuma longa* rhizome, a member of the ginger family *Zingiberaceae*, whose healing properties have been used in Chinese and Indian natural medicine for centuries [9]. Curcumin has properties that regulate the intensity of the inflammatory process, one of the most important being its ability to reduce the production of cytokines released by monocytes and macrophages, which play a major role in the enhancement of the inflammatory response of the body [13]. This is the body's first reaction in response to the factor that causes the wound. The persistent inflammatory process prevents wound granulation and therefore has the ability to regulate it, making curcumin a valuable substance important in the healing process [11]. Furthermore, curcumin also has antioxidant properties and stimulates angiogenesis and cell proliferation processes, so it is used particularly frequently and easily to produce therapeutic dressings for wounds that arise in the course of diabetes [12,13].

Resveratrol is a natural polyphenol present in the highest amounts on the skin of grapes and red wine. It has a strong antioxidant, anti-inflammatory, antifungal and antibacterial effect as well as cardio- and neuroprotective properties [14]. Numerous studies also show its effectiveness against skin, prostate, lung, colon and liver cancer cells [15,16]. Furthermore, resveratrol has the ability to induce cell proliferation and accelerate wound closure in in vivo models in studies conducted on rats [21]. In vitro studies have shown protective effects on fibroblasts by reducing oxidative stress. Due to its antioxidant properties, resveratrol can stabilize cell proliferation, improve migration quality and ultrastructural behavior [18] Furthermore, in vivo results revealed significantly improved wound healing after resveratrol treatment based on antioxidant activity [17]. Angiogenesis also plays a key role in wound healing, and resveratrol is discussed as an important factor that influences neovascularization [19]. This process is essential for tissue regeneration and is mainly regulated by vascular endothelial growth factor (VEGF), whose expression can be significantly increased by resveratrol [20]. The effect of resveratrol on the production of pro-inflammatory cytokines, which are released in large amounts during the inflammation that accompanies wound formation and healing, was also investigated. The presence of cytokines such as interleukin (IL)-1β, IL-6, C-reactive protein (CRP) and TNF-α2 prolongs the inflammatory phase and delays the healing process. Studies have shown that patients who received resveratrol during treatment had lower levels of these mediators and their wounds healed faster [21,22]. Therefore, it seems promising to carry out more studies on the possibilities of wound therapy using an external application of resveratrol due to its multifaceted effect.

Baicalin is a flavonoid extracted from the roots of *Scutellaria baicalensis*, a plant that is used in traditional Chinese medicine. It is widely known for its anticancer, antimicrobial and antioxidant properties [23–25]. Studies also show its potential use as an angiogenesis-regulating agent, which can be successfully used in the wound environment for tissue regeneration and vascularization [24] Research conducted on the wound healing process in immunocompromised dogs has shown that they have a slower healing ability compared to their non-immunocompromised counterparts. Digital analysis data showed that wounds treated with a dressing containing baicalin, β-sitosterol and berberine as active ingredients are characterized by an enhanced epithelialization process, faster contraction and smaller wound area compared to honey-treated wounds alone [26]. Baicalin also has the ability to reduce serum blood glucose levels and oxidative stress markers in rats with experimentally induced *diabetes mellitus*. The study showed that baicalin upregulated the expression of, e.g., VEGF-c, TGF-β, Tie-2 and SMAD2/3, implicating its potential antidiabetic and wound healing properties. Thus, baicalin can be emphasized as a potential candidate for the treatment of chronic wounds [27].

In this study, the effects of selected bioflavonoids on the in vitro wound healing process were examined. The influence of different concentrations of curcumin, resveratrol and baicalin on cell viability (MTT Assay) and cell migration (scratch assay) was evaluated. The use of mathematical modeling is designed to determine the most effective concentrations of selected substances that support the fibroblast proliferation process. So far, no studies have been published that would use the Brian and Cousens model to describe the mitochondrial or cellular response to applied doses of bioflavonoids. The results obtained can be helpful in developing a modern healing dressing based on natural medicinal products.

The cell lines used in the study are well characterized. Furthermore, fibroblasts are one of the foundations of the healing process. These cells multiply and create a matrix for the developing tissue. It is the fibroblasts that are involved in scar formation. It seems natural to use them in the study of substances that are supposed to have a wound-healing effect. Supporting the proliferation of fibroblasts in the wound has an impact on the improvement in the healing process.

2. Results and Discussion

2.1. Model Fit and Statistical Analysis for MTT Test Results

The results of the MTT are presented in Figure 1 respectively. The values of the estimated parameters of the Brian and Cousens model for MTT results can be found in Table 1. The graphs show the prediction of the model and the maximum of the function corresponding to the highest cell viability. Only the mean values of the cell responses obtained are shown to maintain the readability of the graph.

It should be noted that low values of R^2 (Table 1) indicate a small difference between the mean value of the data and the prediction of the model. A low value of RMSE indicates a good fit of the model.

The *t* test was performed to indicate statistical differences between the mean values of the samples, which were suspected to show the stimulation effect and the mean in the control. One of the assumptions of *t* test is that both samples are approximately normally distributed. The normality of the distribution was analyzed using the Anderson–Darling test, and the results are available in the supporting information. The hypothesis that the data come from a population with a normal distribution was not rejected for most of the samples tested at $\alpha = 0.025$. The null hypothesis was rejected only for samples obtained from L929 cell line with 3 mg/L curcumin and 0.5 mg/L baicalin at $\alpha = 0.001$. Therefore, these two samples were not analyzed with the *t* test. The results of the *t* tests, obtained for the experimental points of the MTT tests, are presented in Table 2.

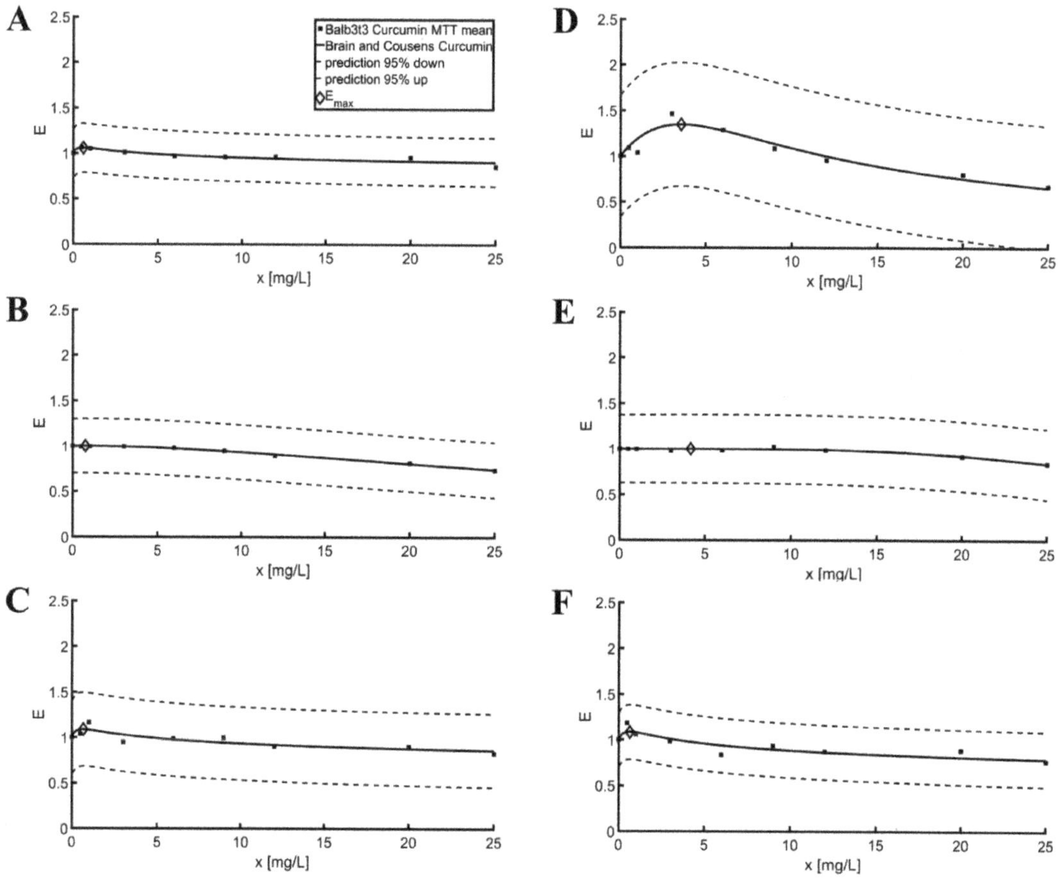

Figure 1. Brian and Cousens model curve fitting with 95% prediction bounds for the MTT assay. (**A**) Curcumin—Balb3t3; (**B**) Resveratrol—Balb3t3; (**C**) Baicalin—Balb3t3; (**D**) Curcumin—L929; (**E**) Resveratrol—L929; (**F**) Baicalin—L929.

Table 1. Estimated Brian and Cousens model parameters and values of the maximum relative effects for MTT assays.

		Parameters					Goodness of Fit	
Cell Line	**Substance**	b	e	f	x_{op} **[mg/L]**	E_{max}	R^2	**RMSE**
Balb3t	Curcumin	1.06	0.61	1.85	0.59	1.06	0.12	0.13
	Resveratrol	1.57	39.07	0.0042	0.76	1.00	0.25	0.15
	Baicalin	1.09	0.74	1.59	0.67	1.09	0.12	0.20
L929	Curcumin	1.66	6.24	0.25	3.55	1.35	0.27	0.34
	Resveratrol	3.53	38.98	0.00032	4.15	1.00	0.06	0.19
	Baicalin	1.12	1.00	1.16	0.67	1.08	0.31	0.15

Table 2. Results of the *t* test. The hypothesis of equal means for samples and equal but unknown variances is: 0 = NOT rejected; 1 = rejected for significance level α = 0.05.

Cell Line	Substance	Dose [mg/L]	*p*-Value	Hypothesis
Balb3t3	Curcumin	0.5	0.073	0
		1	0.102	0
	Resveratrol	0.5	0.890	0
		1	0.921	0
	Baicalin	0.5	0.356	0
		1	0.002	1
L929	Curcumin	3	Not tested	
		6	0.009	1
	Resveratrol	3	0.708	0
		6	0.749	0
	Baicalin	0.5	Not tested	
		1	0.117	0

2.2. Model Fit for Scratch Assay Tests

After confirmation of the absence of cytotoxicity with the MTT tests, it is possible to proceed to the study of the pro-proliferative effect of selected bioflavonoids with the ST test. The results of the experiments are shown in Figure 2, while the parameters of the Brian and Cousens model are presented in Table 3.

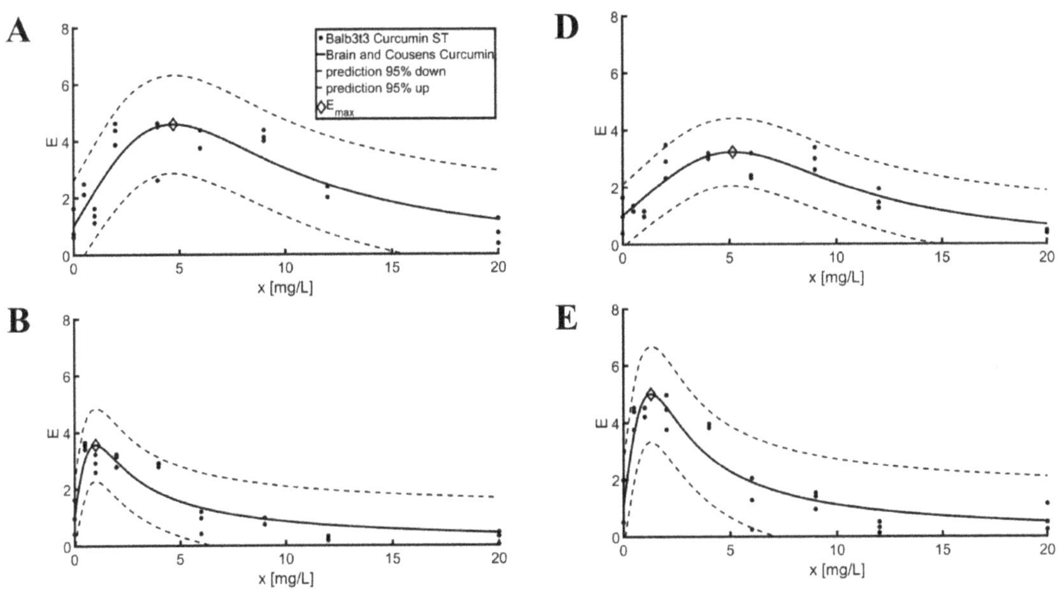

Figure 2. *Cont.*

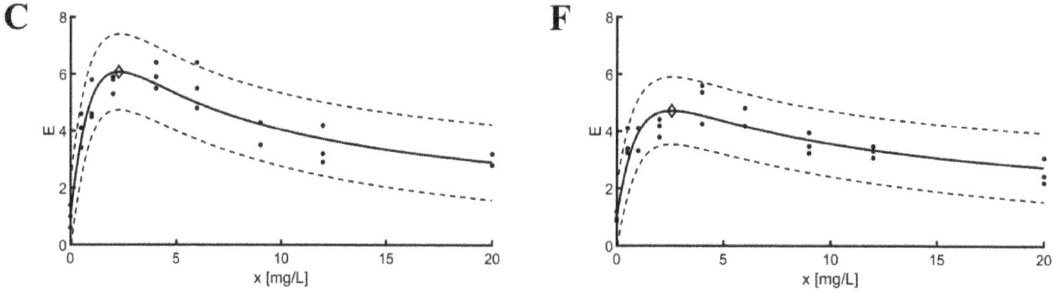

Figure 2. Brian and Cousens model curve adjustment for ST test. (**A**) Curcumin—Balb3t3; (**B**) Resveratrol—Balb3t3; (**C**) Baicalin—Balb3t3; (**D**) Curcumin—L929; (**E**) Resveratrol—L929; (**F**) Baicalin—L929.

Table 3. Estimated Brian and Cousens model parameters and values of maximum relative effects for ST tests.

		Parameters					Goodness of Fit	
Cell Line	**Substance**	b	e	f	x_{op}	E_{max}	R^2	**RMSE**
Balb3t3	Curcumin	2.57	6.21	1.24	4.73	4.59	0.74	0.78
	Resveratrol	1.91	1.15	5.31	1.01	3.56	0.82	0.57
	Baicalin	1.53	1.69	6.44	2.28	6.07	0.87	0.60
L929	Curcumin	2.96	7.34	0.65	5.16	3.23	0.76	0.53
	Resveratrol	2.09	1.49	5.98	1.29	5.01	0.84	0.74
	Baicalin	1.43	1.68	4.82	2.57	4.72	0.81	0.54

3. Discussion

3.1. Model Fit and Statistical Analysis for MTT Test Results

Based on the results of the MTT tests, it can be concluded that none of the substances tested showed a cytotoxic effect on the Balb3t3 and L929 fibroblast cell lines in the concentration range of 0 to 20 mg/L (Figure 1 and Table 1). The greatest negative effect on viability was observed for the L929 cell line for a curcumin concentration of 25 mg/L. Fibroblast cell viability for this concentration was 67.15 ± 5.01%. According to the ISO 10993-5 standard, a substance in a given concentration should be considered to have a cytotoxic potential if cell viability is <70% [28].

Due to the Brian and Cousens model, the half-maximum effective concentrations (EC50) were determined for selected bioflavonoids. The highest values in both lines were obtained for resveratrol; they were an order of magnitude higher than for curcumin and baicalin. It shows a slight influence of resveratrol on fibroblast mitochondrial activity. Parameter b was in a similar range of values for the bioflavonoids used regardless of the cell line used, excluding the combination of resveratrol and L929, where it was highest (3.53), indicating the steepest slope of the model curve.

The lowest values of f were determined for resveratrol. Furthermore, E_{max} values in the range of 1.00 suggest that this particular bioflavonoid does not have a stimulating effect on mitochondrial activity in L929 and Balb3t3 cell lines in tested time intervals. For curcumin and baicalin, the E_{max} values did not exceed 1.35. It may suggest that these substances have a relatively low stimulation effect on fibroblast cell activity after 24 h of exposure. The f parameter could not directly provide information about the E_{max} but it should be read with calibrated x_{op}. The low parameter f and the low x_{op} for resveratrol in both cell lines allowed E_{max} values greater than 1.00, but, on the other hand, the relatively low f and the high x_{op} for L929 curcumin resulted in the value of $Emax$ at the highest level of 1.35.

Increased mitochondrial activity can be correlated with growth rate. The higher the growth rate, the higher the mitochondrial activity. If cell divisions occur more rapidly in the first hours of incubation, it is possible that they were associated with much higher Emax values than those recorded after 24 h.

The observed cytotoxic effect is consistent with the observations of other researchers, e.g., Alqahtani et al. [29]. In the range of curcumin concentrations tested in the MTT assay (2–64 μM) on the human keratinocyte line (HuCaT), the cytotoxic effect was detected for a curcumin concentration greater than 32 μM. Our studies carried out in the mouse fibroblast lines Balb3t3 and L292 cover the concentration range of up to 25 μg/mL (about 67.86 μM) and at the highest concentration of this bioflavonoid, a decrease in cell viability could be observed. Another study carried out in human gingival fibroblasts (HGF) also shows that 0.1–20 μM curcumin solutions did not decrease cell viability, while solutions greater than 30 to 50 μM showed a cytotoxicity effect related to increasing concentration [30,31].

Researchers Lantto et al. [32] did not observe any resveratrol cytotoxicity in the range of 100 μM (22.8 mg/L) for SH-SY5Y (neuroblastoma cells) and CV1-P (fibroblasts) cell lines. A cytotoxic effect was observed for the CV1-P line at concentrations of 300 μM (68.5 mg/L) and 400 μM (91.3 mg/L). Similar studies were also carried out for curcumin, but here the cytotoxic effect was observed at concentrations greater than 25 μM (9.2 mg/L) for SH-SY5Y cell lines, while for the CV1-P line the cytotoxic effect was not observed at concentrations greater than 100 μM (36.8 mg/L). No cytotoxic effect was also observed in research on human dermal fibroblast cells in resveratrol concentrations in the range of 5.55 μM to 150 μM (1.3 to 34.2 mg/L) [33].

Experiments on the effect of baicalin on 3T3 fibroblasts carried out by Manconi et al. [34] also did not show a cytotoxic effect on baicalin concentration in PBS in the concentration range 0.1–20 mg/L. Experiments in rat lung fibroblasts also confirmed that there was no cytotoxic effect in mass concentrations of 20 to 80 mg/L with an addition of 20 mg/L of bleomycin. No cytotoxic effect was also observed in nasal fibroblasts up to 50 μM (22.3 mg/L) of baicalin [35,36].

The observed effect could be explained by a higher sensitivity of cancer cells compared to fibroblast cells to natural phenolic substances [32]. Our research seems to support reports that natural bioflavonoids do not have cytotoxic efficacy on fibroblast cells in the concentrations examined.

Based on the t tests (Table 2), statistically significant differences indicating the stimulating effect on cell viability were observed only for Balb3t3 cell line samples with 1 mg/L baicalin and L929 cell line samples with 6 mg/L curcumin. Although the administered MTT test could not exclude the stimulating effect of curcumin, resveratrol and baicalin on the L929 and Balb3t3 fibroblast cell lines. To fully understand the impact of the examined bioflavonoids on mitochondrial activity, different exposition times should be examined. However, our research appears to support reports that natural bioflavonoids do not have cytotoxic efficacy on fibroblast cells at the concentrations examined.

3.2. Model Fit for Scratch Assay Tests

Regardless of the cell lines tested, a stimulating effect of selected bioflavonoids was observed on the rate of cell division (Figure 2 and Table 3). It should be noted that the ST test provides information on the cumulative increase in the amount of new cells during the incubation period, while the MTT test provides information on the approximate instantaneous (2 h) mitochondrial activity.

In the case of curcumin, the maximum cell division rate for the concentration of 4.73 mg/L is approximately 4.5 times higher than in samples in which no bioflavonoid was added for the Balb3t3 line and more than three times higher than in the control sample for the concentration of 5.15 mg/L for the L929 line.

In both cell lines, a stimulating effect of resveratrol-supplied medium was observed in the range of 0.5–4 mg/L. The maximum cell division rate determined for resveratrol according to the calculated model is more than 3.5 times higher for the Balb3t3 line at

1.01 mg/L and approximately 5 times higher for the L929 line at 1.29 mg/L than for controls. At higher concentrations, a negative effect of resveratrol can be observed on the ability of fibroblasts to divide.

The maximum cell division rate observed for baicalin is 6 times higher for the Balb3t3 line for a concentration of 2.28 mg/L and more than 5.4 times for the L929 line for a concentration of 2.57 mg/L than for the relevant control samples. Unlike the remaining bioflavonoids for higher concentrations of baicalin (above 12 mg/L), a 2.5-fold stimulation of fibroblasts was still observed. This may indicate low toxicity of a high concentration of baicalin in the tested fibroblast lines.

The Brian and Cousens model was successfully fitted to all combinations of bioflavonoid cell lines for ST. The highest effect of the compound tested was observed for the combination of baicalin—Balb3t3 and the lowest for curcumin—L929. The coefficient of determination (R^2) did not drop below 0.74, while the highest RMSE value determined was 0.78. The corresponding slope values (b) and inflection point values (e) for the same substance differ for different cell lines by a maximum of 15% and 30%, respectively. For the same bioflavonoid, the models show the maximum stimulation of cell division at concentrations of the test substance that differ by a maximum of 0.4 mg/L. In all cases, the x_{op} was greater for L929 fibroblasts. This may indicate a very similar mode of action of the bioflavonoid in cells regardless of the type of fibroblast lineage.

For curcumin, Alqahtani et al. observed an increased proliferation effect in the L929 fibroblast cell line [29]. Studies suggest that curcumin-loaded lignin nanoparticles have a stronger stimulative effect than 50 µM (18.4 mg/L). Mirzahosseinipour et al. also observed the wound healing and antimicrobial properties of 50 mg/L curcumin in HDF fibroblast cells [37]. In this case, the form that delivers curcumin encapsulated in silica nanoparticles was also more effective than that of the bioflavonoid solution. Similar to the previous study, researchers did not present results for other concentrations of bioflavonoid solutions.

The process of cutaneous wound healing is extremely complex and depends on an intricate interplay between several highly regulated factors that work together to restore injured skin to repaired barrier function. The ideal dressing whose application would support and accelerate wound healing is faced with more and more challenges. Numerous studies are being conducted on various auxiliary substances and their applications that would meet all requirements, including protection against bacterial infection [38–40], reduction of the inflammatory process [41,42] and acceleration of cell proliferation aimed at reconstructing damaged tissues [43,44].

The substances selected for this study, curcumin, resveratrol and baicalin, have already been shown to have positive effects on wound healing [13,17,19,25,45]. Many studies have shown in which amount and application forms exhibit the most effective supportive effects [5,14,19,20,23–25,28,35–41,46] Understanding the optimal dose of these substances is essential for multiple goals and, above all, their complex role in the inflammatory response in wound repair needs to be addressed before further clinical development.

4. Materials and Methods

4.1. Bioflavonoids

In the presented study, the following bioflavonoids were used: curcumin, resveratrol and baicalin. All substances were sourced from Sigma-Aldrich (St. Louis, MO, USA).

4.2. Cell Lines

The study presented was carried out on L929 and Balb3t3 cell lines. Cell lines were obtained from Sigma-Aldrich (St. Louis, MO, USA). Both cell lines were cultured at 37 °C, 5% CO_2 and the relative humidity was set at 95%. Cell lines were passed twice a week and experiments were performed on cells between passages 15 and 25. The culture medium was changed every 48 h. Each dictation was performed according to the presented procedure: after removing the supernatant from L929 and Balb3t3 cells, they were washed with PBS (phosphate buffered saline), then treated with TrypLE Express solution (Gibco, Thermo

Fisher Scientific, Waltham, MA, USA) and incubated for 5 min at 37 °C. Next, the cells were transferred to a centrifuge tube, complete medium (to inactivate TrypLE Express) was added (to inactivate the TrypLE Express), and cells were centrifuged for 5 min at 1000× *g*. The supernatant was removed and cells were resuspended in fresh medium. The viability of a cell line was checked every day by microscopy observation of the cell culture morphology.

4.2.1. L929

Mice fibroblast L929 cells (subclone of parental strain L, strain L was derived from normal subcutaneous areolar and adipose tissue of a 100 day old male C3H/An mouse) were obtained from Sigma-Aldrich (St. Louis, MO, USA) and cultured in Minimum Essential Medium Eagle (EMEM).

4.2.2. Balb3t3

Mice fibroblast Balb/3T3 cells (clone A31 from a mouse embryo donor) were obtained from Sigma-Aldrich (St. Louis, MO, USA) and cultured in Minimum Essential Medium (MEM).

4.3. Cell Viability

The MTT-3-(4,5-dimethylthiazol-2-yl)-2,5-diphenyltetrazolium bromide assay (Sigma-Aldrich, St. Louis, MO, USA) was used to evaluate the effect of the bioflavonoids chosen on cell viability according to the ISO 10993 standard, part V [28]. The MTT assay was performed on commercial L929 and Balb3t3 cell lines.

The test stocks were prepared by the following procedure: to the bioflavonoids, DMSO (dimethyl sulfoxide) was added to the final concentration set at 10 mM. The stock solutions were stored at −80 °C paying attention that the storage time does not exceed 6 months. The stock solutions were dissolved every time before the planned biological assay with appropriate culture media. The culture medium used was reduced to the FBS level, up to 5%. During the test, it was crucial to set the DMSO concentration level lower than 1% in the highest bioflavonoid concentration of the test.

Each cell line was seeded in 96-well plates at a density of 1×10^4 cells/mL per well. The plates were incubated for 24 h to allow the cells to attach to the bottom of the plate. After this time, each line, in addition to the control, was exposed to different concentrations of bioflavonoids tested. The concentrations examined were: 0.5, 1, 3, 6, 9, 12, 15, 20, 25 mg/L. The exposure time to the test substances was set at 24 h. At the end of the exposition time, the medium was removed and 50 µL of 1 mg/mL of MTT solution was added to each well and then incubated at 37 °C for another 2 h. At this time, crystals of formazan were created. Finally, the supernatant was removed and the formazan crystals formed were dissolved in 100 µL of isopropanol (30 min incubation) for spectrophotometric evaluation. Absorbance was measured with a Victor2 microplate reader (PerkinElmer, Waltham, MA, USA) at 570 nm. The formazan concentration in each sample was expressed as a relative value of the mean formazan concentration in the control and used in further analysis. Rav results can be find in the supplementary material (Tables S1–S6).

4.4. Scratch Assay

A scratch test (ST) was used to perform a wound healing evaluation under in vitro conditions. This procedure allows us to study the collective migration of cells in a two-dimensional confluent monolayer under test conditions [47]. ST was performed as follows:

Cell lines were seeded in 6-well culture plates. The cell was incubated at 37 °C, 5% CO_2, relative humidity 95% for 24 to create a confluent monolayer. After the cell monolayer was achieved, the scratch-making procedure was performed. A sterile plastic micropipette tip was used to simulate an in vivo wound by creating a cell-free zone with a straight edge across the cell monolayer in each well. A gap width of 0.7 mm allows observation at 4 or 10 magnifications. After the scratches were made, the wells were washed with basal medium to remove cell debris and a complete medium was added. Test bioflavonoids at the following concentrations were added to the appropriate wells: 0.5, 1, 3, 6, 9, 12, 20 mg/L. The control sample was not exposed to bioflavonoids. Finally, the tested systems were incubated for 24 h under the following conditions: 37 °C, 5% CO_2, relative humidity 95%. After incubation, each wound was scored at 4 and 10× magnification. The width of the lesion was measured in 3 places. Each defect was measured two times: T0, at the time of wound execution and T24, after 24 h of incubation. The mean rate of the cell gap bridge was determined over the course of 24 h. The results were expressed as relative values of the bridging rate in the control sample. Rav results can be find in the supplementary material (Tables S7–S12).

4.5. Model Fit and Statistical Analysis

The Brian and Cousens model was used to analyze the influence of bioflavonoids on cell viability and cell migration [46,48]. The model can be used to describe the effects of inhibition and stimulation.

$$E = c + \frac{d - c + fx}{1 + \exp(b(ln(x) - ln(e)))} \tag{1}$$

where E—relative effect; x—a concentration of bioflavonoid [mg/L]; e—inflection point equal to EC50 for $c = 0$ and $d = 1$ [mg/L]; b—parameter which determines the slope; and c and d—limit at $x \to 0$ and limit at $x \to \infty$ equal to 0 and 1, respectively; f—stimulation parameter.

The values of the parameters of the Brian and Cousens model were estimated using the nonlinear least squares method in MATLAB. To obtain a more reliable model fit, some additional constraints were provided: $b > 1$ and $f > 0$ for all cases and $e > 1$ for the MTT assay for cell lines L929 and baicalin. For every estimated parameter, the 95% non-simultaneous prediction bounds for new observations were obtained. The goodness of fits was characterized by the coefficient of determination (R^2) and the root mean squared error (RMSE).

The Nelder–Mead Simplex Method implemented in MATLAB was used to find the concentration of bioflavonoids x_{op} for which maximum value of the relative effect E_{max} is reached by maximizing the value of the Brian and Cousens model (1) for each set of estimated parameters.

Based on determined E_{max}, the experimental data sets obtained for the concentration of bioflavonoids next to x_{op} were chosen for further statistical analysis. The Anderson–Darling test was performed to check whether the experimental data are normally distributed at significance levels of 5%, 2.5% and 1%. The two-sample t test was performed to indicate the statistical difference between the mean values of the relative effect of the experimental data chosen and the control samples at the 5% significance level [49]. Both the Anderson–Darling and the t test were performed in MATLAB. Anderson – Darling test results and t-test results for all bioflavonoids can be found in the supplementary material (Tables S13 and S14).

5. Conclusions

This article examined the cytotoxicity of natural bioflavonoids and their effect on mitochondrial and proliferation activity in L929 and Balb3t3 cell lines. The experiments confirmed the lack of cytotoxicity of the selected substances in the concentration range tested in the Balb3t3 and L929 fibroblast lines. The selected bioflavonoids curcumin, resveratrol and baicalin showed a simulative effect on the proliferative capacity of both cell lines. The Brian and Cousens model could be used to describe a stimulative effect of selected bioflavonoids. As a result of the obtained results, all of the examined substances raise hopes that they may be used in difficult-to-heal wound treatment.

Supplementary Materials: The following supporting information can be downloaded at: https://www.mdpi.com/article/10.3390/ph16010082/s1.; Table S1: MTT results for curcumin – Balb3t3, Table S2: MTT results for resveratrol – Balb3t3, Table S3: MTT results for baicalin – Balb3t3, Table S4: MTT results for curcumin – L929, Table S5: MTT results for resveratrol – L929, Table S6: MTT results for baicalin – L929, Table S7: ST results for curcumin – Balb3t3, Table S8: ST results for resveratrol – Balb3t3, Table S9: ST results for baicalin – Balb3t3, Table S10: ST results for curcumin – L929, Table S11: ST results for resveratrol – L929, Table S12: ST results for baicalin – L929, Table S13. Anderson – Darling test results, Table S14. T-test results for all bioflavonoids.

Author Contributions: Conceptualization, K.J., O.U., E.K.-K. and K.M.; methodology, K.J., K.M., E.K.-K.; software, K.J., K.M., M.J.; validation, K.M., B.W., P.K.-R., E.K.-K.; formal analysis, K.M., B.W., P.K.-R., E.K.-K.; investigation, O.U., B.W., P.K.-R., E.K.-K.; resources, K.J., O.U., E.K.-K. and K.M.; methodology, K.J., K.M., E.K.-K.; data curation, K.J., K.M.; writing—original draft preparation, K.J., O.U.; writing—review and editing, K.J., O.U., K.M., E.K.-K.; visualization, K.J.; supervision, K.J., K.M.; project administration, K.J.; funding acquisition, K.J. All authors have read and agreed to the published version of the manuscript.

Funding: This research received no external funding.

Institutional Review Board Statement: Not applicable.

Informed Consent Statement: Not applicable.

Data Availability Statement: Data is contained within the article or supplementary material.

Conflicts of Interest: The authors confirm that there are no conflicts of interest.

References

1. Frykberg, R.G.; Banks, J. Challenges in the Treatment of Chronic Wounds. *Adv. Wound Care* **2015**, *4*, 560–582. [CrossRef] [PubMed]
2. Beers, E.H. Palliative Wound Care: Less Is More. *Surg. Clin. N. Am.* **2019**, *99*, 899–919. [CrossRef] [PubMed]
3. Veith, A.P.; Henderson, K.; Spencer, A.; Sligar, A.D.; Baker, A.B. Therapeutic Strategies for Enhancing Angiogenesis in Wound Healing. *Adv. Drug Deliv. Rev.* **2019**, *146*, 97–125. [CrossRef] [PubMed]
4. Wilkinson, H.N.; Hardman, M.J. Wound Healing: Cellular Mechanisms and Pathological Outcomes: Cellular Mechanisms of Wound Repair. *Open Biol.* **2020**, *10*, 200223. [CrossRef] [PubMed]
5. Kuhnke, J.L.; Keast, D.; Rosenthal, S.; Evans, R.J. Health Professionals' Perspectives on Delivering Patient-Focused Wound Management: A Qualitative Study. *J. Wound Care* **2019**, *28*, S4–S13. [CrossRef] [PubMed]
6. Bowers, S.; Franco, E. Chronic Wounds: Evaluation and Management. *Am. Fam. Physician* **2020**, *101*, 159–166.
7. Atkin, L. Chronic Wounds: The Challenges of Appropriate Management. *Br. J. Community Nurs.* **2019**, *24*, S26–S32. [CrossRef]
8. Tashkandi, H. Honey in Wound Healing: An Updated Review. *Open Life Sci.* **2021**, *16*, 1091–1100. [CrossRef]
9. Mohanty, C.; Sahoo, S.K. Curcumin and Its Topical Formulations for Wound Healing Applications. *Drug Discov. Today* **2017**, *22*, 1582–1592. [CrossRef]
10. Shah, A.; Amini-Nik, S. The Role of Phytochemicals in the Inflammatory Phase of Wound Healing. *Int. J. Mol. Sci.* **2017**, *18*, 1068. [CrossRef]
11. Akbik, D.; Ghadiri, M.; Chrzanowski, W.; Rohanizadeh, R. Curcumin as a Wound Healing Agent. *Life Sci.* **2014**, *116*, 1–7. [CrossRef]
12. Kant, V.; Gopal, A.; Pathak, N.N.; Kumar, P.; Tandan, S.K.; Kumar, D. Antioxidant and Anti-Inflammatory Potential of Curcumin Accelerated the Cutaneous Wound Healing in Streptozotocin-Induced Diabetic Rats. *Int. Immunopharmacol.* **2014**, *20*, 322–330. [CrossRef] [PubMed]
13. Kant, V.; Gopal, A.; Kumar, D.; Pathak, N.N.; Ram, M.; Jangir, B.L.; Tandan, S.K.; Kumar, D. Curcumin-Induced Angiogenesis Hastens Wound Healing in Diabetic Rats. *J. Surg. Res.* **2015**, *193*, 978–988. [CrossRef] [PubMed]
14. Cakmak, G.K.; Irkorucu, O.; Ucan, B.H.; Tascilar, O.; Emre, A.U.; Karakaya, K.; Bahadir, B.; Acikgoz, S.; Pasaoglu, H.; Ankarali, H.; et al. The Effects of Resveratrol on the Healing of Left Colonic Anastomosis. *J. Investig. Surg.* **2009**, *22*, 353–361. [CrossRef] [PubMed]
15. Günal, M.Y.; Ayla, Ş.; Bedri, N.; Beker, M.Ç.; Çağlayan, A.B.; Aslan, İ.; Özdemir, E.M.; Yeşilada, E.; Kılıç, Ü. The Effects of Topical Liposomal Resveratrol on Incisional and Excisional Wound Healing Process. *Turkderm. Turk. Arch. Dermatol. Venereol.* **2019**, *53*, 128–134. [CrossRef]
16. Brâkenhielm, E.; Cao, R.; Cao, Y. Suppression of Angiogenesis, Tumor Growth, and Wound Healing by Resveratrol, a Natural Compound in Red Wine and Grapes. *FASEB J.* **2001**, *15*, 1798–1800. [CrossRef] [PubMed]
17. Huang, X.; Sun, J.; Chen, G.; Niu, C.; Wang, Y.; Zhao, C.; Sun, J.; Huang, H.; Huang, S.; Liang, Y.; et al. Resveratrol Promotes Diabetic Wound Healing via SIRT1-FoxO1-c-Myc Signaling Pathway-Mediated Angiogenesis. *Front. Pharm.* **2019**, *10*, 421. [CrossRef]

18. Yurdagul, A.; Kleinedler, J.J.; McInnis, M.C.; Khandelwal, A.R.; Spence, A.L.; Orr, A.W.; Dugas, T.R. Resveratrol Promotes Endothelial Cell Wound Healing under Laminar Shear Stress through an Estrogen Receptor-α-Dependent Pathway. *Am. J. Physiol. Heart Circ. Physiol.* **2014**, *306*, 797–806. [CrossRef]
19. Hecker, A.; Schellnegger, M.; Hofmann, E.; Luze, H.; Nischwitz, S.P.; Kamolz, L.P.; Kotzbeck, P. The Impact of Resveratrol on Skin Wound Healing, Scarring, and Aging. *Int. Wound J.* **2022**, *19*, 9–28. [CrossRef]
20. Pignet, A.L.; Schellnegger, M.; Hecker, A.; Kohlhauser, M.; Kotzbeck, P.; Kamolz, L.P. Resveratrol-Induced Signal Transduction in Wound Healing. *Int. J. Mol. Sci.* **2021**, *22*, 12614. [CrossRef]
21. Berman, A.Y.; Motechin, R.A.; Wiesenfeld, M.Y.; Holz, M.K. The Therapeutic Potential of Resveratrol: A Review of Clinical Trials. *NPJ Precis. Oncol.* **2017**, *1*, 35. [CrossRef] [PubMed]
22. Khodarahmian, M.; Amidi, F.; Moini, A.; Kashani, L.; Salahi, E.; Danaii-mehrabad, S.; Nashtaei, M.S.; Mojtahedi, M.F.; Esfandyari, S.; Sobhani, A. A Randomized Exploratory Trial to Assess the Effects of Resveratrol on VEGF and TNF-α 2 Expression in Endometriosis Women. *J. Reprod. Immunol.* **2021**, *143*, 103248. [CrossRef] [PubMed]
23. Moore, O.A. The Extraction, Anticancer Effect, Bioavailability, and Nanotechnology of Baicalin. *J. Nutr. Med. Diet. Care* **2016**, *2*, 1–12. [CrossRef]
24. You, J.; Cheng, J.; Yu, B.; Duan, C.; Peng, J. Baicalin, a Chinese Herbal Medicine, Inhibits the Proliferation and Migration of Human Non-Small Cell Lung Carcinoma (NSCLC) Cells, A549 and H1299, by Activating the SIRT1/AMPK Signaling Pathway. *Med. Sci. Monit.* **2018**, *24*, 2126–2133. [CrossRef] [PubMed]
25. Zhang, K.; Lu, J.; Mori, T.; Smith-Powell, L.; Synold, T.W.; Chen, S.; Wen, W. Baicalin Increases VEGF Expression and Angiogenesis by Activating the ERRα/PGC-1α Pathway. *Cardiovasc. Res.* **2011**, *89*, 426–435. [CrossRef]
26. Alshehabat, M.; Hananeh, W.; Ismail, Z.B.; Rmilah, S.A.; Abeeleh, M.A. Wound Healing in Immunocompromised Dogs: A Comparison between the Healing Effects of Moist Exposed Burn Ointment and Honey. *Vet. World* **2020**, *13*, 2793–2797. [CrossRef] [PubMed]
27. Mao, X.; Li, Z.; Li, B.; Wang, H. Baicalin Regulates MRNA Expression of VEGF-c, Ang-1/Tie2, TGF-β and Smad2/3 to Inhibit Wound Healing in Streptozotocin-Induced Diabetic Foot Ulcer Rats. *J. Biochem. Mol. Toxicol.* **2021**, *35*, e22893. [CrossRef]
28. *ISO 10993:5*; Tests for In Vitro Cytotoxicity. International Organization for Standardization: Geneva, Switzerland, 2009.
29. Alqahtani, M.S.; Alqahtani, A.; Kazi, M.; Ahmad, M.Z.; Alahmari, A.; Alsenaidy, M.A.; Syed, R. Wound-Healing Potential of Curcumin Loaded Lignin Nanoparticles. *J. Drug Deliv. Sci. Technol.* **2020**, *60*, 102020. [CrossRef]
30. Celen, C.; Keçeciler, C.; Yapar, E.A.; Gökçe, E.H.; Nalbantsoy, A. Evaluation of Resveratrol Organogels Prepared by Micro-Irradiation: Fibroblast Proliferation through in Vitro Wound Healing. *Turk. J. Biochem.* **2018**, *43*, 385–392. [CrossRef]
31. Rujirachotiwat, A.; Suttamanatwong, S. Curcumin Upregulates Transforming Growth Factor-B1, Its Receptors, and Vascular Endothelial Growth Factor Expressions in an in Vitro Human Gingival Fibroblast Wound Healing Model. *BMC Oral Health* **2021**, *21*, 535. [CrossRef]
32. Lantto, T.A.; Colucci, M.; Závadová, V.; Hiltunen, R.; Raasmaja, A. Cytotoxicity of Curcumin, Resveratrol and Plant Extracts from Basil, Juniper, Laurel and Parsley in SH-SY5Y and CV1-P Cells. *Food Chem.* **2009**, *117*, 405–411. [CrossRef]
33. Eroğlu, I.; Gökçe, E.H.; Tsapis, N.; Tanriverdi, S.T.; Gökçe, G.; Fattal, E.; Özer, O. Evaluation of Characteristics and in Vitro Antioxidant Properties of RSV Loaded Hyaluronic Acid-DPPC Microparticles as a Wound Healing System. *Colloids Surf. B Biointerfaces* **2015**, *126*, 50–57. [CrossRef] [PubMed]
34. Manconi, M.; Manca, M.L.; Caddeo, C.; Cencetti, C.; di Meo, C.; Zoratto, N.; Nacher, A.; Fadda, A.M.; Matricardi, P. Preparation of Gellan-Cholesterol Nanohydrogels Embedding Baicalin and Evaluation of Their Wound Healing Activity. *Eur. J. Pharm. Biopharm.* **2018**, *127*, 244–249. [CrossRef] [PubMed]
35. Zhao, H.; Li, C.; Li, L.; Liu, J.; Gao, Y.; Mu, K.; Chen, D.; Lu, A.; Ren, Y.; Li, Z. Baicalin Alleviates Bleomycin-Induced Pulmonary Fibrosis and Fibroblast Proliferation in Rats via the PI3K/AKT Signaling Pathway. *Mol. Med. Rep.* **2020**, *21*, 2321–2334. [CrossRef] [PubMed]
36. Shin, J.M.; Kang, J.H.; Lee, S.A.; Park, I.H.; Lee, H.M. Baicalin Down-Regulates IL-1β-Stimulated Extracellular Matrix Production in Nasal Fibroblasts. *PLoS ONE* **2016**, *11*, e0168195. [CrossRef]
37. Mirzahosseinipour, M.; Khorsandi, K.; Hosseinzadeh, R.; Ghazaeian, M.; Shahidi, F.K. Antimicrobial Photodynamic and Wound Healing Activity of Curcumin Encapsulated in Silica Nanoparticles. *Photodiagnosis Photodyn. Ther.* **2020**, *29*, 101639. [CrossRef]
38. Wang, C.; Wang, M.; Xu, T.; Zhang, X.; Lin, C.; Gao, W.; Xu, H.; Lei, B.; Mao, C. Engineering Bioactive Self-Healing Antibacterial Exosomes Hydrogel for Promoting Chronic Diabetic Wound Healing and Complete Skin Regeneration. *Theranostics* **2019**, *9*, 65–76. [CrossRef]
39. Zhou, L.; Xi, Y.; Xue, Y.; Wang, M.; Liu, Y.; Guo, Y.; Lei, B. Injectable Self-Healing Antibacterial Bioactive Polypeptide-Based Hybrid Nanosystems for Efficiently Treating Multidrug Resistant Infection, Skin-Tumor Therapy, and Enhancing Wound Healing. *Adv. Funct. Mater.* **2019**, *29*, 1806883. [CrossRef]
40. Qiu, W.; Han, H.; Li, M.; Li, N.; Wang, Q.; Qin, X.; Wang, X.; Yu, J.; Zhou, Y.; Li, Y.; et al. Nanofibers Reinforced Injectable Hydrogel with Self-Healing, Antibacterial, and Hemostatic Properties for Chronic Wound Healing. *J. Colloid Interface Sci.* **2021**, *596*, 312–323. [CrossRef]
41. Dev, S.K.; Choudhury, P.K.; Srivastava, R.; Sharma, M. Antimicrobial, Anti-Inflammatory and Wound Healing Activity of Polyherbal Formulation. *Biomed. Pharmacother.* **2019**, *111*, 555–567. [CrossRef]

42. Tewtrakul, S.; Tungcharoen, P.; Sudsai, T.; Karalai, C.; Ponglimanont, C.; Yodsaoue, O. Antiinflammatory and Wound Healing Effects of *Caesalpinia sappan* L. *Phytother. Res.* **2015**, *29*, 850–856. [CrossRef] [PubMed]
43. Lukiswanto, B.S.; Miranti, A.; Sudjarwo, S.A.; Primarizky, H.; Yuniarti, W.M. Evaluation of Wound Healing Potential of Pomegranate (Punica Granatum) Whole Fruit Extract on Skin Burn Wound in Rats (Rattus Norvegicus). *J. Adv. Vet. Anim. Res.* **2019**, *6*, 202–207. [CrossRef] [PubMed]
44. Marquele-Oliveira, F.; da Silva Barud, H.; Torres, E.C.; Machado, R.T.A.; Caetano, G.F.; Leite, M.N.; Frade, M.A.C.; Ribeiro, S.J.L.; Berretta, A.A. Development, Characterization and Pre-Clinical Trials of an Innovative Wound Healing Dressing Based on Propolis (EPP-AF®)-Containing Self-Microemulsifying Formulation Incorporated in Biocellulose Membranes. *Int. J. Biol. Macromol.* **2019**, *136*, 570–578. [CrossRef] [PubMed]
45. Qu, J.; Zhao, X.; Liang, Y.; Zhang, T.; Ma, P.X.; Guo, B. Antibacterial Adhesive Injectable Hydrogels with Rapid Self-Healing, Extensibility and Compressibility as Wound Dressing for Joints Skin Wound Healing. *Biomaterials* **2018**, *183*, 185–199. [CrossRef] [PubMed]
46. Cedergreen, N.; Ritz, C.; Streibig, J.C. Improved Empirical Models Describing Hormesis. *Environ. Toxicol. Chem.* **2005**, *24*, 3166–3172. [CrossRef] [PubMed]
47. Liang, C.C.; Park, A.Y.; Guan, J.L. In Vitro Scratch Assay: A Convenient and Inexpensive Method for Analysis of Cell Migration in Vitro. *Nat. Protoc.* **2007**, *2*, 329–333. [CrossRef]
48. Brain, P.; Cousens, R. An Equation to Describe Dose Responses Where There Is Stimulation of Growth at Low Doses. *Weed Res.* **1989**, *29*, 93–96. [CrossRef]
49. Calabrese, E.J.; Stanek, E.J.; Nascarella, M.A. Evidence for Hormesis in Mutagenicity Dose-Response Relationships. *Mutat. Res.* **2011**, *726*, 91–97. [CrossRef]

pharmaceuticals

MDPI

Article

Physical Properties and pH Environment of Foam Dressing Containing *Eclipta prostrata* Leaf Extract and Gelatin

Sukhontha Hasatsri [1,*], Jariya Suthi [2], Nattaporn Siriwut [3] and Onjira Charoensappakit [4]

1 Department of Pharmacy Practice, College of Pharmacy, Rangsit University, Pathum Thani 12000, Thailand
2 Sunpasitthiprasong Hospital, Ubon Ratchathani 34000, Thailand
3 NorthEastern Institute of Child and Adolescent Mental Health, Khon Kaen 40000, Thailand
4 Chularat Cholvaej Hospital, Chonburi 20000, Thailand
* Correspondence: sukhontha.h@rsu.ac.th

Abstract: *Eclipta prostrata (E. prostrata)* has several biological activities, including antibacterial and anti-inflammatory activities, that improve wound healing. It is well known that physical properties and pH environment are crucial considerations when developing wound dressings containing medicinal plant extracts in order to create an appropriate environment for wound healing. In this study, we prepared a foam dressing containing *E. prostrata* leaf extract and gelatin. Chemical composition was verified using Fourier-transform infrared spectroscopy (FTIR) and pore structure was obtained using scanning electron microscopy (SEM). The physical properties of the dressing, including absorption and dehydration properties, were also evaluated. The chemical properties were measured to determine the pH environment after the dressing was suspended in water. The results revealed that the *E. prostrata* dressings had a pore structure with an appropriate pore size (313.25 ± 76.51 μm and 383.26 ± 64.45 μm for the *E. prostrata* A and *E. prostrata* B dressings, respectively). The *E. prostrata* B dressings showed a higher percentage of weight increase in the first hour and a faster dehydration rate in the first 4 h. Furthermore, the *E. prostrata* dressings had a slightly acidic environment (5.28 ± 0.02 and 5.38 ± 0.02 for the *E. prostrata* A and *E. prostrata* B dressings at 48 h, respectively).

Keywords: *Eclipta prostrata*; gelatin; foam dressing; wound dressing; physical property; absorption; dehydration; pH environment

1. Introduction

Plant-based biomaterials have several benefits over synthetic materials, including cost-effectiveness, safety for humans, and their environmentally friendly composition [1]. Developing novel wound dressings containing medicinal plant extracts can improve clinical outcomes and increase plant value [2,3]. In this study, we examined *Eclipta prostrata* L. (*E. prostrata* L.) due to its pharmacological properties. *E. prostrata* L., commonly known as False daisy, Ink plant, Bhringraj, Bhumiraj, Aali jhar, or Nash jhar, is a herbaceous plant that belongs to the family Asteraceae [4]. It is a weed that grows in moist places such as rivers, marshes, or the edge of rice fields [4,5]. It is found in many parts of the world, including Thailand, China, India, Nepal, and Brazil [4]. It has been long used in the treatment of several diseases, including coronary heart disease, diabetes, gastrointestinal diseases, respiratory diseases, skin diseases, and wounds [5]. The leaves have various biological activities, including antibacterial, antifungal, and anti-inflammatory activities, that improve wound healing [6–9]. Therefore, a wound dressing containing *E. prostrata* L. extract could be used for treating infection and inflammation in wound healing. Kang et al. [10] suggest that *E. prostrata* L. extract is a potential treatment for inflammatory skin conditions such as atopic dermatitis. The *E. prostrata* L. extract improved the allergic inflammation of the skin by restoring the skin barrier dysfunction, decreasing epidermis/dermis thickness, and regulating the immune balance [10]. Raoul et al. evaluated wound healing in rats after applying an ointment containing *E. prostrata* leaf extract [11]. The results showed that the wounds treated with medicinal ointment completely healed faster than when treated with Vaseline® and Cicatryl® [11]. Babu et al. [12] developed a hydrogel containing *E. prostrata* leaf extract and evaluated its physical properties, including pH, viscosity, and spreadability. However, no studies have yet developed a wound dressing containing *E. prostrata* leaf extract in sheet form or as foam dressings. Wound dressing selection is based on the wound's cause, location, healing phase, exudate level, pain, odor, infection, size, and depth [13]. For deep or tunneling wounds, packing wounds with dressing in the form of rope is essential for promoting wound healing from the inside [14]. On the other hand, superficial or partial-thickness wounds require dressing in the form of a sheet to cover the wound and facilitate wound function [15]. In addition, choosing the physical characteristics of wound dressings according to the exudate level will provide the optimum environment for facilitating wound healing.

The development of foam dressing for wound healing applications should focus on physical properties. According to ideal wound dressing properties, the wound dressings should be able to absorb wound exudate in order to prevent maceration (softening and breaking down of the surrounding skin due to prolonged exposure to moisture), malodor, local wound infection, and delayed wound healing [15–19]. However, different absorption properties of wound dressings are appropriate for different types of wounds [16,20,21]. For example, a wound dressing with a high absorption capacity should be selected for wounds with a high level of exudate. Additionally, the dehydration rate of wound dressing is also an important property that maintains a moist wound-healing environment [22]. A moist wound environment has several benefits, including increased keratinocyte migration and re-epithelialization, increased collagen synthesis, increased autolytic debridement, reduced pain, and decreased inflammation [23,24].

Elevated exudate pH correlates with an increased risk of infection and delayed wound healing [25,26]. Therefore, the ideal wound dressing should not provide an alkaline wound environment. Foam dressing's porous structure is also an essential factor in the wound-healing process [27,28]. The wound-healing process is a complex biological process that seeks to recover damaged tissues and restore the skin's normal function. The wound-healing process consists of four continuous and overlapping phases: hemostasis, inflammation, proliferation, and remodeling [29]. The appropriate pore size of the porous structure is essential for the proliferative phase. Both natural and synthetic polymers are used in wound dressings, and each type of polymer can help to produce a porous structure. Natural polymers are commonly chosen for wound dressing development, including chitosan, cellulose, hyaluronic acid, collagen, alginate, and gelatin [30]. Gelatin could be used to produce porous structures via the freeze-drying technique [31,32]. Porous gelatin materials support cell migration and the development of new tissue [33]. Interestingly, gelatin could also provide biodegradable and biocompatible material [31,34]. Thus, the present study aimed to develop a foam dressing containing *E. prostrata* leaf extract and gelatin; the physical properties and pH wound environment of the dressing were subsequently evaluated. The results from this study could deliver the profile of physical characteristics and pseudo-wound environment after being treated with foam dressing containing *E. prostrata* leaf extract and gelatin.

2. Results

2.1. Thickness Test

The composition of prepared foam dressings containing *E. prostrata* leaf extract and gelatin is shown in Table 1. The *E. prostrata* A dressing had a lower concentration of *E. prostrata* leaf extract than the *E. prostrata* B dressing. The *E. prostrata* dressings were soft and flexible. The *E. prostrata* A dressing had a thickness of 4.236 ± 0.0519 mm; the *E. prostrata* B dressing had a thickness of 3.945 ± 0.1403 mm. The *E. prostrata* A dressing was thicker than the *E. prostrata* B dressing.

Table 1. FTIR peak values and functional groups of the *Eclipta prostrata (E. prostrata)* leaf extract and the *E. prostrata* A and B dressings.

Functional Groups	Peak Values		
	E. prostrata **Leaf Extract**	***E. prostrata*** **A Dressings**	***E. prostrata*** **B Dressings**
Alkane	1376.65 2877.87 2931.46 2971.77	1378.70 2933.99 2973.15	1378.60 2933.97 2973.45
Alkene	1654.70	1646.91	1647.22
Halo compound	802.76 837.70	837.56	837.51

2.2. Fourier-Transform Infrared Spectroscopy (FTIR)

Table 1 shows the FTIR peak values and functional groups of the *E. prostrata* leaf extract and the *E. prostrata* A and B dressings. Figure 1 shows the FTIR spectra of the *E. prostrata* leaf extract. Figure 2 shows the FTIR spectra of the *E. prostrata* A and B dressings. After mixing gelatin and *E. prostrata* leaf extract and then lyophilization or freeze drying, there was an increased intensity in the functional groups (as seen in Figure 2), including amide I (1646.91 cm^{-1} and 1647.22 cm^{-1} for the *E. prostrata* A and B dressings, respectively), and amide II (1553.43 cm^{-1} and 1554.20 cm^{-1} for the *E. prostrata* A and B dressings, respectively). The amide I (mainly related to the C=O stretching vibration) and II (mainly related to the N-H bending vibration and the C-N stretching vibration) bands are associated with the presence of gelatin [35,36].

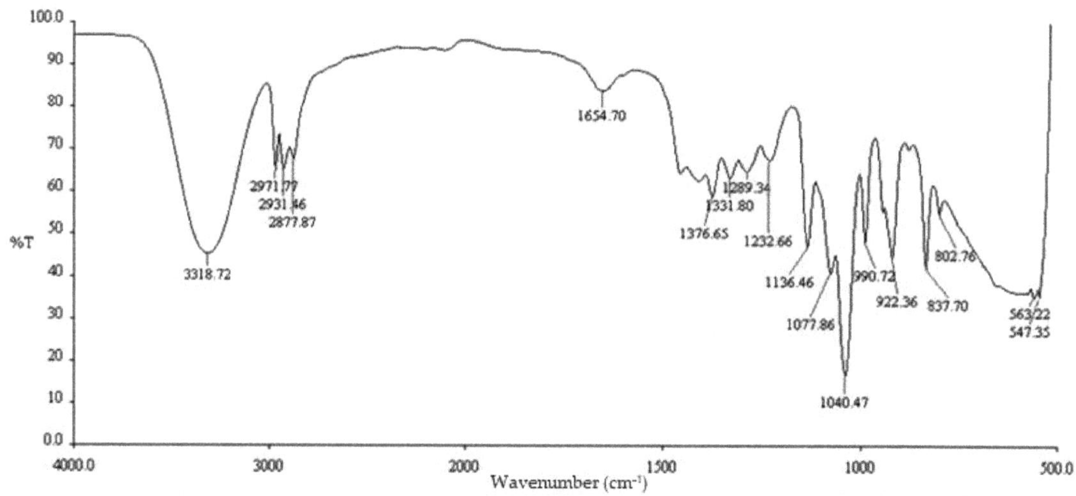

Figure 1. FTIR spectra of the *Eclipta prostrata (E. prostrata)* leaf extract.

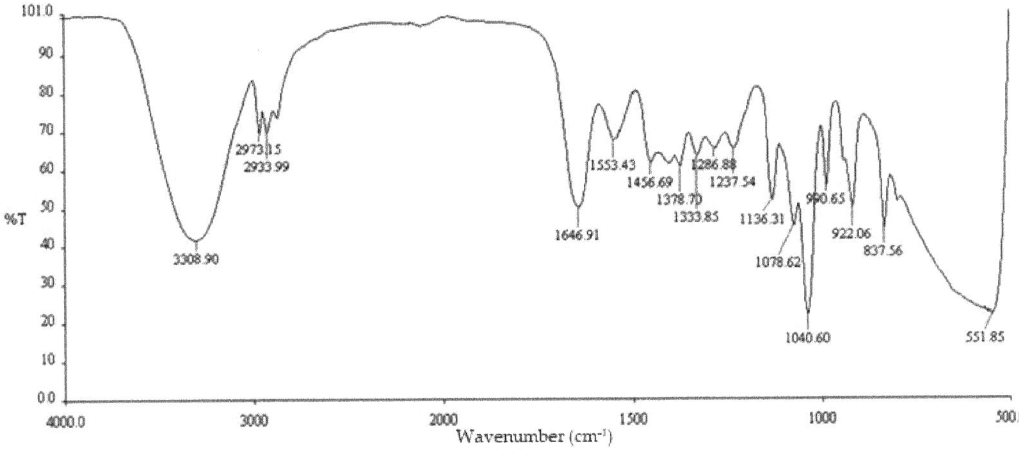

(a)

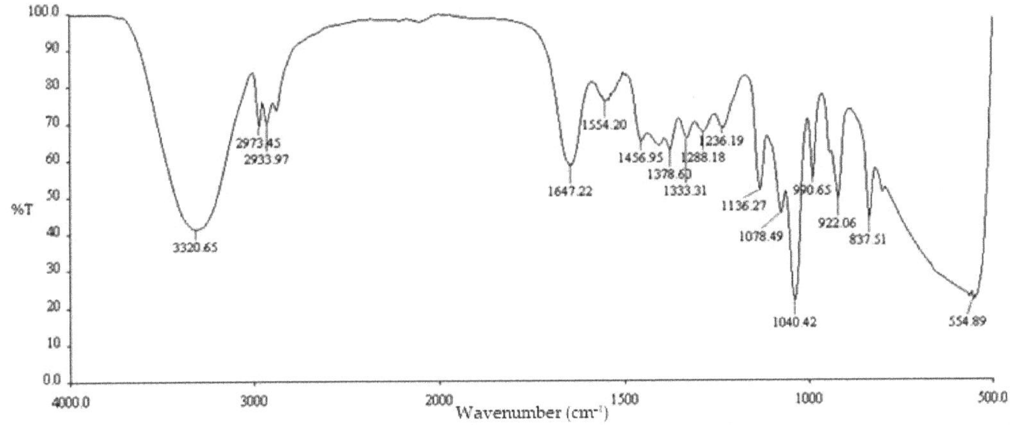

(b)

Figure 2. FTIR spectra of the (**a**) *E. prostrata* A dressing and (**b**) *E. prostrata* B dressing.

2.3. Morphological Properties

The surface and cross-sectional morphologies of *E. prostrata* dressings were observed using SEM (Figure 3). The size, shape, and distribution of pores are shown in Figure 3b. The average pore sizes were 313.25 ± 76.51 μm and 383.26 ± 64.45 μm for the *E. prostrata* A and B dressings, respectively (Figure 3b). The *E. prostrata* B dressing had more consistent porosity than *E. prostrata* A dressing.

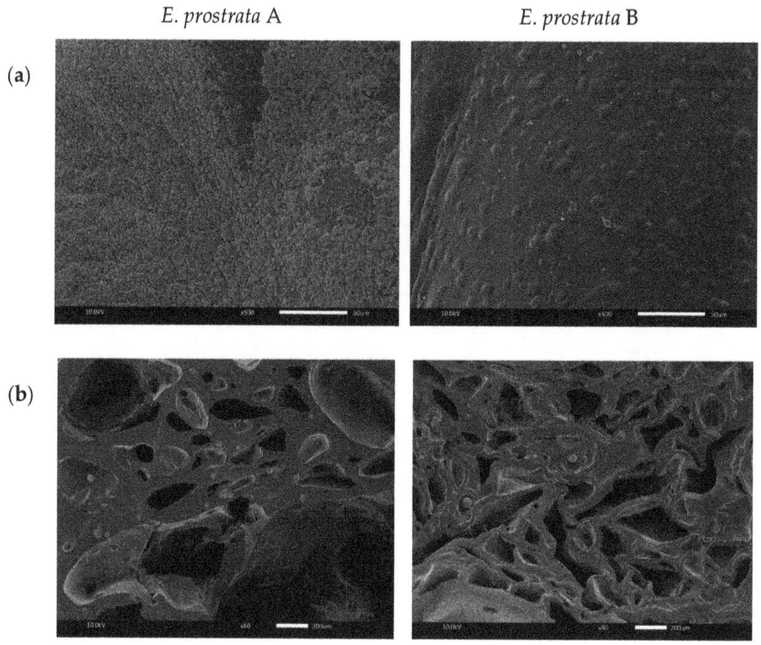

Figure 3. Morphological observation of (**a**) surface and (**b**) cross-section of *E. prostrata* dressings by SEM.

2.4. Absorption Properties

The absorption properties of the dressing determine how well it can manage wound exudate and promote wound healing. The percentage of weight increase of the *E. prostrata* dressing for different periods is shown in Figure 4. The *E. prostrata* A dressing showed a lower percentage of weight increase than the *E. prostrata* B dressing. The higher *E. prostrata* leaf extract promotes the higher absorption capacity.

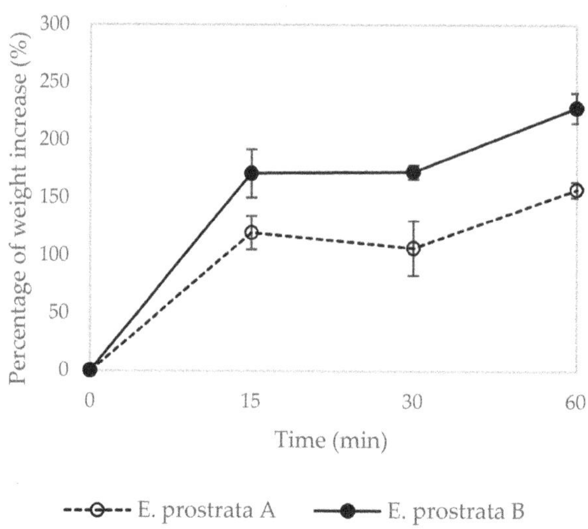

Figure 4. Absorption properties of *E. prostrata* A and B dressings.

2.5. Dehydration Properties

The dehydration rate of the *E. prostrata* dressing for different periods is presented in Figure 5. The *E. prostrata* B dressing showed a higher dehydration rate in the first 4 h than the *E. prostrata* A dressing. The higher *E. prostrata* leaf extract promotes the higher dehydration rate.

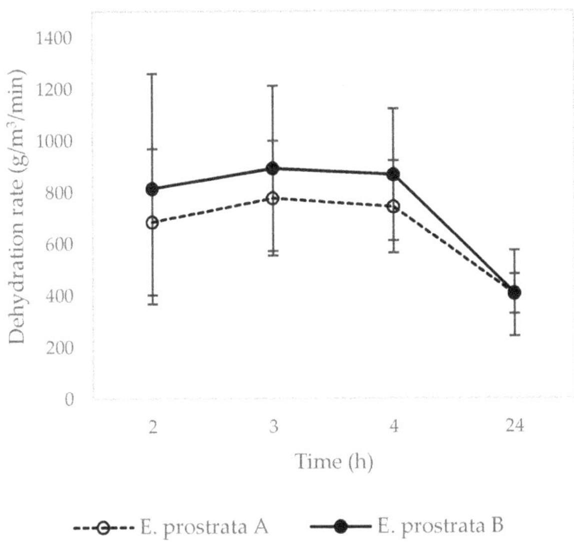

Figure 5. Dehydration properties of *E. prostrata* A and B dressings.

2.6. pH Measurement

Figure 6 demonstrates the pH of deionized water after the *E. prostrata* dressings were submerged in it. The pH of the deionized water with the submerged *E. prostrata* A dressing decreased from 7.55 ± 0.16 to 5.28 ± 0.02. In the same way, the pH of deionized water with the submerged *E. prostrata* B dressing decreased from 7.69 ± 0.24 to 5.38 ± 0.02.

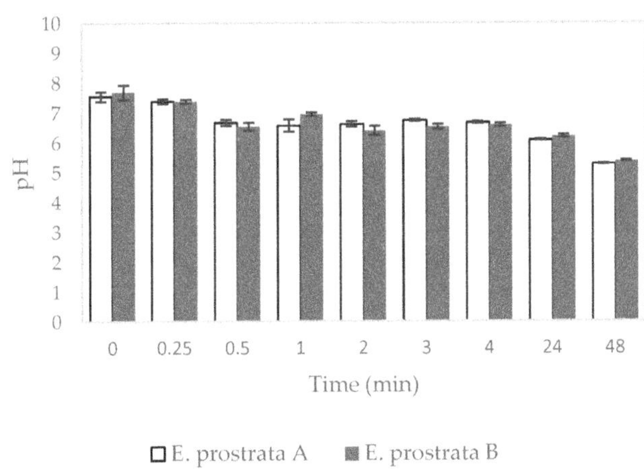

Figure 6. The pH of deionized water with the submerged *E. prostrata* A and B dressings.

2.7. Dispersion Characteristics

The dispersion characteristics of the *E. prostrata* dressings are shown in Figures 7 and 8. The *E. prostrata* A and B dressings did not change much from their original structure after they were immersed in pseudo-wound exudate for 60 s at 100 revolutions per minute (Figure 7). However, the spectra of the pseudo-wound exudate after the *E. prostrata* A and B dressings were submerged in it were not similar to those of the pseudo-wound exudate (Figure 8).

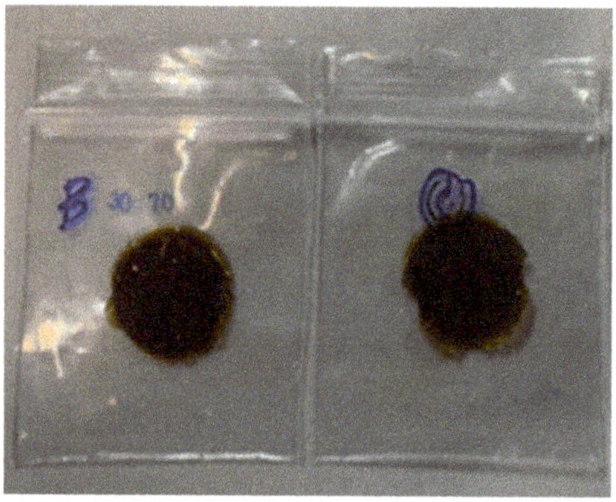

Figure 7. Dispersion Characteristics of (**left**) *E. prostrata* A and (**right**) *E. prostrata* B dressings.

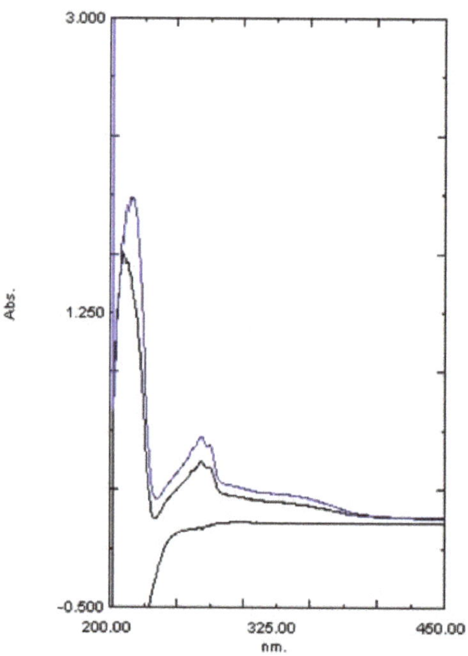

Figure 8. Dispersion Characteristics compared with a pseudo-wound exudate. Spectrum of (**bottom line in black**) $NaCl/CaCl_2{\cdot}H_2O$ solution, (**blue line**) $NaCl/CaCl_2{\cdot}H_2O$ solution after with the *E. prostrata* A dressing were submerged, and (**upper line in black**) $NaCl/CaCl_2{\cdot}H_2O$ solution after with the *E. prostrata* B dressing were submerged.

3. Discussion

E. prostrata leaf extract has been studied for its potential wound-healing benefits, including its antimicrobial and anti-inflammatory properties [6–9]. Prior studies examining the development of wound healing products containing *E. prostrata* focus only on ointment and hydrogel formulations [11,12]. No studies have developed wound dressings containing *E. prostrata* leaf extract in sheet form or foam dressings. Developing wound dressing in sheet form has several advantages, including preventing trauma, minimizing external contamination, absorbing exudate, and keeping a wound in an optimally moist environment [16].

In this study, a foam dressing containing *E. prostrata* extract and gelatin was developed to evaluate the physical properties and pH wound environment. The *E. prostrata* dressings were soft and flexible. These properties help to maintain a moist wound environment, reduce the risk of maceration, and allow use in the movement areas, such as the knee or elbow [37]. The *E. prostrata* A dressing was thicker than the *E. prostrata* B dressing. This is explained as the high protein content in bovine gelatin increased the polymer matrix's solids content. Hence, the increase in gelatin or protein concentration has induced an increase in the thickness of the foam dressing [38]. However, the thickness was unrelated to the absorption and dehydration properties, as shown in Figures 4 and 5.

The FTIR spectra are used to identify the functional groups present in the *E. prostrata* dressing, as compared to the *E. prostrata* leaf extract. It was found that the FTIR spectra of *E. prostrata* dressing had an increased intensity in the functional groups, including amide I and II (Figure 2). The amide I and II bands in the FTIR spectra are commonly used to identify the presence of gelatin [35,36]. The amide I band in FTIR spectra is a strong absorption peak that corresponds to the stretching vibration of the C=O bond in the peptide backbone [39]. This band of gelatin appears in the region of 1600–1700 cm^{-1} [35]. As shown in Figure 2, the amide I band was around 1646–1648 cm^{-1}, indicating the presence of a predominantly random coil structure [39]. The amide II band in the FTIR spectra I also provide information on the vibrational bands of the protein backbone [39]. This band corresponds to the bending vibration of the N-H bond (40–60% of the potential energy) and the stretching vibration of the C-N bond (18–40%) in the protein backbone [39]. In the case of gelatin, the amide II band appears in the region of 1565–1520 cm^{-1} [35]. As shown in Figure 2, the amide II band was around 1553–1555 cm^{-1}. The amide II band is often used in combination with the amide I band to confirm the presence of gelatin. Therefore, it indicates that our process to develop an *E. prostrata* dressing did not affect the structural property of gelatin. Gelatin could provide a porous structure and produce biodegradable and biocompatible material [31,34].

The resulting SEM image provides information about the morphology or porous structure of the *E. prostrata* dressing (Figure 3). A porous structure is crucial in wound healing because it allows cell migration and proliferation [28,40]. When a wound occurs, the first phase of wound healing is hemostasis, with vascular constriction, platelet aggregation, degranulation, and fibrin clot formation [29]. Hemostasis helps to stop bleeding, and inflammatory cells (neutrophils, monocytes, macrophages, and lymphocytes) migrate into the wound, triggering the inflammatory response (also known as the "inflammatory phase") [29]. The next phase is proliferation, with re-epithelialization, angiogenesis, collagen synthesis, and extracellular matrix (ECM) formation; this generally overlaps with the inflammatory phase [29]. The porous structure supports this phase. Fibroblasts and endothelial cells need to migrate into the wound bed in order to proliferate and form granulation tissue at the site of injury [29]. A porous structure allows for these cells to migrate into the wound bed, promoting efficient wound healing. Following cell proliferation, the final phase is remodeling (collagen remodeling and vascular maturation) and regression [29]. A previous study by Murphy et al. [41] showed that a mean pore size of 325 μm facilitated the highest cell attachment and proliferation when compared with pores in the 85–190 μm range. As seen in Figure 3b, our SEM images of the cross-section show an average pore size of around 300 μm. This ensured that the *E. prostrata* A and B dressings had an appropriate pore size for efficient wound healing. Nevertheless, the *E. prostrata* B dressing had a more consistent porosity than the *E. prostrata* A dressing. The effect of this difference in porosity between the *E. prostrata* A and B dressings could result in differences in absorption ability.

We developed the *E. prostrata* dressing, which was designed with a porous structure, in order to increase absorption ability. In this study, absorption ability was obtained by using pseudo-wound exudate. The *E. prostrata* B dressing exhibited a stronger absorption ability than the *E. prostrata* A dressing (Figure 4). The absorption ability of the *E. prostrata* B dressing was derived from a higher-density porous structure (Figure 3b). The ideal wound dressing must absorb excess wound exudate and provide a moist environment [18,21,22,42]. Wound exudate or wound drainage is the fluid that discharges from a wound during the healing process [43]. The mechanism of exudate formation is usually due to inflammation or infection [43]. The amount of exudate produced can vary depending on the type and severity of the wound. A moist wound environment is necessary for the wound-healing process to occur effectively. An optimal moisture level enhances cell migration and proliferation, reduces pain and discomfort, and reduces infection rates [22,23]. Macerated peri-wound skin can lead to an increased risk of infection, whereas desiccated peri-wound skin can lead to decreased epithelial migration and cell death [22,44]. Therefore, the selection of absorbent wound dressing depends on the amount of exudate to prevent both maceration and desiccation. Moreover, a moist environment promotes autolysis or breakdown of necrotic tissue, called autolytic debridement [23,45]. In our previous work [20], the commercial hydrocolloid dressing and hydrocolloid with foam layer dressing had the lowest absorption capacity. Therefore it is an appropriate dressing for wounds with a low amount of exudate. In this study, both the *E. prostrata* A and B dressings had absorption characteristics similar to commercial hydrocolloid dressings and hydrocolloid with foam layer dressings [20]. These absorption characteristics meant that both the *E. prostrata* A and B dressings could be chosen for wounds with low exudate.

Dehydration rate is also essential to control the moisture balance of the wound and enhance wound healing as a result of water-retaining properties [22,46]. This can be achieved through the use of appropriate wound dressings that are designed to manage moisture levels and prevent dehydration. In addition, the selection of wound dressing also depends on the amount of exudate produced by the wound. The *E. prostrata* B dressing showed a higher dehydration rate than the *E. prostrata* A dressing. This can be explained by the higher-density porous structure of the *E. prostrata* B dressing (Figure 3b). Therefore, the *E. prostrata* B dressing can dehydrate exudate to rapidly create a moist wound-healing environment.

The pH of the wound environment is an essential factor for wound healing. The pH of healthy human skin is in the range of 5.4 to 5.9, which is slightly acidic. [47]. Propionibacterium is commonly found on human skin. Propionibacterium grow well at pH 6.00–6.50 [48]. *Staphylococcus aureus* is a pyogenic bacterium [49]. *S. aureus* prefers a neutral pH environment for optimal growth and survival [50]. Thus, an acidic environment is not favorable for harmful bacterial growth. In addition, the pH environment of chronic wounds exists at a range of 7.15 to 8.90; this is alkaline and chronic wounds are characterized by excessive protease activity [51–55]. Sim et al. found that faster recovery of wounded tissues was observed in wounds treated by pH 4 buffers when compared to pH 6 buffers [25]. A previous study by Leveen et al. showed that a slightly acidic environment significantly inhibits protease activity and may potentially enhance the healing of cutaneous wounds [56]. Previous studies reported fibroblast proliferation and migration behaviors associated with the acidic environment [57,58]. It means rapid wound healing occurs in an acidic environment [25,54]. We found that the *E. prostrata* A and B dressings showed similar pH decreases continuously over the period. Our *E. prostrata* dressings tended to create a slightly acidic environment. Hence, it was supposed that the *E. prostrata* A and B dressings would not interfere with the wound healing process.

The dispersion of the wound dressing refers to how well the dressing covers the wound surface. In this study, the spectra of the pseudo-wound exudate after the *E. prostrata* A and B dressings were submerged in it were not similar to those of the pseudo-wound exudate (Figure 8). In our previous study, commercial alginate dressings had the spectra of the pseudo-wound exudate after the dressings were submerged was also not similar to those of the pseudo-wound exudate [20]. Nevertheless, after interacting with the pseudo-wound exudate, the *Eclipta prostrata* A and B dressings did not change substantially from their original structure (Figure 7). It means that the *E. prostrata* dressing will not be difficult to remove. According to the spectra of the pseudo-wound exudate after the dressings were submerged, our *E. prostrata* dressings have an immediate-release formulation. The *E. prostrata* dressing should be further modified for controlled release applications by crosslinking techniques with a crosslinker, such as glutaraldehyde [59,60].

4. Materials and Methods

4.1. Materials

Gelatin (from bovine skin, gel strength 225, Type B) was purchased from Sigma–Aldrich, Inc. (St. Louis, MO, USA). *E. prostrata* leaf extract was purchased from SK Herb Co., Ltd. (Samut Sakhon, Thailand). Sodium chloride and calcium chloride dihydrate were purchased from VWR International bvba (Leuven, Belgium).

4.2. Preparation of Foam Dressing Containing E. prostrata Extract and Gelatin

The gelatin solution (10% w/v) was prepared by dissolving the gelatin in deionized water at 40 °C and stirring continuously for 1 h. Then, the *E. prostrata* dressing was prepared by mixing gelatin solution and *E. prostrata* leaf extract, as shown in Table 2. The mixture was stirred for 1 h to obtain a homogeneous solution. After stirring, the solution was sonicated to eliminate air bubbles and then poured into plastic plates. The plastic plates were placed into a freezer at −80 °C and frozen for 24 h. The frozen solution was then lyophilized in a freeze-dryer (SHM 021) for 48 h to become a sponge. Finally, the sponge (*E. prostrata* dressing) was slowly removed from the plastic plate. In order to prevent contamination, the *E. prostrata* dressings were then stored inside an airtight container. The composition with *E. prostrata* leaf extract of more than 40% could not prepare foam dressing.

Table 2. Composition of prepared foam dressings containing *E. prostrata* extract and gelatin.

E. prostrata	*E. prostrata* Leaf Extract: Gelatin (v/v)
A	3:7
B	2:3

4.3. Thickness Test

After lyophilization, a thickness test was performed using the Mitutoyo Dial Thickness Gauge, which provided an accuracy of 0.001 mm. Thickness was measured at five different positions (one in the center and four in the middle of each side).

4.4. Fourier Transform Infrared Spectroscopy (FTIR)

The *E. prostrata* leaf extracts and the *E. prostrata* dressings were recorded on a spectrum 100 FTIR Spectrometer (PerkinElmer Inc., Waltham, MA, USA) FTIR spectra were recorded from
500 to 4000 cm^{-1}.

4.5. Morphological Properties

At a voltage of 10 kV, the *E. prostrata* dressings were examined using a Scanning Electron Microscope (SEM, JSM-IT300 JEOL). SEM with an Energy Dispersive X-ray Spectrometer (EDS) was used to analyze the dressings with the surface (500×) and cross-sectional (60×) images. The *E. prostrata* dressing was first prepared by attaching it to the aluminium stubs and then coating it with gold. This process helps to improve the conductivity of the dressing, allowing for better imaging results. The pore sizes were measured using the Image J® software (National Institutes of Health, Bethesda, MA, USA).

4.6. Absorption Properties

The absorption properties of the *E. prostrata* dressing were examined using BS EN 13726-1: 2002, Part 1: the aspects of absorbency, Section 3.2: free swell absorptive capacities with slight modifications [61]. The *E. prostrata* dressing (2 cm × 2 cm) was prepared and weighed. A test solution (8.298 g of NaCl (0.142 mol/L) and 0.367 g of $CaCl_22H_2O$ (0.0025 mol/L)) was added to one liter of deionized water, representing a pseudo-wound exudate. The *E. prostrata* dressing was immersed in the test solution and then incubated at 37 °C. At different periods, the dressing was removed and weighed.

4.7. Dehydration Properties

The *E. prostrata* dressing (2 cm × 2 cm) was prepared and weighed. The *E. prostrata* dressing was immersed in the test solution (pseudo-wound exudate) for 30 min. Then, the dressing was removed, weighed, and incubated at 37 °C. At different periods, the dressing was weighed [62].

4.8. pH Measurement

The *E. prostrata* dressing (2 cm × 2 cm) was suspended in deionized water at a ratio of 1:25 (w/v). At different periods, the deionized water was measured using a pH meter (pH 700) [62].

4.9. Dispersion Characteristics

The dispersion characteristics of the *E. prostrata* dressing were examined using BS EN 137262: 2002, Part 1: the aspects of absorbency, Section 3.6: dispersion characteristics with slight modifications [63]. The *E. prostrata* dressing (2 cm × 2 cm) was prepared and immersed in the test solution and shaken for 60 s at 100 revolutions per minute. Then, the absorbance of the collected test solution was measured using a UV-spectrophotometer (UV-2501PC) by scanning between a wavelength of 200 and 450 nm.

4.10. Statistical Analysis

The experiments were performed in triplicate and represented in a mean ± standard deviation.

5. Conclusions

This study is the first development of wound dressing sheets containing *E. prostrata* leaf extract and gelatin. Our study investigated the physical properties and pH pseudo-wound environment of the *E. prostrata* dressing. Both the *E. prostrata* A and B dressings had an appropriate pore size (313.25 ± 76.51 µm and 383.26 ± 64.45 µm, respectively) for cell migration and proliferation in the wound healing process. Greater *E. prostrata* leaf extract produces a higher-density porous structure of foam dressing, resulting in a higher absorption capacity and faster dehydration rate. The *E. prostrata* dressings are designed for the low level of exudate due to their absorption capacity. In addition, the *E. prostrata* dressings make the environment slightly acidic. Therefore, it was supposed that our *E. prostrata* dressings would not provide favorable conditions for bacterial growth. Our results provide the wound dressing profiles that are essential for the decision of physicians to select the appropriate wound dressing according to the amount of exudate. Further experimental studies should focus on release patterns, pharmacological properties, such as antibacterial and anti-inflammatory activities, and wound healing assays.

Author Contributions: Conceptualization, S.H.; methodology, S.H.; investigation, J.S., N.S. and O.C.; resources, S.H.; data curation, S.H., J.S., N.S. and O.C.; writing—original draft preparation, S.H.; supervision, S.H.; funding acquisition, S.H. All authors have read and agreed to the published version of the manuscript.

Funding: This research was funded by the College of Pharmacy, Rangsit University, Thailand.

Institutional Review Board Statement: Not applicable.

Informed Consent Statement: Not applicable.

Data Availability Statement: Data is contained within the article.

Acknowledgments: Authors would like to thank the Department of Pharmacology, Pharmaceutical Chemistry, and Manufacturing Pharmacy, College of Pharmacy, Rangsit University, Thailand, for providing the laboratory equipment used for experiments.

Conflicts of Interest: The authors declare no conflict of interest.

References

1. Kepekçi, R.A.; Yener İlçe, B.; Demir Kanmazalp, S. Plant-derived biomaterials for wound healing. In *Studies in Natural Products Chemistry*; Elsevier: Amsterdam, The Netherlands, 2021; pp. 227–264.
2. Martin, C.; Low, W.L.; Amin, M.C.I.M.; Radecka, I.; Raj, P.; Kenward, K. Current trends in the development of wound dressings, bio-materials and devices. *Pharm. Pat. Anal.* **2013**, *2*, 341–359. [CrossRef] [PubMed]
3. Yazarlu, O.; Iranshahi, M.; Kashani, H.R.; Reshadat, S.; Habtemariam, S.; Iranshahy, M.; Hasanpour, M. Perspective on the application of medicinal plants and natural products in wound healing: A mechanistic review. *Pharm. Res.* **2021**, *174*, 105841. [CrossRef] [PubMed]
4. Timalsina, D.; Devkota, H.P. *Eclipta prostrata* (L.) L. (Asteraceae): Ethnomedicinal uses, chemical constituents, and biological activities. *Biomolecules* **2021**, *11*, 1738. [CrossRef] [PubMed]
5. Feng, L.; Zhai, Y.Y.; Xu, J.; Yao, W.F.; Cao, Y.D.; Cheng, F.F.; Bao, B.H.; Zhang, L. A review on traditional uses, phytochemistry and pharmacology of *Eclipta prostrata* (L.) L. *J. Ethnopharmacol.* **2019**, *245*, 112109. [CrossRef]
6. Gurrapu, S.; Mamidala, E.; Mamidala, E.; Mamidala, E. In vitro Antibacterial Activity of Alkaloids Isolated from Leaves of Eclipta alba Against Human Pathogenic Bacteria. *Pharmacogn. J.* **2017**, *9*, 573–577. [CrossRef]
7. Nahid, A.; Neelabh, C.; Navneet, K.; Kumar Navneet, C. Evaluation of antioxidant and antimicrobial potentials of *Eclipta prostrata* collected from the Nepal region. *Pharma Innov. J.* **2017**, *6*, 4–7.
8. Singh, L.; Antil, R.; Kumar, D.; Dahiya, P. Phytochemical analysis and In-vitro assays for antimicrobial and antioxidant activity of Bhringraj herb *Eclipta prostrata* (L.). *J. Pharm. Phytochem.* **2019**, *8*, 4527–4533.
9. Arunachalam, G.; Subramanian, N.; Pazhani, G.P.; Ravichandran, V. Anti-inflammatory activity of methanolic extract of *Eclipta prostrata* L. (Astearaceae). *Afr. J. Pharm. Pharmacol.* **2009**, *3*, 97–100.
10. Kang, Y.M.; Kim, H.M.; Lee, H.; Lee, D.S.; An, H.J. Anti-inflammatory effects of *Eclipta prostrata* Linné on house dust mite-induced atopic dermatitis in vivo and in vitro. *J. Ethnopharmacol.* **2022**, *292*, 115233. [CrossRef]
11. Raoul, A.; CyrJonas, M.; MatokoChristevyRommelle, S.; ItouDeGardeRomaric, E.; Martin, D.; AngeAntoine, A. Antidiabetic and Wounds Healing Activities of *Eclipta prostrata* (Asteraceae) Leaves. *Int. J. Adv. Res.* **2018**, *6*, 393–398. [CrossRef]
12. Babu, I.S.; Bhramaramba, R.; Tegjaswini, S.S.N. Formulation and Evaluation of Herbal Gel containing Eclipta alba Linn., leaves extract. *Int. J. Adv. Pharm. Biol. Chem.* **2015**, *4*, 496–500.
13. Edwards, H.; Gibb, M.; Finlayson, K.; Jensen, R. *Wound Dressing Guide*; Institute of Health and Biomedical Innovation: Kelvin Grove, Australia, 2013; pp. 1–49.
14. Dabiri, G.; Damstetter, E.; Phillips, T. Choosing a Wound Dressing Based on Common Wound Characteristics. *Adv. Wound Care* **2016**, *5*, 32–41. [CrossRef] [PubMed]
15. Vivcharenko, V.; Przekora, A. Modifications of wound dressings with bioactive agents to achieve improved pro-healing properties. *Appl. Sci.* **2021**, *11*, 4114. [CrossRef]
16. Broussard, K.C.; Powers, J.G. Wound dressings: Selecting the most appropriate type. *Am. J. Clin. Dermatol.* **2013**, *14*, 449–459. [CrossRef]
17. Cutting, K.F.; White, R.J. Maceration of the skin and wound bed. 1: Its nature and causes. *J. Wound Care* **2002**, *11*, 275–278. [CrossRef] [PubMed]
18. Rezvani Ghomi, E.; Khalili, S.; Nouri Khorasani, S.; Esmaeely Neisiany, R.; Ramakrishna, S. Wound dressings: Current advances and future directions. *J. Appl. Polym. Sci.* **2019**, *136*, 47738. [CrossRef]
19. Gardner, S. Managing high exudate wounds. *Wound Essent.* **2012**, *7*, 1–3.
20. Hasatsri, S.; Pitiratanaworanat, A.; Swangwit, S.; Boochakul, C.; Tragoonsupachai, C. Comparison of the Morphological and Physical Properties of Different Absorbent Wound Dressings. *Dermatol. Res. Pract.* **2018**, *2018*, 9367034. [CrossRef]
21. Dhivya, S.; Padma, V.V.; Santhini, E. Wound dressings—A review. *BioMedicine* **2015**, *5*, 24–28. [CrossRef]

22. Butcher, M. Moist wound healing, exudate and management of the wound bed. *J. Wound Care* **2013**, *19* (Suppl. S5), 10–13. [CrossRef]
23. Nuutila, K.; Eriksson, E. Moist Wound Healing with Commonly Available Dressings. *Adv. Wound Care* **2021**, *10*, 685–698. [CrossRef]
24. Sharman, D. Moist Wound Healing: A Review of Evidence, Application and Outcome. *Diabet. Foot.* **2003**, *6*, 112–120.
25. Sim, P.; Strudwick, X.L.; Song, Y.M.; Cowin, A.J.; Garg, S. Influence of Acidic pH on Wound Healing In Vivo: A Novel Perspective for Wound Treatment. *Int. J. Mol. Sci.* **2022**, *23*, 13655. [CrossRef]
26. Aly, R.; Shirley, C.; Cunico, B.; Maibach, H.I. Effect of prolonged occlusion on the microbial flora, pH, carbon dioxide and transep-idermal water loss on human skin. *J. Investig. Dermatol.* **1978**, *71*, 378–381. [CrossRef]
27. Toker-Bayraktar, M.; Erenay, B.; Altun, B.; Odabaş, S.; Garipcan, B. Plant-derived biomaterials and scaffolds. *Cellulose* **2023**, *30*, 2731–2751. [CrossRef]
28. Karageorgiou, V.; Kaplan, D. Porosity of 3D biomaterial scaffolds and osteogenesis. *Biomaterials* **2005**, *26*, 5474–5491. [CrossRef] [PubMed]
29. Guo, S.; DiPietro, L.A. Factors affecting wound healing. *J. Dent. Res.* **2010**, *89*, 219–229. [CrossRef] [PubMed]
30. Evren Okur, M.; Karantas, I.D.; Enyi, S.; Üstünda, N.; Siafaka, P.I. Recent trends on wound management: New therapeutic choices based on polymeric carriers. *Asian J. Pharm. Sci.* **2020**, *15*, 661–684. [CrossRef]
31. Sultana, N.; Hassan, M.I.; Ridzuan, N.; Ibrahim, Z.; Soon, C.F. Fabrication of gelatin scaffolds using thermally induced phase separation technique. *Int. J. Eng. Trans. B Appl.* **2018**, *31*, 1302–1307.
32. Annabi, N.; Nichol, J.W.; Zhong, X.; Ji, C.; Koshy, S.; Khademhosseini, A.; Dehghani, F. Controlling the Porosity and Microarchitecture of Hydrogels for Tissue Engineering. *Tissue Eng.* **2010**, *16*, 371–383. [CrossRef]
33. Ndlovu, S.P.; Ngece, K.; Alven, S.; Aderibigbe, B.A. Gelatin-based hybrid scaffolds: Promising wound dressings. *Polymers* **2021**, *13*, 2959. [CrossRef] [PubMed]
34. Naomi, R.; Bahari, H.; Ridzuan, P.M.; Othman, F. Natural-based biomaterial for skin wound healing (Gelatin vs. collagen): Expert review. *Polymers* **2021**, *13*, 2319. [CrossRef] [PubMed]
35. Cebi, N.; Durak, M.Z.; Toker, O.S.; Sagdic, O.; Arici, M. An evaluation of Fourier transforms infrared spectroscopy method for the classification and discrimination of bovine, porcine and fish gelatins. *Food Chem.* **2016**, *190*, 1109–1115. [CrossRef] [PubMed]
36. Mahmoud, A.A.; Osman, O.; Eid, K.; Ashkar, E.A.; Okasha, A.; Atta, D.; Eid, M.; Aziz, Z.A.; Fakhry, A. FTIR Spectroscopy of Natural Bio-Polymers Blends. *Middle East. J. Appl. Sci.* **2014**, *4*, 816–824.
37. Thomas, M.; Hamdan, M.; Hailes, S.; Walker, M. An investigation into the conformability of wound dressings. *Wounds UK* **2011**, *7*, 14–24.
38. Said, N.S.; Sarbon, N.M. Physical and Mechanical Characteristics of Gelatin-Based Films as a Potential Food Packaging Material: A Review. *Membranes* **2022**, *12*, 442. [CrossRef]
39. Sadat, A.; Joye, I.J. Peak fitting applied to fourier transform infrared and raman spectroscopic analysis of proteins. *Appl. Sci.* **2020**, *10*, 5918. [CrossRef]
40. Chaudhari, A.A.; Vig, K.; Baganizi, D.R.; Sahu, R.; Dixit, S.; Dennis, V.; Singh, S.R.; Pillai, S.R. Future prospects for scaffolding methods and biomaterials in skin tissue engineering: A review. *Int. J. Mol. Sci.* **2016**, *17*, 1974. [CrossRef]
41. Murphy, C.M.; Haugh, M.G.; O'Brien, F.J. The effect of mean pore size on cell attachment, proliferation and migration in colla-gen-glycosaminoglycan scaffolds for bone tissue engineering. *Biomaterials* **2010**, *31*, 461–466. [CrossRef]
42. Shi, C.; Wang, C.; Liu, H.; Li, Q.; Li, R.; Zhang, Y.; Liu, Y.; Shao, Y.; Wang, J. Selection of Appropriate Wound Dressing for Various Wounds. *Front. Bioeng. Biotechnol.* **2020**, *8*, 182. [CrossRef]
43. World Union of Wound Healing Societies (WUWHS) Consensus Document. Wound exudate: Effective assessment and management. *Wounds Int.* **2019**, 1–34.
44. Ennis, W.J.; Hill, D. Wound Healing: A Comprehensive Wound Assessment and Treatment Approach. In *Skin. Tissue Engineering and Regenerative Medicine*; Elsevier Inc.: Amsterdam, The Netherlands, 2016; pp. 239–263.
45. Rippon, M. Tissue Viability. *Br. J. Nurs.* **2016**, *25*, 1–8.
46. Negut, I.; Dorcioman, G.; Grumezescu, V. Scaffolds for Wound Healing Applications. *Polymers* **2020**, *12*, 2010. [CrossRef] [PubMed]
47. Braun-Falco, O.; Korting, H. Normal pH value of human skin. *Hautarzt* **1986**, *37*, 126–129.
48. Wallace, L.A.; Gwynne, L.; Jenkins, T. Challenges and opportunities of pH in chronic wounds. *Ther. Deliv.* **2019**, *10*, 719–735. [CrossRef]
49. Ekawati, E.R.; Darmanto, W.; Wahyuningsih, S.P.A. Detection of Staphylococcus aureus in wound infection on the skin surface. In *IOP Conference Series: Earth and Environmental Science*; Institute of Physics Publishing: Bristol, UK, 2020.
50. Iyer, V.; Raut, J.; Dasgupta, A. Impact of pH on growth of Staphylococcus epidermidis and Staphylococcus aureus in vitro. *J. Med. Microbiol.* **2021**, *70*, 001421. [CrossRef]
51. Romanelli, M.; Schipani, E.; Piaggesi, A.; Barachini, P. Evaluation of Surface pH on Venous Leg Ulcers Under Allevyn Dressings. In *Evidence-Based Wound Care*; Smith and Nephew: London, UK, 1997; pp. 57–60.
52. Tsukada, K.; Tokunaga, K.; Iwama, T.; Mishima, Y. The pH changes of pressure ulcers related to the healing process of wounds. *Wounds* **1992**, *2*, 16–20.
53. Wilson, I.; Henry, M.; Quill, R.; Byrne, P. The pH of varicose ulcer surfaces and its relationship to healing. *Vasa* **1979**, *8*, 339–342.

54. Gethin, G. The significance of surface pH in chronic wounds. *Wounds* **2007**, *3*, 52–56.
55. McCarty, S.M.; Percival, S.L. Proteases and Delayed Wound Healing. *Adv. Wound Care* **2013**, *2*, 438–447. [CrossRef]
56. Leveen, H.H.; Falk, G.E.; Borek, B.; Diaz, C.A.; Lynfield, Y.; Wynkoop, B.J.; Mabunda, G.A.; Rubricius, J.L.; Christoudias, G.C. Chemical Acidification of Wounds An Adjuvant to Healing and the Unfavorable Action of Alkalinity and Ammonia. *Ann. Surg.* **1973**, *178*, 745–753. [CrossRef] [PubMed]
57. Lengheden, A.; Jansson, L. pH effects on experimental wound healing of human fibroblasts in vitro. *Eur. J. Oral Sci.* **1995**, *103*, 148–155. [CrossRef] [PubMed]
58. Sim, P.; Song, Y.; Yang, G.N.; Cowin, A.J.; Garg, S. In Vitro Wound Healing Properties of Novel Acidic Treatment Regimen in Enhancing Metabolic Activity and Migration of Skin Cells. *Int. J. Mol. Sci.* **2022**, *23*, 7188. [CrossRef] [PubMed]
59. Welz, M.M.; Ofner, C.M. Examination of self-crosslinked gelatin as a hydrogel for controlled release. *J. Pharm. Sci.* **1992**, *81*, 85–90. [CrossRef]
60. Liu, S.; Zhang, H.; Ahlfeld, T.; Kilian, D.; Liu, Y.; Gelinsky, M.; Hu, Q. Evaluation of different crosslinking methods in altering the properties of extrusion-printed chitosan-based multi-material hydrogel composites. *Bio-Des. Manuf.* **2023**, *6*, 150–173. [CrossRef]
61. *BS EN 13726-1*; Part 1; Aspects of Absorbency. Section 3.2—Free Swell Absorptive Capacities. Test. Methods for Primary Wound Dressings. British Standards Institution: London, UK, 2002.
62. Parsons, D.; Bowler, P.G.; Myles, V.; Jones, S. Silver antimicrobial dressings in wound management: A comparison of antibacterial, physical and chemical characteristics. *Wounds* **2005**, *17*, 222–232.
63. *BS EN 13726-1*; Part 1; Aspects of Absorbency. Section 3.6—Dispersion Characteristics. Test. Methods for Primary Wound Dressings. British Standards Institution: London, UK, 2002.

pharmaceuticals

Article

Thermosensitive Polyurethane-Based Hydrogels as Potential Vehicles for Meloxicam Delivery

Ioana-Alexandra Plugariu [1], Luiza Madalina Gradinaru [1,*], Irina Rosca [1], Loredana Elena Nita [1], Claudia Maxim [2] and Maria Bercea [1,*]

[1] "Petru Poni" Institute of Macromolecular Chemistry, 41-A Grigore Ghica Voda Alley, 700487 Iasi, Romania; plugariu.ioana@icmpp.ro (I.-A.P.); mavadanei@icmpp.ro (M.A.); rosca.irina@icmpp.ro (I.R.); lnazare@icmpp.ro (L.E.N.)
[2] Faculty of Chemical Engineering and Environmental Protection "Cristofor Simionescu", "Gheorghe Asachi" Technical University of Iasi, 73A, D. Mangeron Blvd., 700050 Iasi, Romania; claudia.maxim@student.tuiasi.ro
* Correspondence: gradinaru.luiza@icmpp.ro (L.M.G.); bercea@icmpp.ro (M.B.)

Abstract: Meloxicam (MX) is a nonsteroidal anti-inflammatory drug (NSAID) used mainly to reduce pain, inflammation, and fever. In the present study, thermosensitive polyurethane (PU)-based hydrogels with various excipients (PEG, PVP, HPC, and essential oil) were prepared and loaded with MX. Rheological investigations were carried out on the PU-based formulations in various shear regimes, and their viscoelastic characteristics were determined. The average size of the PU micelles was 35.8 nm at 37 °C and slightly increased at 37 nm in the presence of MX. The zeta potential values of the hydrogels were between −10 mV and −11.5 mV. At pH = 6 and temperature of 37 °C, the formulated PU-based hydrogels loaded with MX could deliver significant amounts of the active substance, between 60% and 80% over 24–48 h and more than 90% within 2 weeks. It was found that anomalous transport phenomena dominated MX's release mechanism from the PU-based networks. The results are encouraging for further studies aiming to design alternative carriers to commercial dosage forms of nonsteroidal anti-inflammatory drugs.

Keywords: polyurethane; hydrogels; molecular docking; viscoelasticity; meloxicam delivery

1. Introduction

Nonsteroidal anti-inflammatory drugs (NSAIDs) are able to reduce pain and inflammation in the treatment of degenerative joint diseases such as arthritis or osteoarthritis (short-term treatment) and rheumatoid polyarthritis or ankylopoietic spondylitis (long-term treatment), and they are used in different pharmaceutical forms, including oral, injected, and topical dosage administration [1,2]. However, orally administered NSAIDs have shown many adverse side effects; they increase the risk of adverse reactions in the gastrointestinal tract [3], cardiovascular or renal failure, osteoporosis, hypophyse and hypothalamus suppression, and water and salt retention [4]. Their long-term use diminishes the life expectancy of patients with rheumatoid arthritis, a chronic inflammation of the synovial tissues affecting cartilage and joints [1].

Meloxicam (MX) is an analgesic and anti-inflammatory drug (NSAID) (4-hydroxy-2-methyl-N-(5-methyl-2-thiazolyl)-2H-1,2-benzothiazine-3-carboxamide-1,1-dioxide) with the ability to selectively inhibit cyclo-oxygenase-2 (COX-2) involved in the inflammatory response. Doses of up to 15 mg MX/day are usually recommended for the treatment of rheumatoid arthritis and osteoarthritis [5,6], with lower therapy costs compared with other NSAIDs (diclofenac or piroxicam) [7].

The main difficulty in the incorporation of MX in suitable delivery vehicles is its poor solubility in water. The prolonged transdermal delivery of MX still represents a challenge. Many efforts have focused on finding a suitable way to avoid the aforementioned gastrointestinal effects and promote local analgesia, providing steady levels in plasma [8,9].

Research in this field has been oriented toward the design of advanced drug delivery systems able to minimize the side effects during the administration of MX doses. This can be achieved by using either injectable or transdermal delivery systems [10–12]. Different organogels (glyceryl monostearate or glyceryl fatty acid ester) and hydrogels based on carbopol 940 or Pluronic F127 were investigated as transdermal delivery systems of MX using oleic acid, Mygliol 812, or Labrasol in a liquid phase [9]. Good release results and anti-inflammatory activity were obtained using organogels (Mygliol 812 and Labrasol). In situ gelling systems, such as Pluronics, can be considered effective vehicles for the delivery of poorly water-soluble drugs [12–14]. Below the lower critical solution temperature (LCST), they behave as liquid-like systems. Above the LCST, hydrophobic interactions increase, determining the formation of micelles with a hydrophilic core and a hydrophobic shell; further temperature and concentration increases make the entropy of mixing unfavorable, and micelle interactions can lead to fast sol–gel transitions [15,16]. Pluronics (F127 and F68, with a concentration of 20–30% in water, *w/w*) in the presence of different additives (poly(vinylmethylether-*co*-maleic anhydride), hydroxypropyl methylcellulose (HPMC), poly(ethylene glycol) 400, dimethyl sulfoxide, and sodium chloride) were tested, and it was found that Pluronic® F127 in combination with HPMC could be considered as a vehicle for MX delivery [13]. However, this formulation is homogeneous at room temperature and tends to precipitate at body temperature. Other disadvantages of these smart temperature-responsive hydrogels (limiting their potential use in drug delivery applications) are their weak mechanical properties, poor biocompatibility, and delayed responses in physiological conditions [17].

Meloxicam was fully released within 20 days from hydrogels containing carboxymethyl chitosan, methylcellulose, and Pluronic. A slower release (in about 37 days) was obtained from hydrogels containing nanoparticles [11]. The cumulative release of MX was about 85% at pH 7.4 within 96 h from the alginate–chitosan–Pluronic composite nanoparticles [10]. Also, nanostructured lipid carriers were used for the enhancement of the transdermal absorption of MX [18].

Polyurethanes (PUs) are a versatile class of polymers that have been used in a wide range of applications [19–22]. Their versatility comes from their chemistry, which allows for the incorporation of various segments and specific functional groups into a polymeric backbone that enables adjustments of their properties. Furthermore, this versatility also opens the path to the design of novel PU-based hydrogels that are able to provide sustained and prolonged drug release or to be used as injectable materials in minimally invasive medicine [23–26]. The use of an amphiphilic polymer as a macrodiol in PU synthesis led to the preparation of stimuli-sensitive PU structures that could be further engineered to develop new formulations with enhanced properties. A poly(ethylene oxide)/poly(propylene oxide)/poly(ethylene oxide) (PEO–PPO–PEO) triblock copolymer (e.g., Pluronic P123) was selected as a macrodiol for the synthesis of PU due to its ability to undergo a lower critical solution temperature. As a result, these aqueous solutions exhibited a sol–gel transition with an increasing temperature (up to physiological values), making them attractive alternative drug delivery systems. Moreover, to further expand the promising biomedical properties of the resultant formulation, an aliphatic diisocyanate (L-lysine ethyl ester diisocyanate) was used.

The aim of the present study was to develop various formulations containing a thermosensitive PU structure and different excipients that could be used for therapeutic agent delivery. In this regard, a nonsteroidal anti-inflammatory drug (MX) was selected, and its release in correlation with gel characteristics was investigated.

2. Results and Discussion

A polyurethane (PU) sample was synthesized and then used as the main component for the development of thermosensitive hydrogels loaded with meloxicam (MX), an anti-inflammatory drug. Our main interest was in preparing PU-based samples in the sol state (low viscosity at a low temperature) for the facile incorporation of drug molecules. Under physiological conditions, the samples undergo gelation, leading to the formation of stable physical networks suitable for topical drug delivery. The pharmacokinetic benefits of these temperature-sensitive hydrogels for NSAID loading and delivery may be significant because a depot formulation can be generated and an anti-inflammatory drug (MX in our study) can be gradually eluted, preserving a constant local concentration of a drug in the surrounding tissues for a long period of time. In addition, they are very versatile, and their networks can be formed in situ, making them suitable for systemic delivery [26–28].

The PU-based formulations were prepared by using a mixture of 9.9 mL physiological serum (concentration of 0.15 M NaCl in aqueous solution) and 0.1 mL solution of NaOH (0.125 M NaOH in water), assuring the complete dissolution of MX. The gradual drug delivery at the targeted site depends on the excipients used. Klucel® hydroxypropylcellulose (HPC) [29] was selected as the main excipient. HPC is a water-soluble cellulose ether that exhibits hydrophilic and hydrophobic interactions, having a lower critical solution temperature (LCST) around 41 °C [30]. It was previously reported that the gel consisting of 2.5% HPC, 0.3% MX, and 5% menthol in propylene glycol:ethanol:water = 1:1:1 can deliver therapeutically relevant doses of MX through the human skin [31]. In this study, two drug adsorption enhancers were used, namely poly(ethylene glycol) (PEG) and poly(vinylpyrrolidone) (PVP), known for their ability to improve the skin permeability [32–35]. The addition of these penetration enhancers influences the thermodynamic activity of MX in the delivery system [31]. PVP is a suitable additive that reduces the particle size to nanometers and prevents the aggregation of nanoparticles, increasing the MX solubility [33,36,37]. PEG is a biocompatible polymer able to enhance the dissolution rate of poor water-soluble drugs due to its hydrophilic and lipophilic properties [38,39].

Also, *Origanum Compactum* essential oil (EO) was incorporated as a skin penetration enhancer for transdermal MX delivery [40]. In addition, EO presents antimicrobial activity [41].

At low temperatures (below 20 °C), the PU-based samples (Table 1) presented liquid-like behavior. This is an important advantage for homogeneous loading of the poor soluble drug into the polymer solution. At physiological temperature, they became gels with solid-like behavior, containing well-dispersed MX into the polymeric matrix. These hydrogels were stable for a long period of time (they were observed for approx. 6 months), being of interest for topical formulations. A syneresis phenomenon occurred for Sample 3 stored for several weeks at room temperature. As a result, a contraction of the gel and an exclusion of a small amount of liquid phase took place. However, when the sample was vigorously mixed, the liquid was again incorporated into the polymer network. We suppose that the hydrophobic environment and dehydration of the PEO corona due to the interactions with PVP are responsive for this behavior [33].

Table 1. The composition of the investigated hydrogels and their rheological characteristics at 37 °C.

Sample Code	PU (% wt.)	Excipient Type	Excipient Content (% wt.)	Solvent (% wt.)	MX (%)	τ_0 [(a)] (Pa)	γ_L (%)	G' [(b)] (Pa)
1	25	-	-	75	1	79.2	31.6	525.5
2	25	PEG	3	72	1	72.8	14.7	456.1
3	25	PEG PVP	3 3	69	1	9.4	3.2	208.6
4	18.75	HPC	6.25	75	1	87.3	10.9	1330
5	12.5	HPC	12.5	75	1	85.6	6.8	1203
6	25	EO	6	69	1	46.1	21.5	474.3

[(a)] continuous flow (imposed shear stress experiment); [(b)] ω = 10 rad/s; γ = 0.1%; PU = polyurethane; MX = meloxicam; PEG = poly(ethylene glycol); PVP = poly(vinylpyrrolidone); HPC = hydroxypropylcellulose; EO = *Origanum Compactum*.

The pH value of the normal skin surface is between 4.5 and 6.0 [42]. It was previously shown that the topical products should be slightly acidified, with an optimum pH value ranging from 4 to 6 [43,44]. Thus, for the present study, the value of pH = 6 was selected.

2.1. FTIR Spectra

Figure 1 presents the FTIR spectra of PU, MX, and PU loaded with MX.

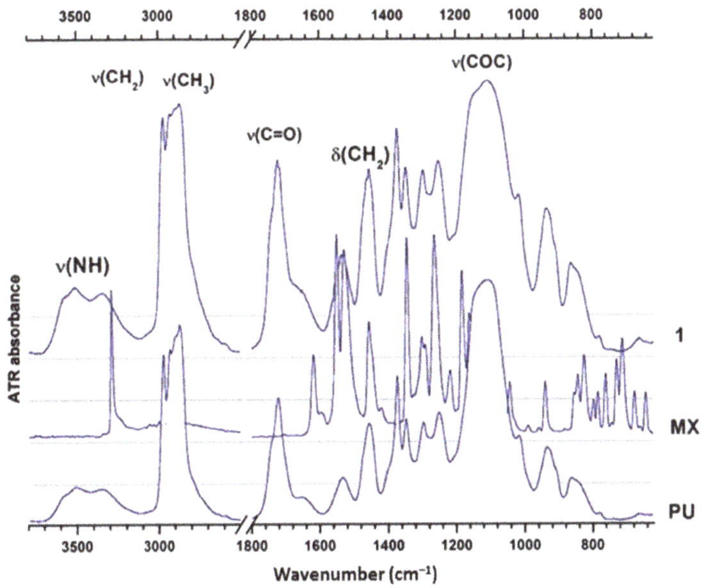

Figure 1. ATR-FTIR spectra of the starting compounds (PU and MX) and of the PU loaded with MX (Sample 1).

The first aspect to point out when making a comparative analysis between the infrared spectrum of the PU and Sample 1 is the high similarity between them, where most bands have the same profile and position. The signals of MX are overlapped by PU's, but nevertheless, some spectral changes in PU may be observed. The ν(NH) region is structured and contains two absorption bands assigned to free –NH at 3585 cm^{-1} and 3514 cm^{-1}. While only the first band is slightly reduced in intensity, it can be deduced that the most available urethane groups for interactions with MX were those located in the interphase. Based on the band intensity, this relocation would involve approx. 23% from the free urethane groups. The vibration of –NH groups that are intermolecularly H-bonded with C=O (3345 cm^{-1}) is not changed.

The deformation and bending vibrations of methyl and methylene groups are also observed as being unchanged at 1453 cm^{-1}, 1372 cm^{-1}, or 1348 cm^{-1}. The ester carbonyl stretching ν(C=O) at 1723 cm^{-1} has a lower intensity than in the initial PU, while the absorption band centered on 1110 cm^{-1} is the most affected. This fact indicates a possible redistribution of the intermolecular interactions between the hard segment of PU (represented mainly by ν(C=O)) and the Pluronic soft segment, which defines the maximum at 1110 cm^{-1}. More precisely, the main peak at 1723 cm^{-1} belongs to free, non-associated C=O groups that could be located in the "disordered" interphase or in the soft regions. For Sample 1, the ν(C=O) band decreased with the simultaneous development of a sub-band around 1680 cm^{-1}. This indicates that, for a fraction of carbonyls located in the interfacial regions, the bonding partner of the –N–H group has changed. Moving from a moderate to a strong –N–H • • • H-bond implies that the ether oxygen atom from the Pluronic segment has been replaced by a carbonyl or sulfone oxygen from MX. The addition of MX into the PU matrix would lead to the breaking of some intramolecular C–H • • • O and S–O • • • H–C H-bonds in MX [45], and it would build intermolecular links with donor or acceptor groups from the PU matrix, such as C=O • • • O–S and C=O • • • H–N (MX). The other carbonyl bands observed around 1740 cm^{-1} (ester carbonyl from the lateral chain of the LDI segment and/or free urethane groups) and 1660 cm^{-1} ("ordered", strongly H-bonded urethane C=O • • • H–N–) have a similar intensity to the native PU.

The complex band centered at 1110 cm^{-1} is the envelope derived from the ester ν(C=O–O) of the hard segment and also from the composite vibration ν_s(COC) + ν(CC) + ν_{as}(COC) in the Pluronic soft segment. Although this band has roughly the same profile as in the initial PU, its lower intensity corresponds to the decrease of ν(C=O) band. This confirms that a part of the interactions between the urethane groups and the Pluronic ether groups have changed. The stable PU–MX matrices were identified by molecular docking, with the binding affinities between −2.9 and −3.1 kcal/mol. The most probable interactions between the PU matrix and MX can be summarized in Figure 2.

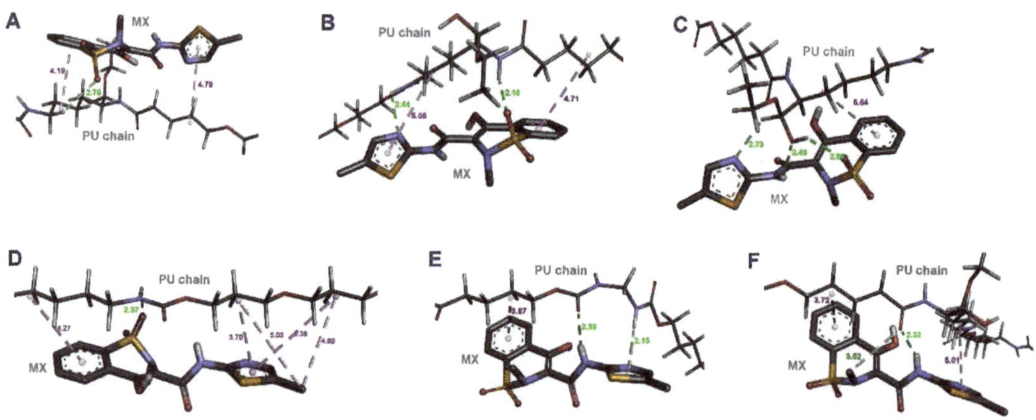

Figure 2. Docking model of the PU–MX matrix, showing the most favorable docking poses of MX: (**A–C**) involving the sulfone group of MX; (**D–F**) mainly hydrophobic interactions at the level of aromatic rings of MX. The two compounds are shown in the stick representation. Color code: magenta—hydrophobic interactions; green—hydrogen bonding. The distance between the donor and acceptor is given in Å.

The addition of PEG into PU matrix (Sample 2) leads to a significant enhancement of the whole ν(NH) band due to the development of a new band around 3430 cm^{-1} at the expense of the free –NH groups from 3585 cm^{-1} and of strongly H-bonded groups from 3345 cm^{-1}. This change accompanies the redshift of the ν(C=O) vibration to 1717 cm^{-1} and its decrease in magnitude, simultaneously with the appearance of new bands around 1665 cm^{-1}, 1630 cm^{-1}, and 1605 cm^{-1}. It can be supposed that some intermolecular associations in the interfacial and disordered regions of PU have been broken upon PEG insertion between the chains. There is a fraction of N–H • • • O< (PEG) links of moderate strength (3430 cm^{-1}) and several kinds of urethane groups with either H-bonded C=O (1630 cm^{-1}) or with free C=O and N–H • • • O=C from an adjacent chain (1665 cm^{-1}). The urethane units having the free C=O and N–H • • • O< (PEG) would absorb at 1717 cm^{-1}.

The infrared spectra of Samples 4 and 5 share different kinds of ν(NH) (3420 cm^{-1}) and ν_s(COC) (Pluronic) + ν(C=O–O) (urethane) (1095 cm^{-1}) bands, due to the contribution of the specific signals of HPC. The free ν(NH) component is missing in both hydrogels. The main ν(C=O) peak is downshifted to 1720 cm^{-1} and a new absorption between 1650 and 1580 cm^{-1} appears, suggesting a reorganization of the strongly H-bonded carbonyls. Involvement of a fraction of urethane –NH groups in the association with –OH groups of HPC also affected the vibration of the C=O bond, lowering it by several cm^{-1}. The lower position of the ν_s(COC) + ν(C=O–O), shifted to 1095 cm^{-1}, is a combination of both Pluronic and HPC maxima. This fact suggests the high compatibility between them, involving a reordering of the Pluronic chains, and the high degree of mixing at the level of PU soft segments. According to the literature, the PVP addition determines a weak secondary bonding between MX and PVP (according to FTIR spectra presented in Figures 6 and 7 from Ref. [34]), whereas MX exhibits a high and fast dissolution rate in PVP-based formulations [33,37].

2.2. Rheological Behavior

2.2.1. Temperature-Induced Gelation Monitored by Rheological Measurements

The rheological measurements were used to delimit the temperature ranges where the samples are in a sol state or gel state for PU-based samples and to characterize the gel behavior at a physiological temperature. Thus, the elastic (G') and viscous (G'') moduli, as well as the loss tangent ($tan\ \delta = G''/G'$), were monitored in various oscillatory tests as a function of temperature, strain amplitude (γ), oscillation frequency (ω), or time.

Sample 1 is in a sol state at low temperature, with a predominantly viscous behavior: $G'' > G'$ and $tan\ \delta > 1$ (Figure 3). A sol–gel transition occurs around 21 °C, and above this temperature the solid-like behavior prevails. The temperature increase determines the intensification of hydrophobic interactions and the formation of micelles with the hydrophobic core and hydrophilic shell. The gelation of PU is attributed to the formation of a polymicellar network structure [46], when a sharp variation in the viscoelastic parameters takes place. In the gel state, $G' > G''$ and $tan\ \delta < 1$. The network strength is not significantly influenced by MX addition or the heating rate, but it is sensibly influenced by the excipients used in the gel formulation (Table 1).

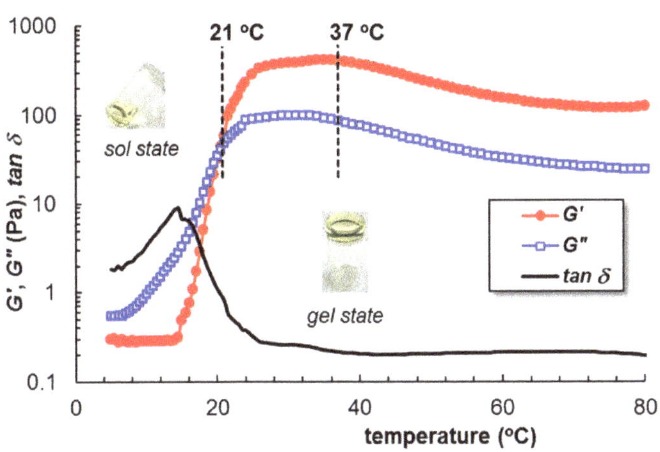

Figure 3. The viscoelastic parameters G', G'', and $tan\ \delta$ as a function of temperature for PU sample loaded with MX and submitted to a heating rate of 0.5 °C/min (γ = 1%, ω = 10 rad/s).

Figure 4 shows the rheological behavior of Samples 1–6 from 20 °C (close to the storage temperature) to 50 °C (above the physiological temperature). PEO and PVP weaken the network, G' decreases, and $tan\ \delta$ increases for Samples 2 and 3. The behavior of Samples 4 and 5 is strongly influenced by HPC addition. The highly entangled HPC chains and PU micelles [46,47] form an interpenetrating network with preponderant hydrophilic interactions at low temperatures, ensuring the homogenization of the polymer mixtures in solution. By raising the temperature, the hydrophobic interactions are developed by both polymers and determine an increase in the viscoelastic moduli. However, above

41 °C, the loss tangent remains almost constant, regardless of the HPC content in the PU/HPC mixture. Sample 6 presents a compact and stable structure at low temperatures, with the oil molecules well dispersed into the amphiphilic micellar network of PU. The network strength decreases above 36 °C, probably due to the decrease in the intermolecular interactions between PU chains and oil molecules.

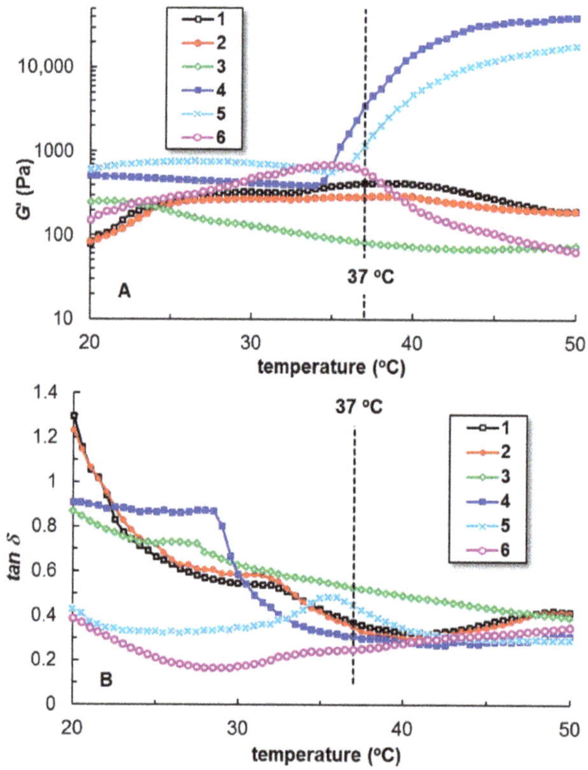

Figure 4. The temperature dependence of (**A**) elastic modulus (G′) and (**B**) loss tangent (*tan δ*) for the hydrogels loaded with MX, heating rate of 1 °C/min, γ = 1%, ω = 1 rad/s.

2.2.2. Linear and Non-Linear Viscoelasticity

Amplitude sweep tests were carried out for all hydrogels loaded with MX in order to determine the limiting strain value (γ_L) (Table 1), at the end of the linear viscoelastic region (VLR), when the viscoelastic moduli start to decrease. For the PU-based hydrogels, γ_L was estimated from G'–γ dependences (Figure 5A) because G'' decreases at higher γ values (Figure 5B). This can be due to the presence of salts that can influence the hydrophilic/hydrophobic balance. γ_L is correlated with the stability of the hydrogel submitted to the action of the external forces. For $\gamma < \gamma_L$, $G' > G''$ and both viscoelastic moduli are independent of strain; for $\gamma > \gamma_L$, the physical network is broken and the sample undergoes viscous flow (permanent and indefinite deformation). Higher γ_L values suggest a higher network resistance to deformation.

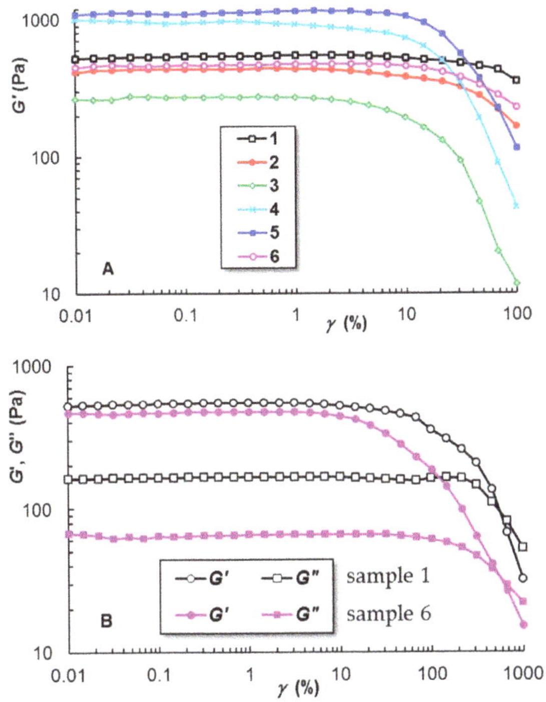

Figure 5. The dependence on the strain amplitude of (**A**) G' for Samples 1–6; (**B**) G' and G'' for Samples 1 and 6 (ω = 10 rad/s, 37 °C).

2.2.3. Self-Healing Behavior

The analysis of the structure recovery after applying large amplitude deformations allows us to discuss the ability of the hydrogel samples to exhibit self-healing behavior. Thus, successive cycles of low strain values (in the linear range of viscoelasticity, according to Figure 5) and high strains ($\gamma > \gamma_L$) were applied to the hydrogels and the viscoelastic parameters were monitored as a function of time (Figure 6).

For Samples 1, 2, and 6, the structure integrity is recovered very quickly (within seconds). In the presence of long HPC chains (Samples 4 and 5), the return to the previous G′ value (before applying high deformation) is slower and time dependent. The structure recovery is very fast for PU micelles (Sample 1), also in the presence of shorter PEO chains (Sample 2) or EO (Sample 6). The addition of PVP in the PU/PEO system (Sample 3) slightly influences the recovery time, but it determines a decrease in G' and other viscoelastic parameters (Table 1). This can be explained by the interactions between C=O groups of PVP chains and C–O–C groups of PEO blocks from micelles corona, influencing the colloidal stability [48,49]. In our case, the increase of PVP content diminishes or even cancels the gelation of PU. PVP chains have a stronger enthalpy of adsorption to micellar corona as compared with PEG [48]; thus, the destabilization of the PU network structure is higher, as can be seen from rheological data. However, both excipients, PEG and PVP are recommended as adsorption enhancers for MX [33,37]. As a result, the composition of Sample 3 was optimized by incorporating a PEG/PVP mixture in the PU sol state. The intermolecular interactions between free PEG and PVP chains in an aqueous saline environment somehow moderate the effect of PVP on PU gelation at an increasing temperature. For Samples 1, 4, and 6, the structure is well recovered after applying high strains (2000% or 5000%, Figure 6A), but for Samples 2, 3, and 5 the network structure fails in the conditions of very high deformations (γ > 1000%).

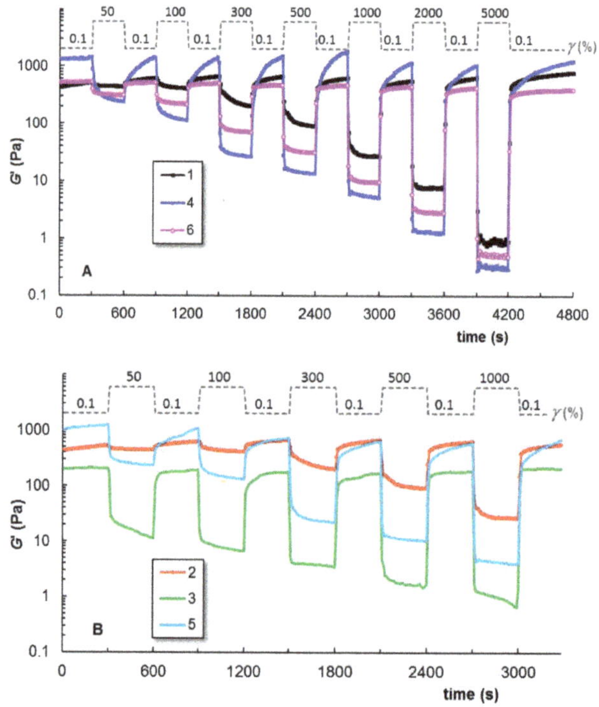

Figure 6. Illustration of self-healing behavior of hydrogels through variation of G' during the experiments carried out at low (linear viscoelastic domain) and high (non-linear domain of viscoelasticity) successive step strains applied every 300 s: (**A**) Samples 1, 4, and 6; (**B**) Samples 2, 3, and 5.

2.2.4. Shear Flow Behavior at 37 °C

Figure 7 shows the dependence of apparent viscosity (η) as a function of the shear rate ($\dot{\gamma}$) for the investigated gel samples. The flow is non-Newtonian and the viscosity scales as $\eta \sim \dot{\gamma}^{-n}$. The flow index n is between 0.78 and 0.82 for Samples 1, 2, and 6, and it takes the value of 0.6 for Sample 3. For $\dot{\gamma} > 10$ s^{-1}, a change in the slope (decrease in n value) was depicted for Samples 4 and 5. For a high HPC content, a pronounced viscosity decrease can be observed. This can be due to the high shear forces that overcome the strong hydrophobic interactions occurring in the presence of HPC chains. The drug release rate from the polymeric matrix is usually inversely proportional to its viscosity [28].

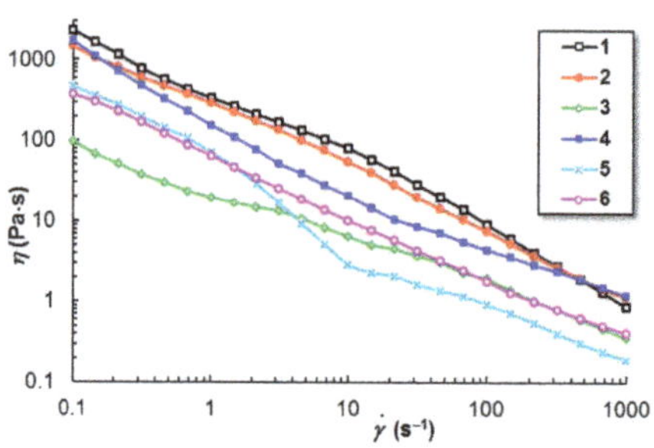

Figure 7. Shear viscosity as a function of shear rate for the hydrogel samples loaded with MX (at temperature of 37 °C).

Generally, the yield stress fluids are able to deform like solids (finite deformation) and to flow only by applying a stress above a critical value [50]. From the equilibrium flow curves (stress-controlled experiments), the yield stress (τ_o) was determined and its values for Samples 1–6 are given in Table 1.

2.2.5. Creep and Recovery Behavior

The analysis of the creep and recovery behavior also allows the evaluation of the viscoelasticity of the gels submitted to the action of a constant shear stress (τ) for 30 s (creep curves) through the strain γ (t) (Figure 8A–C) or compliance $J(t)$ (Figure 8D) variation in time. When the shear stress is removed, the recovered strain is monitored until the equilibrium state is reached (recovery curves). The creep compliance is correlated with the strain as:

$$J(t) = \frac{\gamma(t)}{\tau} \tag{1}$$

Below 100 Pa, the hydrogels undergo viscoelastic behavior (as shown in Figure 8 for Samples 1, 4, and 6). During the creep test (τ = 0), the transient response consists of fast (γ_{el}) and delayed (γ_d) elastic strains followed by a viscous flow (γ_v). The recovery takes place in the same order: γ_{el}–γ_d–γ_v, and the recovery process (the required time and the value of the irreversible component, γ_v, at equilibrium) depends on the applied τ value. For $\tau < \tau_o$, the creep compliance, $J(t)$, decreases with increasing shear stress for PU hydrogels in the presence of other polymeric excipients (Samples 1–5). For $\tau > \tau_o$, $J(t)$ changes its trend and starts to increase due to the preponderance of the viscous flow. Similar behavior was reported for PU/peptide systems [46]. However, an anti-creep behavior was observed for Sample 6 (Figure 8D) due to the EO presence.

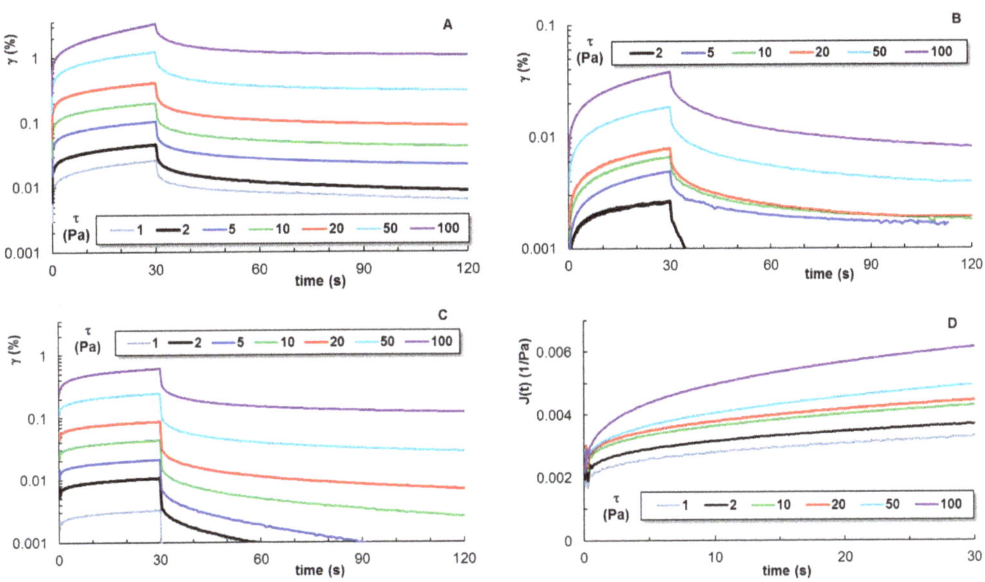

Figure 8. The strain evolution during the creep at different shear stress (τ) values applied for 30 s and the strain recovery (τ = 0) for (**A**) Sample 1; (**B**) Sample 4; (**C**) Sample 6; (**D**) creep compliance for Sample 6.

2.3. Zeta Potential and Average Diameter of PU Micelles

PU, PEG, and HPC used for hydrogel formulation are neutral polymers. Due to the ions resulting from the salts dissolved in an aqueous solution and used as a solvent for MX, the values of the zeta potential of the hydrogels are negative and range between

−10 ± 0.3 mV and −11.5 ± 0.345 mV. The presence of MX determines a slow increase in the number of negative charges in the environment. In the solvent used in hydrogel formulation, the mean hydrodynamic diameter (D_H) of PU micelles increases from 32.8 nm to 35.8 nm when the temperature increases from 25 °C to 37 °C. The interaction with MX contributes to a slight rise in the D_H value of PU micelles (Figure 9). A value of 37 nm was registered at 37 °C for PU in the presence of MX. The values of the polydispersity index (PDI) are below 0.4, indicating a low polydispersity and a monomodal distribution peak (Table 2).

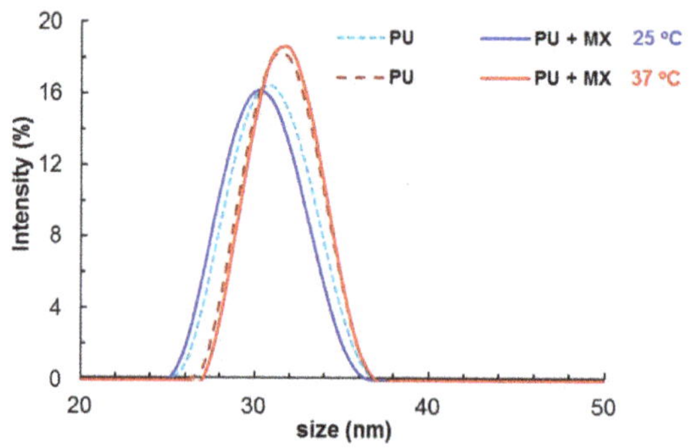

Figure 9. The size distribution for the PU micelles in the presence (continuous line) and absence (dashed line) of MX at 25 °C (blue line) and 37 °C (red line).

Table 2. The particle size (expressed as the mean hydrodynamic diameter, D_H) and polydispersity index (PDI) for PU micelles and PU loaded with MX at 25 °C and 37 °C.

Sample	Temperature (°C)	D_H ± SD * (nm)	PDI
PU	25	32.8 ± 0.98	0.120
PU loaded with MX	25	31.6 ± 0.94	0.132
PU	37	35.8 ± 1.06	0.245
PU loaded with MX	37	37.0 ± 1.10	0.246

* SD is the standard deviation.

It was shown that the drug loading capacity and therapeutic properties are improved when the network used as a carrier is composed of micelles with an average size lower than 200 nm [51]. Due to the nanomicellar structure of the PU matrix with a hydrophobic core and hydrophilic shell, these hydrogels are able to encapsulate both hydrophilic and hydrophobic compounds for the local delivery of different active principles in a single matrix. The incorporation of poor water-soluble MX into the PU nanomicellar hydrogels enhanced the solubility of the drug, bioavailability, and formulation stability.

2.4. *Meloxicam Delivery from PU-Based Hydrogels*

Figure 10 presents the MX release profiles for the six hydrogel samples. The cumulative drug release during the first 24 h reaches levels between 40% and 70%, depending on the sample composition. The maximum efficiency is registered for Samples 1 (PU hydrogel) and 6 (PU hydrogel containing essential oil). These two formulations are suitable as gels for topical applications. The polymeric excipients addition improves the delivery profile for a longer period of time (Samples 2–4); thus, these gels could be considered appropriate materials for wound-dressing applications. Sample 5, with a high HPC content, releases less than 50% MX during 24 h. Then, a slow MX release is registered for two weeks until the delivered MX reaches about 80%.

Similar delivery profiles were reported for alginate–chitosan–Pluronic composite nanoparticles, with 85% of the cumulative MX released within 96 h at pH = 7.4. In such systems, the mean dissolution time was about 9 h [10]. The advantage of our formulation is the rapid dissolution of MX in the saline solutions and then the PU is easily dissolved at a low temperature (5 °C) in a sol state. In this way, the homogeneous distribution of the drug in the network is ensured during gelation. At room temperature, the gel is formed and the MX molecules remain immobilized in the gel, without any separation in time.

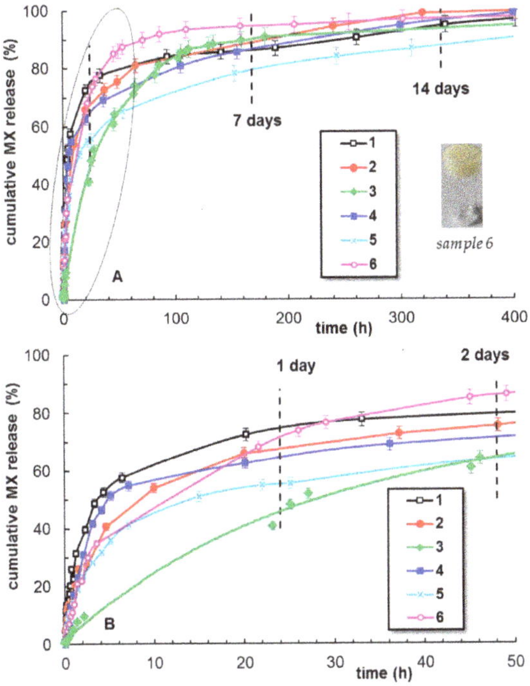

Figure 10. Kinetics of meloxicam delivery from PU-based hydrogels (37 °C, pH = 6): (**A**) cumulative release of MX during 400 h; (**B**) details of the release curves during the first 50 h (gray ellipse from Figure (**A**)). The lines are a guide to the eye.

The MX delivery from the hydrogel samples can be discussed by using different mathematical models. Among them, first-order [52] and Higuchi [53] models allow the discussion of the delivery data through the first-order and Higuchi release rate constants, k_{11} and k_H, respectively:

First-order: $$ln(1 - M_t/M_\infty) = -k_{11}\, t \quad (2)$$

Higuchi: $$M_t/M_\infty = k_H\, t^{1/2} \quad (3)$$

where M_t/M_∞ represents the fraction of the drug released at the time t.

The most versatile approaches were developed by Peppas and coworkers [54,55] and they are suitable for drug delivery from various hydrogels:

Korsmeyer-Peppas: $$M_t/M_\infty = k\, t^n \quad (4)$$

Peppas-Sahlin: $$M_t/M_\infty = k_1\, t^m + k_2\, t^{2m} \quad (5)$$

k, k_1, k_2 are the release rate constants, which depend on the matrix and drug characteristics. Equation (4), applied for the first drug-release periods until 60% of the maximum level is reached, gives the release exponent n. The n value allows the discussion of the drug-release mechanism from the network, i.e., the Fickian or non-Fickian contributions to the diffusion during the drug delivery process [55]. For the PU-based hydrogels in the presence or absence of excipients, $0.45 < n < 0.89$ (Table 3), suggesting the occurrence of anomalous transport phenomena, controlled by the drug diffusion through the network [54,56,57].

Topical gels loaded with MX exhibit reduced systemic side effects and a better performance against pain and inflammation as compared with other NSAID gels (diclofenac or piroxicam) [58]. The homogeneous incorporation and delivery of poor water-soluble MX into PU-based hydrogels make them promising topical gels. The thermosensitive PU matrix (Sample 1) appears as a suitable carrier for short-term meloxicam delivery. The addition of a small amount of polymeric excipients (Samples 2–5) improves the long-term drug delivery. Furthermore, the incorporation of the essential oils (Sample 6) offers multiple other benefits in controlling the drug release, improving the biological activity and transdermal drug delivery [40,41,59], and reducing the ulcerative side effect associated with MX [60]. The selected essential oil was extracted from *Origanum Compactum* and presents antimicrobial and antifungal properties.

Table 3. The parameters that describe the kinetics of MX release from hybrid hydrogels according to Equations (2)–(5) (37 °C, pH = 6). The values of standard deviations were below ±3%.

Sample Code	First Order Equation (2)		Higuchi Equation (3)		Korsmeyer-Peppas Equation (4)		Peppas-Sahlin Equation (5)			
	$10^2 \cdot k_{11}$ (min^{-1})	AIC	$10^2 \cdot k_h$ ($min^{-1/2}$)	AIC	n	AIC	$10 \cdot k_1$ (min^{-m})	$10^2 \cdot k_2$ (min^{-2m})	m	AIC
1	2.250	−78.600	2.588	−73.785	0.831	−34.492	1.446	0.778	0.465	−108.299
2	0.984	−71.619	1.294	−111.686	0.863	−31.354	1.896	3.274	0.744	−51.282
3	3.274	−84.467	1.422	−150.85	0.672	−37.223	1.659	2.642	0.186	−109.711
4	0.431	−46.850	7.428	−44.058	0.806	−41.852	2.337	1.678	0.713	−90.105
5	2.590	−42.543	7.328	−46.382	0.835	−43.257	2.352	2.190	0.843	−116.873
6	1.375	−89.8648	2.040	−96.243	0.770	−74.9818	5.061	6.918	0.120	−105.87

In conclusion, the developed PU-based systems can fulfill some of the basic requirements for a matrix that can easily encapsulate and efficiently deliver the anti-inflammatory drug. Also, the selected excipients can act as delivery enhancers or therapeutic agents, ensuring the optimal MX concentration over time or, in addition, can provide antimicrobial activity to the formulation. Further studies will be focused on improving the biological properties of the PU-based hydrogels, as alternative carriers to commercial dosage forms of nonsteroidal anti-inflammatory drugs.

3. Materials and Methods

3.1. Materials

3.1.1. Chemicals

Poly(ethylene oxide)$_{20}$–*b*–poly(propylene oxide)$_{70}$–*b*–poly(ethylene oxide)$_{20}$ (PEO–*b*–PPO–*b*–PEO), $M_n = 5.8 \times 10^3$ g/mol, poly(vinylpyrrolidone) (PVP), $M = 4 \times 10^4$ g/mol, and 1,4-butane-diol (BD) were purchased from Sigma Aldrich (Steinheim, Germany). L-lysine ethyl ester diisocyanate, 97%, (LDI) was obtained from Alfa Aesar (Kandel, Germany) and was freshly distilled before synthesis. Poly(ethylene glycol) (PEG), $M = 4 \times 10^2$ g/mol, sodium hydroxide (NaOH), and sodium chloride (NaCl) were purchased from Fluka Chemie GmbH (Switzerland). A sample of Klucel™ hydroxypropylcellulose (HPC) with $M = 9.5 \times 10^4$ g/mol was kindly offered by Ashland Aqualon [29].

The oregano essential oil used for preparing sample 6, extracted from *Origanum Compactum* (family *Lamiaceae*, species native from Morocco), was provided by Euflora

Company (Iasi, Romania) and contains mainly carvacrol (53%), tymol (28%), paracymene (26%), and terpinene gamma (20%).

The meloxicam sample (99%, M = 351.4 g/mol) was purchased from Thermo Fisher Scientific (Leicestershire, UK).

The structures of the commercial chemicals and drug used in the present study are given in Scheme 1.

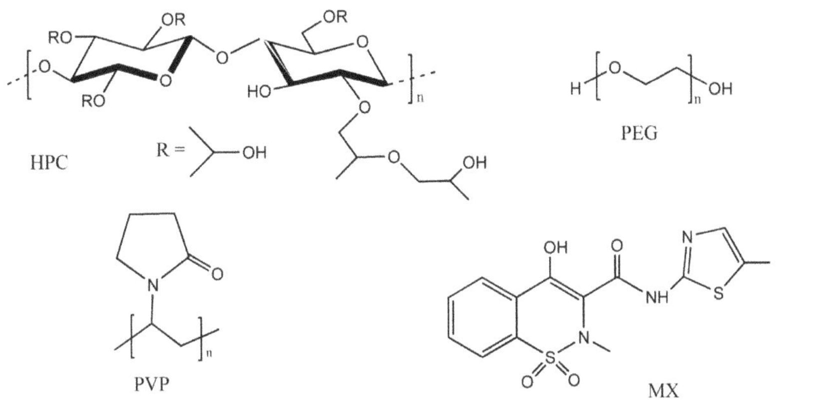

Scheme 1. Structure of the commercial polymers and the investigated drug.

3.1.2. Synthesis of Thermoresponsive Polyurethane

The polyurethane (PU) sample was synthesized according to a procedure recently reported [46], via a standard two-step prepolymer method. In brief, the copolymer (PEO–*b*–PPO–*b*–PEO) sample was firstly dehydrated and then reacted with an excess of LDI for 4 h at 80 °C, without any catalyst. Then, the BD chain extender was added to the prepolymer and allowed to react for another period of 6 h. The reaction was carried out using an NCO:OH molar ratio of 1:1. The resulting PU structure is presented in Scheme 2.

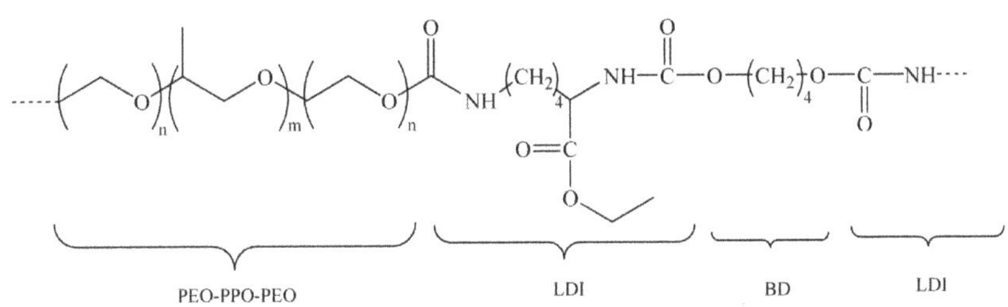

Scheme 2. Structure of the synthetized thermoresponsive polyurethane.

3.1.3. Preparation of Thermoresponsive PU-Based Hydrogels

Firstly, the appropriate amount of MX was dissolved in the physiological serum of pharmaceutical use (0.15 M NaCl aqueous solution) at room temperature. The pH was fine-adjusted by using an aqueous solution of 0.125 M NaOH until the complete dissolution of the drug (0.1 mL NaOH solution was required for 9.9 mL physiological serum). Then, the PU was added and the mixture was stored in the refrigerator and mixed from time to time by using a roller mixer at a low rotation speed. The excipients were added to the sample in the sol state and the final formulations were homogenized by further mixing and then stored at room temperature. The syneresis appearance (as observed for PVP containing sample stored for a long time) can be avoided by using a small amount of organic salts [61].

3.2. Methods

3.2.1. Attenuated Total Reflectance-Fourier Transform Infrared Spectroscopy

ATR-FTIR spectra were recorded using a Bruker Vertex 70 type spectrometer (Bruker, Germany), equipped with a diamond ATR device (Golden Gate, Bruker, Germany) and software for spectral processing. Spectra were obtained in absorbance mode in the range of 4000–500 cm^{-1}, averaging over 64 scans at a resolution of 2 cm^{-1}.

3.2.2. In Silico Investigations of Polymer-Drug Binding

The most probable binding sites of MX with the PU matrix have been explored through a ligand flexible docking study. The 2D model of the PU chain has been drawn in Marvin JS by Chemaxon [62]. Associated SMILES were used to build the 3D model and to optimize it by using USCF Chimera [63]. The input files for docking were prepared by using USCF Chimera and AutoDock Tools 1.5.7 packages (Molecular Graphics Lab, La Jolla, CA, USA). The blind docking experiment was performed with AutoDock Vina 1.2.0 [64]. The final pose of every docked MX has been selected from the top-binding conformations with the highest binding score. The PU–MX interactions were visualized and the structural figures were drawn in BIOVIA Discovery Studio [65].

3.2.3. Rheology

Rheological measurements were carried out by using an MCR 302 Anton-Paar rheometer (Gratz, Austria), equipped with plane–plane geometry of 50 mm (the selected gap was of 500 μm) and a Peltier device for temperature control.

The temperature-induced gelation was monitored through the viscoelastic parameters, firstly for Sample 1 at a heating rate of 0.5 °C/min from 5 °C to 80 °C. Then, all samples were tested with a heating rate of 1 °C/min for the temperature range of interest (from 20 °C to 50 °C). The elastic (G') and viscous (G'') moduli were registered as the amount of stored and dissipated energy during one cycle of deformation, respectively. The loss tangent ($tan\ \delta = G''/G'$) expresses the degree of viscoelasticity: $tan\ \delta < 1$–solid-like behavior and $tan\ \delta > 1$–liquid-like behavior.

The gels thermostatted at 37 °C were investigated in various shear conditions. Amplitude sweep tests were carried out to determine the upper limit of strain, γ_L, for the linear viscoelastic regime (37 °C, ω = 10 rad/s). The thixotropic tests were carried out in oscillatory regime for ω = 10 rad/s and step strains successively changed every 300 s from low (0.1%, value of strain in the linear viscoelastic domain) to high values (50%, 100%, 300%, 500%, 1000%, 2000%, and 5000%, that belong to nonlinear range of viscoelasticity) and again at the low step of strain (0.1%). The shear viscosity was determined as a function of shear rate ($\dot{\gamma}$) from 0.1 s^{-1} to 1000 s^{-1}. Yield stress (τ_o) was determined from the stress-controlled experiments carried out in stationary shear flow conditions. The creep and recovery curves were monitored at different shear stress (τ) values applied for 30 s during the creep test and then, for τ = 0, the strain recovery was monitored over time.

3.2.4. Zeta Potential and Average Diameter

Zeta potential (ζ) and hydrodynamic diameter (D_H) values were determined by using Zetasizer Nano ZS instrument (Malvern Instruments, UK, equipped with 633 nm laser He/Ne and Peltier device), according to the following relationships:

$$\zeta = \frac{\eta\,\mu}{\varepsilon} \quad \text{(Smoluchowski equation)} \tag{6}$$

and

$$D_H = \frac{k\,T}{6\,\pi\,\eta\,D} \quad \text{(Mie method)} \tag{7}$$

where: η is the viscosity; μ—electrophoretic mobility; ε—dielectric constant; k—Boltzmann constant; T—absolute temperature; D—diffusion coefficient.

Each measurement was performed 3 times and the average values were considered.

3.2.5. Meloxicam Delivery

The drug-loaded hydrogels were prepared by adding 1% wt. MX to the polymer solutions prepared as shown above (Section 3.1.3). In vitro drug release behavior in the physiological serum environment was evaluated by the dialysis method. About 0.5 g sample was introduced in a dialysis bag (the molecular weight cut-off being 10 kDa), immersed in a closed bottle containing 15 mL of salted solution (pH = 6), and placed in a thermostatic chamber at a constant temperature of 37 °C. At different time intervals, aliquots of 1 mL were withdrawn from the release medium and replaced by 1 mL pre-heated solution, in order to maintain a constant volume. The quantity of drug in the release medium was determined by UV spectrophotometry, using a standard calibration curve (a linear dependence of absorbance versus drug concentration was determined). The absorbance was recorded at 362 nm using a Libra UV–Vis spectrophotometer (Biochrom Libra S35PC, Cambridge, UK). The drug-release studies were performed in triplicate. The experimental data were analyzed using OriginPro 8.5 software and the values obtained for the minimum values of the residual sum of the squares (RSS) were considered [66]. However, the number of parameters (p) involved in a given model influences RSS values. The Akaike Information Criterion (AIC) [67] was used for the statistical analysis of the drug-release mechanism, being independent of the number of parameters introduced by each model:

$$\mathrm{AIC} = N \ln(SSR) + 2\,p \tag{8}$$

where N represents the number of experimental data.

According to this criterion, the model with the smallest AIC value is taken into consideration as the best fitting model to describe the drug-release mechanism.

4. Conclusions

In this study, PU-based hydrogel carriers were successfully developed, capable of incorporating specific functional groups and imparting new functionalities that can be exploited in the design of smart materials, used to ensure a sustained and prolonged drug release. Different formulations of the thermal-sensitive PU-based hydrogels loaded with MX were prepared as a minimally invasive alternative for drug administration. The influence of several excipients, such as HPC, PEO, PVP, and oregano essential oil, was analyzed. FTIR spectra revealed the established interactions and rheological data indicated some particular behaviors depending on the composition of the system. The delivery of the active substance in the physiological serum environment was investigated at 37 °C and the process was dominated by anomalous transport phenomena. The main conclusion is that the PU-based hydrogels containing only PU or PU in the presence of a small amount of PEG or essential oil (with antimicrobial activity) are suitable for reducing local inflammation and pain during a period of 24 h to 48 h. On the other hand, the addition of a PEO/PVP mixture or low HPC content allows the design of suitable MX vehicles for wound-dressing applications with extended anti-inflammatory drug release. The use of natural therapeutic agents (essential oils with antimicrobial activity) as excipients presents a high potential for the development of new PU-based carriers for MX delivery.

Further studies are required to analyze the ability to deliver therapeutically relevant amounts of MX and the evaluation of the anti-inflammatory effect induced by oil addition.

Author Contributions: Conceptualization, L.M.G. and M.B.; methodology, I.-A.P. and M.B.; validation, L.M.G., M.A., I.R. and L.E.N.; formal analysis, I.-A.P., I.R. and C.M.; investigation, I.-A.P., L.M.G., M.A., I.R., L.E.N. and M.B.; resources, L.M.G. and M.B.; writing—original draft, I.-A.P., L.M.G., M.A. and M.B.; writing—review and editing, I.-A.P., L.M.G., M.A. and M.B.; supervision, I.-A.P., L.M.G., M.A. and M.B. All authors have read and agreed to the published version of the manuscript.

Funding: This research received no external funding.

Institutional Review Board Statement: Not applicable.

Informed Consent Statement: Not applicable.

Data Availability Statement: The data are available on request.

Acknowledgments: The authors thank R.V. Gradinaru for the validation of the drug delivery data.

Conflicts of Interest: The authors declare no conflict of interest.

References

1. Deshmukh, R. Rheumatoid arthritis: Pathophysiology, current therapeutic strategies and recent advances in targeted drug delivery system. *Mater. Today Commun.* **2023**, *35*, 105877. [CrossRef]
2. Luger, P.; Daneck, K.; Engel, W.; Trummlitz, G.; Wagner, K. Structure and physicochemical properties of meloxicam, a new NSAID. *Eur. J. Pharm. Sci.* **1996**, *4*, 175–187. [CrossRef]
3. Sostres, C.; Gargallo, C.J.; Lanas, A. Nonsteroidal anti-inflammatory drugs and upper and lower gastrointestinal mucosal damage. *Arthritis Res. Ther.* **2013**, *15* (Suppl. 3), S3. [CrossRef]
4. Gerwin, N.; Hops, C.; Lucke, A. Intraarticular drug delivery in osteoarthritis. *Adv. Drug Deliv. Rev.* **2006**, *58*, 226–242. [CrossRef] [PubMed]
5. Noble, S.; Balfour, J.A. Meloxicam. *Drugs* **1996**, *51*, 424–432. [CrossRef]
6. Fleischmann, R.; Iqbal, I.; Slobodin, G. Meloxicam. *Expert Opin. Pharmacother.* **2002**, *3*, 1501–1512. [CrossRef]
7. Tavakoli, M. Modelling therapeutic strategies in the treatment of osteoarthritis: An economic evaluation of meloxicam versus diclofenac and piroxicam. *Pharmacoeconomics* **2003**, *21*, 443–454. [CrossRef]
8. Beetge, E.; du Plessis, J.; Muller, D.G.; Goosen, C.; van Rensburg, F.J. The influence of the physicochemical characteristics and pharmacokinetic properties of selected NSAIDs on their transdermal absorption. *Int. J. Pharm.* **2000**, *193*, 261–264. [CrossRef]
9. Fetih, G. Meloxicam formulations for transdermal delivery: Hydrogels versus organogels. *J. Drug Deliv. Sci. Technol.* **2010**, *20*, 451–456. [CrossRef]
10. Fattahpour, S.; Shamanian, M.; Tavakoli, N.; Fathi, M.; Sheykhi, S.; Fattahpour, S. Design and optimization of alginate-chitosan-pluronic nanoparticles as a novel meloxicam drug delivery system. *Appl. Polym. Sci.* **2015**, *132*, 42241. [CrossRef]
11. Sadeghi-Aliabadi, H.; Sheykhi, S.R.; Fesharaki, M.; Fattahpour, S. An injectable carboxymethyl chitosan-methylcellulose-pluronic hydrogel for the encapsulation of meloxicam loaded nanoparticles. *Int. J. Biol. Macromol.* **2020**, *151*, 220–229. [CrossRef]
12. Kolawole, O.M.; Cook, M.T. In situ gelling drug delivery systems for topical drug delivery. *Eur. J. Pharm. Biopharm.* **2023**, *184*, 36–49. [CrossRef] [PubMed]
13. Inal, O.; Yapar, E.A. Effect of mechanical properties on the release of meloxicam from poloxamer gel bases. *Indian J. Pharm. Sci.* **2013**, *75*, 700–706. [PubMed]
14. McKenzie, M.; Betts, D.; Suh, A.; Bui, K.; Kim, L.D.; Cho, H. Hydrogel-based drug delivery systems for poorly water-soluble drugs. *Molecules* **2015**, *20*, 20397–20408. [CrossRef]
15. Lupu, A.; Gradinaru, L.M.; Rusu, D.; Bercea, M. Self-healing of Pluronic® F127 hydrogels in the presence of various polysaccharides. *Gels* **2023**, *9*, 719. [CrossRef]
16. Lupu, A.; Rosca, I.; Gradinaru, R.; Bercea, M. Temperature induced gelation and antimicrobial properties of Pluronic F127 based systems. *Polymers* **2023**, *15*, 355. [CrossRef]
17. Khan, B.; Arbab, A.; Khan, S.; Fatima, H.; Bibi, I.; Chowdhry, N.P.; Ansari, A.Q.; Ursani, A.A.; Kumar, S.; Hussain, J.; et al. Recent progress in thermosensitive hydrogels and their applications in drug delivery area. *MedComm-Biomater. Appl.* **2023**, *2*, e55. [CrossRef]
18. Khurana, S.; Jain, N.K.; Bedi, P.M.S. Development and characterization of a novel controlled release drug delivery system based on nanostructured lipid carriers gel for meloxicam. *Life Sci.* **2013**, *93*, 763–772. [CrossRef]
19. Wendels, S.; Aveous, L. Biobased polyurethanes for biomedical applications. *Bioact. Mater.* **2021**, *6*, 1083–1106. [CrossRef]
20. Joseph, J.; Patel, R.M.; Wenham, A.; Smith, J.R. Biomedical applications of polyurethane materials and coatings. *Trans. IMF* **2018**, *96*, 121–129. [CrossRef]
21. Das, A.; Mahanwar, P. A brief discussion on advances in polyurethane applications. *Adv. Ind. Eng. Polym. Res.* **2020**, *3*, 93–101. [CrossRef]
22. Wang, J.; Dai, D.; Xie, H.; Li, D.; Xiong, G.; Zhang, C. Biological effects, applications and design strategies of medical polyurethanes modified by nanomaterials. *Int. J. Nanomed.* **2022**, *17*, 6791–6819. [CrossRef] [PubMed]
23. Boffito, M.; Pontremoli, C.; Fiorilli, S.; Laurano, R.; Ciardelli, G.; Vitale-Brovarone, C. Injectable thermosensitive formulation based on polyurethane hydrogel/mesoporous glasses for sustained co-delivery of functional ions and drugs. *Pharmaceutics* **2019**, *11*, 501. [CrossRef] [PubMed]
24. Laurano, R.; Boffito, M.; Cassino, C.; Liberti, F.; Ciardelli, G.; Chiono, V. Design of injectable bioartificial hydrogels by green chemistry for mini-invasive applications in the biomedical or aesthetic medicine fields. *Gels* **2023**, *9*, 59. [CrossRef] [PubMed]
25. Huynh, C.T.; Nguyen, M.K.; Jeong, I.K.; Kim, S.W.; Lee, D.S. Synthesis, characteristics and potential application of poly(β-amino ester urethane)-based multiblock copolymers as an injectable, biodegradable and pH/temperature-sensitive hydrogel system. *Biomater. Sci. Polym. Ed.* **2012**, *23*, 1091–1106. [CrossRef]
26. Gradinaru, L.M.; Ciobanu, C.; Vlad, S.; Bercea, M.; Popa, M. Thermoreversible poly(isopropyl lactate diol)-based polyurethane hydrogels: Effect of isocyanate on some physical properties. *Ind. Eng. Chem. Res.* **2012**, *51*, 12344–12354. [CrossRef]

27. Yu, Y.; Cheng, Y.; Tong, J.; Zhang, L.; Wei, Y.; Tian, M. Recent advances in thermo-sensitive hydrogels for drug delivery. *J. Mater. Chem. B* **2021**, *9*, 2979–2992. [CrossRef]
28. Hoare, T.R.; Kohane, D.S. Hydrogels in drug delivery: Progress and challenges. *Polymer* **2008**, *49*, 1993–2007. [CrossRef]
29. Available online: https://www.ashland.com/file_source/Ashland/Product/Documents/Pharmaceutical/PC_11229_Klucel_HPC.pdf (accessed on 28 September 2023).
30. Gao, J.; Haidar, G.; Lu, X.; Hu, Z. Self-association of hydroxypropylcellulose in water. *Macromolecules* **2001**, *34*, 2242–2247. [CrossRef]
31. Jantharaprapap, R.; Stagni, G. Effects of penetration enhancers on in vitro permeability of meloxicam gels. *Int. J. Pharm.* **2007**, *343*, 26–33. [CrossRef]
32. Chen, J.; Yunhua Gao, Y. Strategies for meloxicam delivery to and across the skin: A review. *Drug Deliv.* **2016**, *23*, 3146–3156. [CrossRef]
33. El-Badry, M.; Fathy, M. Enhancement of the dissolution and permeation rates of meloxicam by formation of its freeze-dried solid dispersions in polyvinylpyrrolidone K-30. *Drug Dev. Ind. Pharm.* **2006**, *32*, 141–150. [CrossRef] [PubMed]
34. Mártha, C.; Kürti, L.; Farkas, G.; Jójárt-Laczkovich, O.; Szalontai, B.; Glässer, E.; Deli, M.A.; Szabó-Révész, P. Effects of polymers on the crystallinity of nanonized meloxicam during a co-grinding process. *Eur. Polym. J.* **2013**, *49*, 2426–2432. [CrossRef]
35. Ochi, M.; Takaki Kawachi, T.; Toita, E.; Hashimoto, I.; Yuminoki, K.; Onoue, S.; Hashimoto, N. Development of nanocrystal formulation of meloxicam with improved dissolution and pharmacokinetic behaviors. *Int. J. Pharm.* **2014**, *474*, 151–156. [CrossRef] [PubMed]
36. Kurti, L.; Kukovecz, A.; Kozma, G.; Ambrus, R.; Deli, M.; Szabó-Révész, P. Study of the parameters influencing the co-grinding process for the production of meloxicam nanoparticles. *Powder Technol.* **2011**, *212*, 210–217. [CrossRef]
37. Shi, X.; Huang, W.; Xu, T.; Fan, B.; Sheng, X. Investigation of drug–polymer miscibility and solubilization on meloxicam binary solid dispersion. *J. Pharm. Innov.* **2020**, *15*, 125–137. [CrossRef]
38. Leuner, C.; Dressman, J. Improving drug solubility for oral delivery using solid dispersions. *Eur. J. Pharm. Biopharm.* **2000**, *50*, 47–60. [CrossRef]
39. Sugimoto, M.; Okagi, T.; Narisawa, S.; Koida, Y.; Nakjima, K. Improvement of dissolution characteristics and bioavailability of poorly water soluble drugs by novel co-grinding method using water soluble polymer. *Int. J. Pharm.* **1998**, *160*, 11–19. [CrossRef]
40. Herman, A.; Herman, A.P. Essential oils and their constituents as skin penetration enhancer for transdermal drug delivery: A review. *J. Pharm. Pharmacol.* **2014**, *67*, 473–485. [CrossRef]
41. Bouyahya, A.; Abrini, J.; Dakka, N.; Bakri, Y. Essential oils of *Origanum Compactum* increase membrane permeability, disturb cell membrane integrity, and suppress quorumsensing phenotype in bacteria. *J. Pharm. Anal.* **2019**, *9*, 301–311. [CrossRef]
42. Kuo, S.H.; Shen, C.J.; Shen, C.F.; Cheng, C.M. Role of pH value in clinically relevant diagnosis. *Diagnostics* **2020**, *10*, 107. [CrossRef] [PubMed]
43. Lukic, M.; Pantelic, I.; Savic, S.D. Towards optimal pH of the skin and topical formulations: From the current state of the art to tailored products. *Cosmetics* **2021**, *8*, 69. [CrossRef]
44. Percival, S.L.; McCarty, S.; Hunt, J.A.; Woods, E.J. The effects of pH on wound healing, biofilms, and antimicrobial efficacy. *Wound Rep. Reg.* **2014**, *22*, 174–186. [CrossRef]
45. Huang, S.; Venables, D.S.; Lawrence, S.E. Pharmaceutical salts of piroxicam and meloxicam with organic counterions. *Cryst. Growth Des.* **2022**, *22*, 6504–6520. [CrossRef] [PubMed]
46. Gradinaru, L.M.; Bercea, M.; Lupu, A.; Gradinaru, V.R. Development of polyurethane/peptide-based carriers with self-healing properties. *Polymers* **2023**, *15*, 1697. [CrossRef] [PubMed]
47. Mandru, M.; Bercea, M.; Gradinaru, L.M.; Ciobanu, C.; Drobota, M.; Vlad, S.; Albulescu, R. Polyurethane/poly(vinyl alcohol) hydrogels: Preparation, characterization and drug delivery. *Eur. Polym. J.* **2019**, *118*, 137–145. [CrossRef]
48. McFarlane, N.L.; Wagner, N.J.; Kaler, E.W.; Lynch, M.L. Poly(ethylene oxide) (PEO) and poly(vinyl pyrolidone) (PVP) induce different changes in the colloid stability of nanoparticles. *Langmuir* **2010**, *26*, 13823–13830. [CrossRef]
49. Kiran Kumar, K.K.; Ravi, M.; Pavani, Y.; Bhavani, S.; Sharma, A.K.; Narasimha Rao, V.V.R. Electrical conduction mechanism in NaCl complexed PEO/PVP polymer blend electrolytes. *J. Non-Cryst. Solids* **2012**, *358*, 3205–3211. [CrossRef]
50. Coussot, P. Yield stress fluid flows: A review of experimental data. *J. Non-Newton. Fluid Mech.* **2014**, *211*, 31–49. [CrossRef]
51. Maya, S.; Sarmento, B.; Nair, A.; Rejinold, N.S.; Nair, S.V.; Jayakumar, R. Smart stimuli sensitive nanogels in cancer drug delivery and imaging: A review. *Curr. Pharm. Des.* **2013**, *19*, 7203–7218. [CrossRef]
52. Peppas, N.A.; Narasimhan, B. Mathematical models in drug delivery: How modeling has shaped the way we design new drug delivery systems. *J. Control. Release* **2014**, *190*, 75–81. [CrossRef] [PubMed]
53. Siepmann, J.; Peppas, N.A. Higuchi equation: Derivation, applications, use and misuse. *Int. J. Pharm.* **2011**, *418*, 6–12. [CrossRef] [PubMed]
54. Korsmeyer, R.W.; Gumy, R.; Doelker, E.; Buri, P.; Peppas, N.A. Mechanisms of solute release from porous hydrophilic polymers. *Int. J. Pharm.* **1983**, *15*, 25–35. [CrossRef]
55. Peppas, N.A.; Sahlin, J.J. A simple equation for the description of solute release. III. Coupling of diffusion and relaxation. *Int. J. Pharm.* **1989**, *57*, 169–172. [CrossRef]

56. Peppas, N.A. Analysis of Fickian and non-Fickian drug release from polymers. *Pharm. Acta Helv.* **1985**, *60*, 110–111. [PubMed]
57. Ritger, P.L.; Peppas, N.A. A simple equation for description of solute release II. Fickian and anomalous release from swellable device. *J. Control. Release* **1987**, *5*, 37–42. [CrossRef]
58. Gupta, S.K.; Bansal, P.; Bhardwaj, R.K.; Jaiswal, J.; Velpandian, T. Comparison of analgesic and anti-inflammatory activity of meloxicam gel with diclofenac and piroxicam gels in animal models: Pharmacokinetic parameters after topical application. *Skin Pharmacol. Physiol.* **2002**, *15*, 105–111. [CrossRef]
59. Chiriac, A.P.; Rusu, A.G.; Nita, L.E.; Chiriac, V.M.; Neamtu, I.; Sandu, A. Polymeric carriers designed for encapsulation of essential oils with biological activity. *Pharmaceutics* **2021**, *13*, 631. [CrossRef]
60. Sindi, A.M.; Hosny, K.M. Lyophilized composite loaded with meloxicam-peppermint oil nanoemulsion for periodontal pain. *Polymers* **2021**, *13*, 2317. [CrossRef]
61. Panja, S.; Dietrich, B.; Adams, D.J. Controlling syneresis of hydrogels using organic salts. *Angew. Chem. Int. Ed.* **2022**, *61*, e202115021. [CrossRef]
62. Available online: https://www.rcsb.org/chemical-sketch (accessed on 10 October 2023).
63. Pettersen, E.F.; Goddard, T.D.; Huang, C.C.; Couch, G.S.; Greenblatt, D.M.; Meng, E.C.; Ferrin, T.E. UCSF Chimera—A visualization system for exploratory research and analysis. *J. Comput. Chem.* **2004**, *25*, 1605–1612. [CrossRef] [PubMed]
64. Trott, O.; Olson, A.J. AutoDock Vina: Improving the speed and accuracy of docking with a new scoring function, efficient optimization, and multithreading. *J. Comput. Chem.* **2010**, *31*, 455–461. [CrossRef] [PubMed]
65. Available online: https://www.3ds.com/products-services/biovia (accessed on 10 October 2023).
66. Unagolla, J.M.; Ambalangodage, C.; Jayasuriya, A.C. Drug transport mechanisms and in vitro release kinetics of vancomycin encapsulated chitosan-alginate polyelectrolyte microparticles as a controlled drug delivery system. *Eur. J. Pharm. Sci.* **2018**, *114*, 199–209. [CrossRef] [PubMed]
67. Yamaoka, K.; Nakagawa, T.; Uno, T. Application of Akaike's information criterion (AIC) in the evaluation of linear pharmacokinetic equations. *J. Pharmacokinet. Biophacodyn.* **1978**, *6*, 165–175. [CrossRef]

pharmaceuticals

MDPI

Article

Wound Healing Performance in a Moist Environment of Crystalline Glucose/Mannose Film as a New Dressing Material Using a Rat Model: Comparing with Medical-Grade Wound Dressing and Alginate

Celine Chia Qi Wong, Kanako Tomura and Osamu Yamamoto *

Graduate School of Science and Engineering, Yamagata University, 4-13-16 Jonan, Yonezawa 992-8510, Yamagata, Japan
* Correspondence: yamamoto@yz.yamagata-u.ac.jp; Tel.: +81-238-26-3366

Abstract: Although medical wound dressings produced using hydrocolloids and alginate were effective in wound healing, adhesion at the wound site and the resulting delayed healing have been a problem. As a new wound dressing material, crystalline wound dressings produced from glucose/mannose were used in this study, which aimed to clarify the properties, adhesion reduction, and wound healing performance of a new wound dressing. Crystalline glucose/mannose films were obtained via alkali treatment using the solution casting method. The structure of the crystalline glucose/mannose films was analogous to the cellulose II polymorph, and the crystallinity decreased with time in hydrated conditions. The crystalline glucose/mannose films had adequate water absorption of 34×10^{-4} g/mm^3 for 5 min. These allowed crystalline glucose/mannose films to remove excess wound exudates while maintaining a moist wound healing condition. This in vivo study demonstrated the healing effects of three groups, which were crystalline glucose/mannose group > alginate group > hydrocolloid group. At 1 week, the crystalline glucose/mannose group was also found to be non-adhesive to the portion of wound healing. This was evidenced by the earlier onset of the healing process, which assisted in re-epithelization and promotion of collagen formation and maturation. These results implied that crystalline glucose/mannose films were a promising candidate that could accelerate the wound healing process, compared with medical-grade wound dressing and alginate.

Keywords: wound healing; wound dressings; glucose/mannose; adhesion; skin regeneration; moist therapy

1. Introduction

The skin is the largest organ of the human body, and its primary function is to serve as the first line of defense against microorganisms. Wound injury occurs when there is a laceration on the skin tissue, leading to the loss of the epidermis layer and some of the connective tissue depending on the wound depth [1]. This increases the risk of wound infection and other complications as wounds act as a port of entry, where microbes are more likely to invade [2]. Therefore, wound dressing is crucial as it serves to protect the wound from any further injuries, prevent bacterial invasion, and provide a conducive environment to promote wound healing.

Before the discovery of moist healing, traditional wound dressing like gauze, lint, plasters, and cotton wool were commonly used to provide basic features. However, these dressings tend to have low absorption and high vapor transmission rates for water. Moreover, it is also found that injured skin tends to have 20 times greater moisture loss than uninjured skin [3–5]. Hence, wounds can easily dry out and these dressings tend to adhere to the granulation tissue, causing pain during removal and slowing wound healing.

Modern wound dressings were then developed in the mid-1980s to overcome these shortcomings. The wound dressings not only protect the wound but also can absorb wound exudates while creating an optimal moist environment. In wound healing, a moist healing environment plays an important role in facilitating the healing process [6,7]. The effect of a moist environment in wound healing has been reported as follows: A moist environment prevents the tissue from drying out and maintains the cell's vitality and functions for carrying out the wound-healing process [8]. Furthermore, it also helps in reducing scars, collagen synthesis and the migration of cells [9,10]. Hence, modern dressing materials containing water such as hydrocolloids, hydrogels, etc. have been developed and commercialized for use in the medical field.

Hydrocolloid dressings with are one of the most used in wound healing [1]. Hydrocolloid dressings are made up of two layers, which are composed of the colloidal layer with a polyurethane outer layer, which is water resistant [11]. The colloidal layer forms hydrated gel upon the absorption of wound exudates [12]. Moreover, hydrocolloid dressings are occlusive, making them impermeable to bacteria, water vapor, and oxygen [13,14]. This creates an environment that is moist and hypoxic, which triggers angiogenesis [15]. However, hydrocolloid dressings containing water are not suitable for highly exudating and deep wounds, because their dressings may lead to the accumulation of wound exudates causing infection and adhesion between wound and dressings [16–18].

In recent years, research on wound dressing using natural polymers such as alginate, chitosan, and gelatin has gained popularity as an alternative to synthetic polymers due to their biocompatibility [19–22]. Alginate is one of the natural polymers that has been extensively studied in the wound-healing region. Alginate dressings are widely known for their high similarity to the extracellular matrix, gel-forming ability, and supreme water absorptivity, making them suitable for moderate to highly exudating wounds [23, 24]. However, alginate dressings are not suitable for dry wounds to have no hydrating properties [25]. Weller C. et al. [26] have reported that insufficient fluid absorption may trigger an inflammatory immune response due to the presence of alginate residues at the wound site.

On the other hand, glucose/mannose is one of the candidates due to its superior properties such as non-toxicity, excellent film formation, biodegradability, and unique swelling and water retention properties [27,28]. These unique water retention properties can regulate an optimum amount of water in a moist environment. Moreover, the evaporation of water provides a microenvironment that has a high concentration of nutrients, proteins, growth factors and electrolytes [9]. This status would give good results for wound healing, which is possible to shorten the healing period [29]. Furthermore, the high content of water in glucose/mannose can relieve pain, and the non-adhesion to granulation tissue can prevent damage to the tissue during the removal of dressings [30].

Although many studies on wound dressings have been reported, there are very few comparative studies in a moist environment. Using a rat model, this study focused on the healing effects of glucose/mannose wound dressings on deep wounds in a moist environment. The present work aimed to compare glucose/mannose wound dressings with medical-grade hydrocolloids and alginate dressings as positive control in a moist environment and to clarify the significance of crystalline glucose/mannose wound dressings on the healing of deep wounds.

2. Results and Discussion

2.1. Characterization of G/M

2.1.1. X-ray Diffraction Measurement

The diffraction patterns of G/M film in dry conditions and at different soaking time intervals of 3 min, 10 min, 1 and 2 weeks are shown in Figure 1. The dry G/M film demonstrated three sharp peaks, which corresponds to the typical diffraction pattern of cellulose type II [31]. When the G/M film was soaked in distilled water, peak broadening occurred. Moreover, the intensity of the diffraction peak further decreases with increasing the soaking time. This peak broadening was largely due to the decrease in crystallinity of the G/M polymer structure. When the G/M film was soaked in water, the water molecules entered the G/M polymer chains and interacted with the hydroxyl groups of the G/M backbone. This interaction caused the polymer backbone to swell and become more disordered, reducing the crystallinity of the G/M chains.

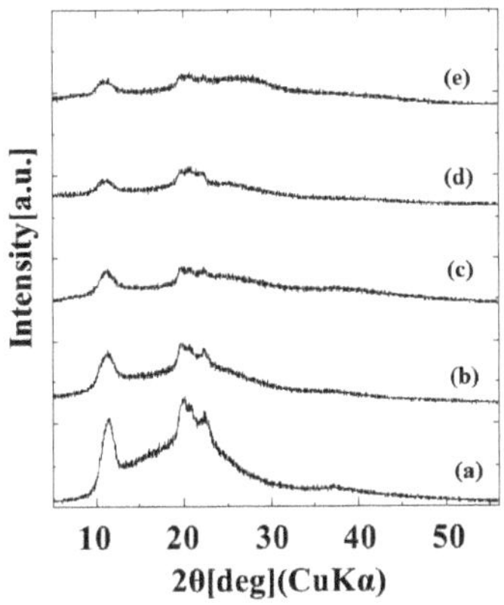

Figure 1. XRD patterns of (**a**) dry G/M and G/M in different soaking time intervals of (**b**) 3 min, (**c**) 10 min, (**d**) 1 week, and (**e**) 2 weeks.

2.1.2. Mass Spectroscopy

MALDI-TOF MS ranging from 800 to 400 m/z was used to identify the degree of polymerization of the G/M film prepared using 0.1 mol/L sodium carbonate. As shown in Figure 2, a peak at approximately 972 m/z corresponded to oligosaccharides of 6 mers [32]. Moreover, a peak at a maximum of 3418 m/z was also detected. According to the mass spectrum, m/z values of 972 to 3418 demonstrated that the G/M film prepared has a degree of polymerization of 6 to 21 mers.

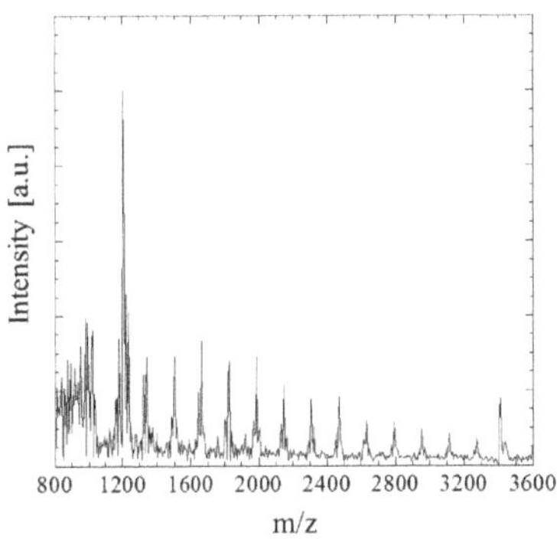

Figure 2. MALDI-TOF MS spectrum of G/M film.

2.1.3. Water Absorption Behavior

The fluid uptake capacity was determined to evaluate the capability of G/M as a wound dressing in absorbing wound exudates. Figure 3 shows the water absorption behavior of G/M at room temperature. When the G/M film was immersed in water for 5 min, the water absorption increased significantly. The water content of G/M film reached 34×10^{-4} g/mm^3. After 5 min, the water absorption increased slightly, showing a maximum absorption capacity of 35.5×10^{-4} g/mm^3 after 20 min of soaking time. As aforementioned, water absorption in G/M film would be achieved by the formation of hydrogen bonding between the water molecules and hydrophilic groups of G/M. The initial steep increase in water content in G/M film is due to the presence of a large amount of vacant hydrophilic groups in G/M chains, hence, leading to the increase in the binding affinity to water molecules [33,34]. G/M film then reaches its maximum swelling capacity when all its vacant hydroxyl groups interact with the water molecules.

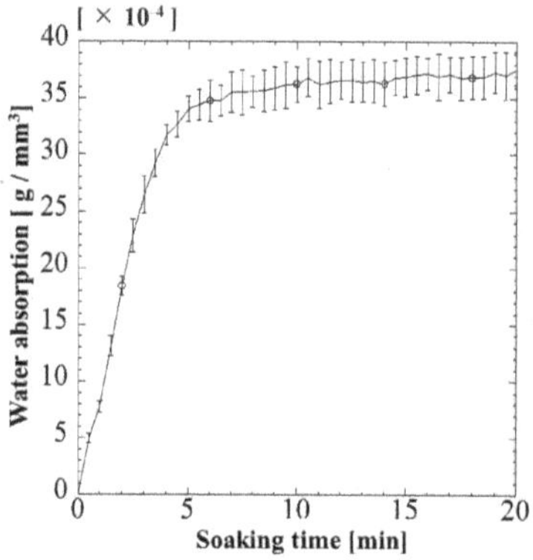

Figure 3. Change in water absorption of G/M film with soaking time at 37 °C.

2.1.4. Water Vapor Transmission Rate

Wound dressing material with optimal water vapor permeability is crucial in providing a conducive healing environment. The water vaporization results of blank control, G/M film, and the G/M film with secondary dressing, which simulates the condition for animal study, are shown in Figure 4. The evaporation volume slightly decreased when the G/M film was present. On the other hand, when secondary dressing was used in combination with G/M film, the amount of evaporation per unit surface area was 31.71 mm^3/mm^2 with a significant reduction.

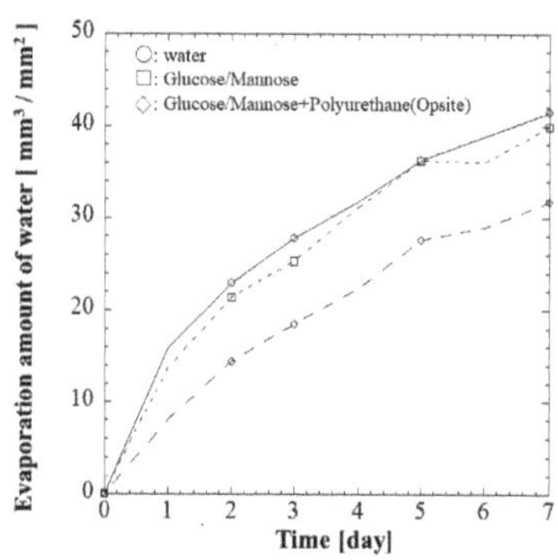

Figure 4. Water vapor transmission rate (WVTR) of (□) G/M and (◇) G/M with secondary dressing over 7 days at 37 °C. Notice: the mark of ○ shows water evaporation under the same conditions.

2.1.5. Surface Roughness

The surface roughness of G/M film in dry and hydrated at 3 and 10 min soaking intervals was determined as shown in Figure 5. The *Ra* of dry G/M film was 0.5627 μm. The surface roughness of dry G/M film decreased drastically with immersing in distilled water above 3 min. There was no significant difference in surface roughness of the G/M films at 3 and 10 min, which had *Ra* of 0.3001 μm and 0.2861 μm, respectively. This decrease in surface roughness was attributed to the swelling of the G/M matrix, which was due to the relaxation of the G/M chains. According to J.C. Doloff. et al. [35], optimal surface roughness is crucial to prevent irritation and persistent inflammatory responses. Therefore, the G/M film was suitable to be used as a dressing material as it demonstrated *Ra* falls within the micron range.

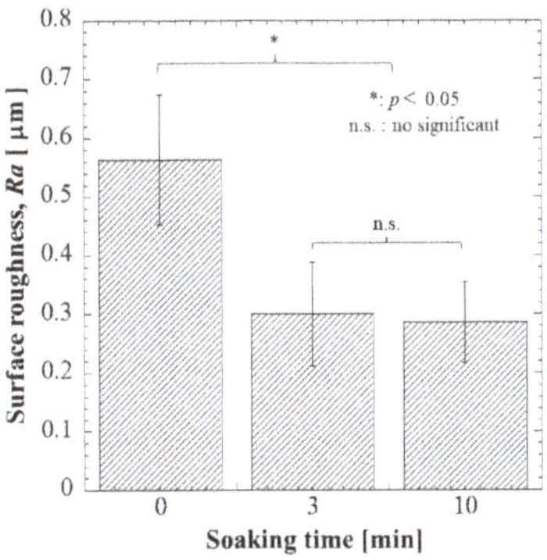

Figure 5. Surface roughness of G/M at different soaking intervals of 0, 3, and 10 min.

2.2. *In Vivo Evaluation of Commercial Hydrocolloid Dressing (Duoactive ET®), Alginate, and G/M*

2.2.1. Macroscopic Evaluation

The wound healing condition of the full-thickness wounds of three treatment groups was evaluated 1 and 2 weeks post-surgery. The adhesiveness of these samples to the wound site was assessed during the removal of these wound dressings. As shown in Figure 6, the commercial hydrocolloid dressing had the most aggressive adhesion to the wound area. The alginate group was slightly adhesive to the wound, whereas G/M film could be removed easily from the wound site; that is, the G/M film was non-adhesive. Moreover, Figure 7 shows the condition of the granulation tissue and residual wound area at 1 and 2 weeks healing. At 1 week, red-colored tissue, which was an indication of the formation of healthy granulation tissue, could be observed in both alginate and G/M groups. However, the observation of red tissue was difficult in the hydrocolloid group. This could be attributed to the strong adhesion of the dressing to the wound, leading to the damage of the fragile tissue [36]. At 2 weeks, wounds of alginate and G/M treatment experienced complete wound closure. On the other hand, there was still incomplete epithelial formation for the hydrocolloid group.

The residual wound area (%) was then identified using ImageJ software Ver.1.51 (Figure 8). At 1 week, the residual wound area of these groups was as stated: hydrocolloid > alginate > G/M, where the G/M group had a significant smaller wound than the hydrocolloid group. The wound area decreased as healing progressed at 2 weeks post-surgery for all groups. Alginate and G/M groups had completed the re-epithelization process, whereas there was still approximately 2.83% residual wound area for the hydrocolloid group. Macroscopic evaluation was insufficient to determine the healing quality of each treatment group. Therefore, histological assessment was conducted for further verification.

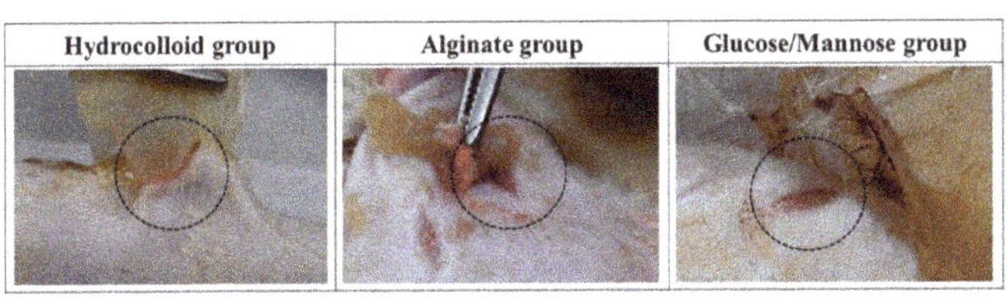

Figure 6. Adhesion status of dressing groups to the wound area and surrounding skin at 1 week.

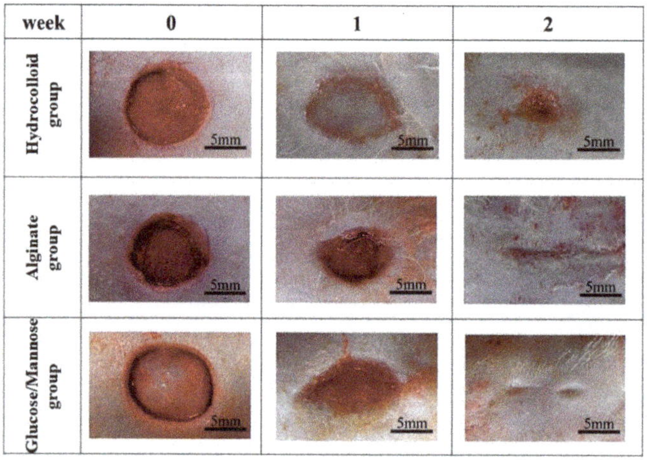

Figure 7. Macroscopic observations of wound status of each dressing group at 0, 1, and 2 weeks post-surgery.

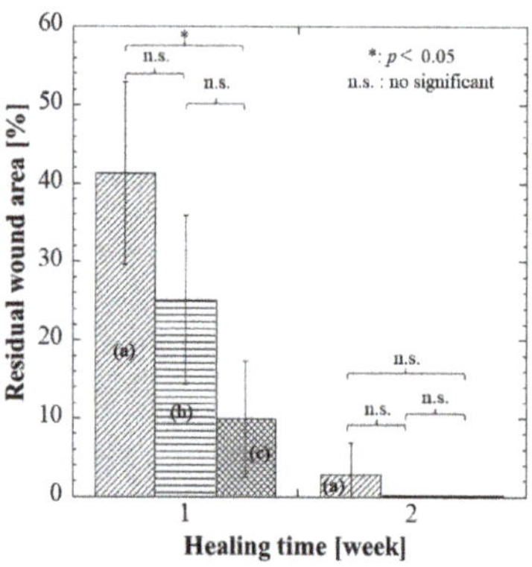

Figure 8. Residual wound area of each dressing group at 1 and 2 weeks. (**a**–**c**) represent hydrocolloid, alginate, and G/M groups, respectively. Notice: Complete wound closure (0 + 0.1%) in (**b**,**c**) groups at 2 weeks.

2.2.2. Histological Evaluation

HE, MT, and PSR staining were conducted for hydrocolloid, alginate, and G/M groups at 1 and 2 weeks healing times to evaluate the healing condition of the wounds. The types of cells present, angiogenesis, collagen deposition, and collagen type were identified and compared between the three groups.

Figure 9 shows HE and MT staining images of the regenerated tissues in each group at 1 and 2 weeks. In HE staining of regenerated and surrounding tissues (Figure 9A), tissue regeneration was observed in all groups at 1 week, but the tissues were immature and there was no epithelialization. Epithelial formation was observed in all groups at 2 weeks, and tissue maturation was particularly remarkable in the G/M group.

At 1 week shown in Figure 9B, the G/M group had a smaller number of neutrophils and macrophages than the alginate and hydrocolloid group. The infiltration of inflammatory cells in the hydrocolloid and alginate groups seemed to be stronger compared to the G/M group. This indicates that the G/M group has the fastest onset for the inflammation process. The collagen synthesis for all three groups had no significant difference, where sparse and thin collagen could be observed in MT staining. Figure 10 shows the PSR staining of normal skin tissue and that of the three treatment groups at 1 and 2 weeks healing. PSR staining indicated the type of collagen present at the wound site, where type III and type I collagen were green and yellow in color, respectively. At 1 week, type III collagen dominated the wound area of all three treatment groups. This result corresponded to the MT staining shown in Figure 9B, as type III collagen was newly deposited collagen at the wound area during the early healing phase.

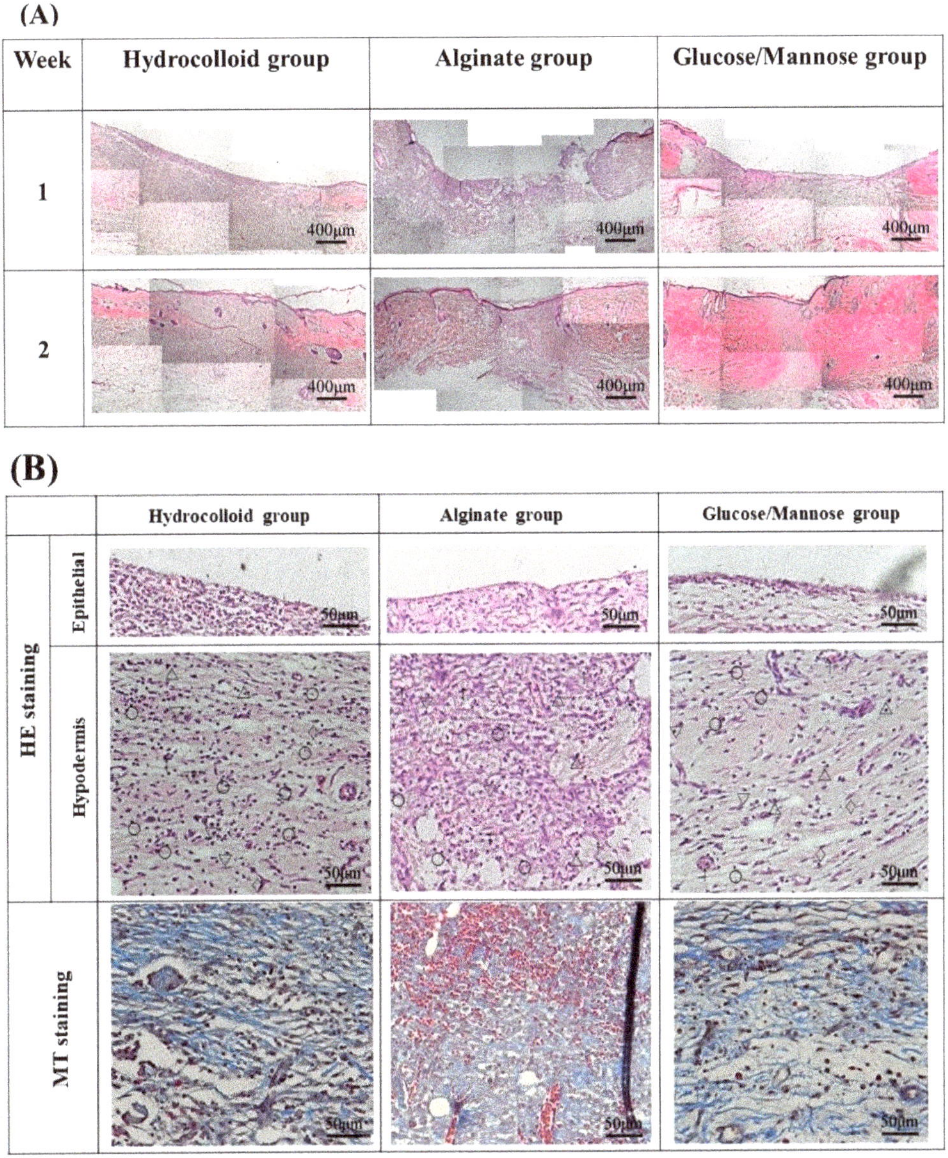

Figure 9. *Cont.*

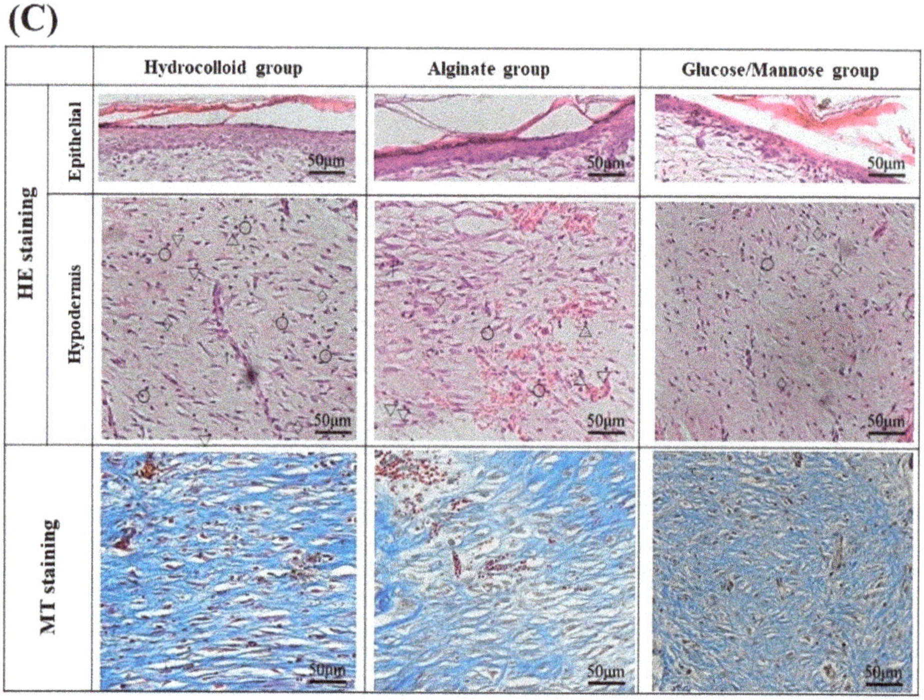

Figure 9. Staining images of the regenerated tissues in each group at 1 and 2 weeks: (**A**) HE staining of regenerated and surrounding tissues at 4× magnification. (**B**) HE and MT staining of 1 week regenerated tissue at 20× magnification. (**C**) HE and MT staining of 2 weeks regenerated tissue at 20× magnification. The symbols of ○, ▽, △, ◇ in HE staining images and ↑ represent lymphocytes, macrophages, neutrophils, fibroblasts, and new blood vessels.

Figure 9C shows the HE and MT staining at 2 weeks of healing. As wound healing progressed, epithelial cells could be observed for all groups. It has been reported that the epidermis layer will become thinner, resembling the thickness of the epidermis layer of uninjured skin when healing continues [37]. G/M and alginate groups demonstrated a thinner epidermal layer, which resembled more of the uninjured skin compared to that of the hydrocolloid group. The number of inflammatory cells for both G/M and alginate groups decreased at 2 weeks, coupled with more fibroblasts being observed. On the other hand, many neutrophils and macrophages could still be observed in the hydrocolloid and alginate groups. In the G/M group, no inflammatory cell infiltration was observed. The density of collagen at the wound site increased for all groups. However, the G/M group demonstrated a tighter and more packed collagen deposition than the alginate and hydrocolloid groups. In PSR staining (Figure 10), the ratio of type I to type III collagen increased at week 2. It could be observed that the G/M group had the most type I collagen deposition compared to other groups. This is evidence that collagen in the G/M group is densely packed. Furthermore, this result may be due to the maturation of type III collagen and its reorientation to the more complex structure of type I collagen for tensile strength recovery.

Angiogenesis, which is the formation of new blood vessels, is an important event in wound healing. The blood vessels found at the wound site are responsible for providing nutrients and oxygen, which are essential for wound healing. Figure 11 presents the number of blood vessels found at each healing time. There was a trend where the number of blood vessels decreased with healing time. At 1 week, there were significant differences in the alginate group to G/M and hydrocolloid groups. This could be explained by the fact that the alginate group induced neovascularization due to severe inflammation, as shown in Figure 9B.

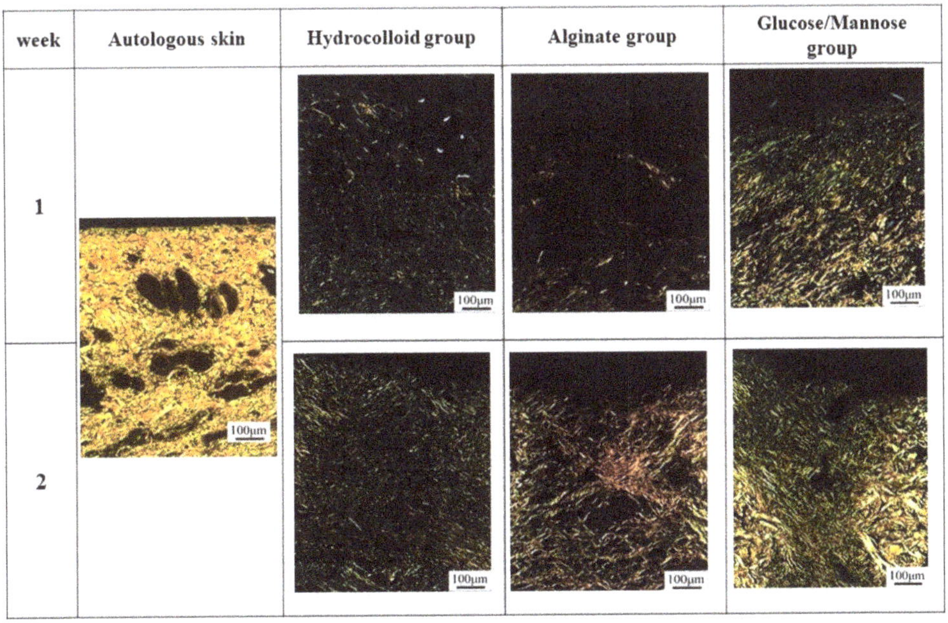

Figure 10. PSR staining of regenerated tissues in each group at 1 and 2 weeks post-surgery.

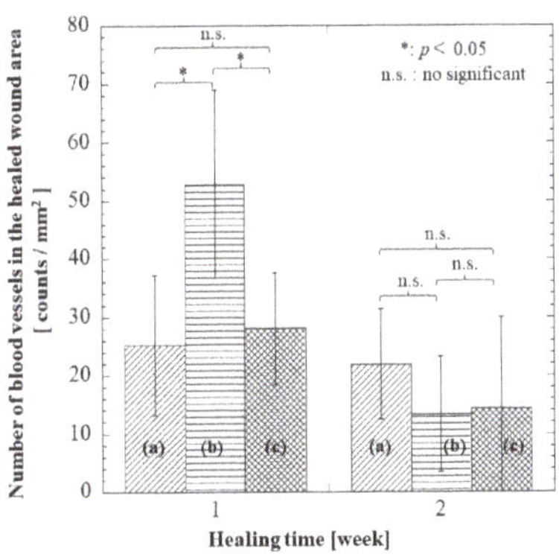

Figure 11. Number of blood vessels at regenerated tissue region in each group at 1 and 2 weeks: (**a**) hydrocolloid group, (**b**) alginate group, and (**c**) G/M group.

2.3. Discussion

Glucose/mannose (G/M) is a natural polysaccharide made up of β-1,4-linked D-mannose and D-glucose. G/M possesses ideal properties for a wound dressing such as good biocompatibility, excellent film formation, unique water absorption, and retention properties [28,38]. Native G/M consists of a low degree of approximately 5–10% of acetyl groups, positioned randomly at C-6 of the sugar units [39]. On the other hand, G/M prepared was treated with Na_2CO_3 in this study. This leads to the deacetylation reaction where the acetyl groups were removed from the G/M structure. This aligned with the

XRD spectra obtained where the alkali-treated G/M dressing prepared demonstrated typical patterns of cellulose type II polymorph, where inter-sheet bonding occurs as G/M strands arranged in an antiparallel configuration [31,40]. It is known that a moist healing environment can promote effective wound healing as it promotes a faster re-epithelization process. In this study, G/M demonstrated good water absorption attributed to the presence of hydrophilic groups and adequate water retention properties, where it can absorb wound exudates while providing a conducive moist wound healing environment. A wound dressing with excellent swelling behavior can absorb excessive blood and wound exudates to prevent the wound from infection and maceration. The wound dressings with a high transmission rate will cause the wound to dehydrate while a relatively low transmission rate will lead to the accumulation and leakage of exudates [41]. Therefore, it is also important for a wound dressing to have adequate water vapor permeation to provide a moist wound-healing environment.

Wound healing is an overlapping process that consists of four phases, including hemostasis, inflammation, proliferation, and remodeling, orchestrated by different cells [42]. Hemostasis begins immediately after trauma and will last for a few hours after the injury to prevent excessive bleeding through the formation of fibrin clots. After bleeding from the wound is stopped, vasodilation occurs. Then, inflammation is initiated due to the flux of inflammatory cells to the wound site. During inflammation, neutrophils will infiltrate the wound area and carry out sanitation of the wound. Macrophages then perform phagocytosis on bacteria and debris to further clean the wound. Acute inflammation usually lasts up to a few days. Simultaneously, the granulation phase, which is the deposition of the extracellular matrix, also occurs. In the proliferation phase, collagen deposition and the formation of new blood vessels continues. Re-epithelization then occurs by the migration of the keratinocytes from the wound periphery to the wound site and proliferate, to form the epidermal layer [43]. The remodeling phase can last up to months after injury, where the newly deposited type III collagen matures and crosslinks to type I collagen to regain tensile strength.

At 1 week, the G/M group demonstrated a significantly smaller residual wound area than the hydrocolloid group. Moreover, the large number of inflammatory cells coupled with some fibroblasts and new blood vessels can be observed in the alginate group. On the other hand, the hydrocolloid group had the highest residual area of 41.30%, in which neutrophils and macrophages were observed. This result suggests that the hydrocolloid group is at the early inflammatory phase whereas the G/M and alginate groups are at the intermediate phase between inflammation and proliferation. At 2 weeks, both G/M and alginate groups had complete epidermis regeneration, which also demonstrated a decrease in inflammatory cells with an increase in fibroblasts. However, type I collagen, which was more organized and tightly packed, could be found more at the wound site in the G/M group than in the alginate group. This result suggests that the G/M group is at the transition phase between proliferation and early remodeling phase, while the alginate group is at the end of the proliferation phase. This statement was further supported by the decrease in the number of blood vessels at 2 weeks. The decrease in the number of blood vessels occurs when wound healing advances through the proliferation and remodeling phase. This phenomenon occurs to facilitate the reorganization of the collagen matrix [44]. Contrarily, the wound for the hydrocolloid group shows an incomplete re-epithelization process. Moreover, many inflammatory cells and type III collagen, with a negligible amount of collagen I, were observed at the wound site. Therefore, it is presumed that the hydrocolloid group is in the early phase of proliferation.

3. Materials and Methods

3.1. Materials

Glucose/mannose powder and sodium carbonate were used for the preparation of crystalline glucose/mannose film (G/M). For the preparation of alginate, sodium alginate powder was used. Glucose/mannose powder (PROPOL® A) was purchased as a raw material from SHIMIZU Chemical Corporation (Hiroshima, Japan), in which the molar ratio (glucose/mannose) was approximately 0.1. Sodium carbonate and sodium alginate (viscosity: 300 cps, 1% solution) were procured from Nacalai Tesque Inc. (Kyoto, Japan). All the materials listed were used as received.

3.2. *Preparation of Glucose/Mannose (G/M) Film*

A total of 50 mL of 0.1 mol/L sodium carbonate (Na_2CO_3) aqueous solution was prepared prior to the preparation of the G/M film, and 1.0 g of G/M powder was dissolved in 100 mL of distilled water. The G/M solution was then stirred with a magnetic stirrer for 100 min at room temperature. After the G/M solution was stirred for 100 min, the prepared Na_2CO_3 aqueous solution was added slowly to the G/M solution. The mixture was then further stirred for 5 min. Next, 20 mL of the reacted mixture was cast onto a circular petri dish (Diameter 100 mm) and dried for 5 days at 26 °C, i.e., solution casting method. The dried G/M film with the thickness of 0.1 mm was further washed with distilled water several times to obtain a film with pH 7.

3.3. *Preparation of Alginate*

A total of 3.0 g of sodium alginate powder was dissolved in 30 mL of distilled water. The alginate solution was then stirred at room temperature until all powder was completely dissolved. After the complete dissolution of the powder, 20 mL of the solution was then cast on a circular petri dish and matured for 5 days at 26 °C to obtain an alginate film with a thickness of 2.0 mm.

3.4. *Characterization of G/M Film*

3.4.1. X-ray Diffraction Measurement (XRD)

The crystalline structure of G/M film in dry and hydrated (in distilled water at different soaking times) conditions was analyzed using an XRD meter (XRD Ultima-IV, Rigaku, Tokyo, Japan). The testing parameters were as stated: Cu Kα radiation (λ = 0.15418 nm) with voltage and current of 40 kV and 40 mA, respectively, over a measurement range of (2θ) 3–60°.

3.4.2. Mass Spectroscopy

The sample solution was prepared by first cutting G/M film into squares of approximately 5 mm and dissolved in distilled water by sonicating at 50 °C, followed by heat treatment at 90 °C. Cationization agent (20 mg/mL sodium trifluoroacetate), sample solution, and 2,5-dihydroxybenzoic acid matrix solution were mixed and deposited onto a MALDI plate and allowed to dry. The sample was then analyzed using MALDI Time of Flight Mass (MALDI-TOF Mass-8020, Shimadzu Corporation, Kyoto, Japan) using a nitrogen laser and a measurement mass range of 800–4000 m/z.

3.4.3. Behavior of Water Absorption in G/M Film

Dry G/M film was cut into square shapes with dimensions of 6.50 $\pm$ 0.07 mm. Next, the thickness of the cut film was measured at three random points using a digital micrometer with a wide range (Mitutoyo, Kanagawa, Japan). The degree of absorption of G/M film was then weighed to obtain the initial mass of dry film (W_o). The dried film was then immersed completely in 50 mL of distilled water. The weight of the absorbed film (W_t) was measured at a time interval of 30 s for 20 min, gently removing excess water on the surface of the film using filter paper. The measurement was conducted in three replications. The water absorption behavior of the G/M film was determined as follows (1):

$$Absorption\ behavior\left(g/mm^3\right) = \frac{w_t - w_o}{v} \quad (1)$$

where W_t represents the weight of swollen film at time t, W_o represents the initial weight of the dried film, and v is the volume of the dried film.

3.4.4. Water Vapor Transmission Rate

The water vapor transmission rate (*WVTR*) analysis consists of three groups, which include i. blank control, ii. G/M and iii. G/M and secondary dressing (Opsite Quick Guard; Smith & Nephew plc, Watford, UK). Dry G/M and secondary dressing were trimmed into rounded shapes, which can be fitted perfectly into the test tube. The trimmed films were then placed into test tubes with fully filled saline solution (h_i) and maintained at a temperature of 37 °C. It is noted that a doughnut-shaped styrofoam ring was placed between the dressing and saline solution to prevent the G/M film from sinking. The change in the level of the saline solution in the test tubes (h_t) was monitored every 24 h for a period of 7 days and further analyzed using ImageJ software (NIH, Bethesda, ML, USA). Each group was repeatedly tested 3 times. The WVTR of all groups was determined as stated (2):

$$WVTR\left(\text{mm}^3/\text{mm}^2\text{ of film}\right) = \frac{(h_t - h_i) \times A}{A_f} \quad (2)$$

where h_i and h_t represent the initial level and level of saline solution at interval t, respectively. A is the area of the test tube and A_f is the area of the film.

3.4.5. Surface Roughness

The surface roughness of G/M film in dry and hydrated (in distilled water) conditions was analyzed using a confocal laser scanning microscope (VK-9700 Violet Laser; Keyence Corporation, Osaka, Japan). Ten measurement points were randomly selected from the film, and the results were reported as the average surface roughness, *Ra*.

3.5. In Vivo Study of Full Thickness Wound

3.5.1. Animal Operation

The G/M film, alginate sheet, and all surgical instruments were sterilized at 121 °C with 120 kPa for 20 min using an autoclave (LBS-245; Tomy Seiko Co. Ltd., Tokyo, Japan) prior to surgery. Regarding wound healing in a moist environment, wet G/M and alginate films containing 35×10^{-4} and 35×10^{-2} g/mm^3 saline to dry film volume, respectively, were used as wound dressings. The following animal experiment has been approved by the animal research committee of Yamagata University. Three treatment groups were evaluated in this study, including i: commercial hydrocolloid wound dressing (Duoactive ET®, Convatec Inc., Bridgewater, NJ, USA), ii: alginate, and iii: G/M. Six male Sprague-Dawley rats (n = 6), weighing 250–300 g, used in this study were anesthetized with a triple anesthetic mixture administered intramuscularly. The amount of the triple anesthetic mixture was as follows based on the rat's body weight (kg), i.e., Medetomidine hydrochloride (NIPPON ZENYAKU KOGYO Co., Ltd., Fukushima, Japan); 0.15 mg/Kg, Midazolam (Astellas Pharma Inc., Tokyo, Japan); 2.0 mg/Kg, Butorphanol tartrate (Meiji Seika pharma Co., Tokyo, Japan); 2.5 mg/Kg. After removing the body hair with clippers, the remaining body hair was completely removed with hair removal cream. The surgical site was then disinfected with 7% povidone-iodine and 70% ethanol. Circular wounds extended to the panniculus muscle were then created on the abdomen of the rats using a 10 mm diameter trephine bar. The wounds were then covered with commercial hydrocolloid dressing, alginate, and G/M, respectively (Figure 12). Notably, alginate and G/M were secured to the wounds by a secondary dressing. Wound healing evaluation was then conducted at 1 and 2 weeks post-surgery.

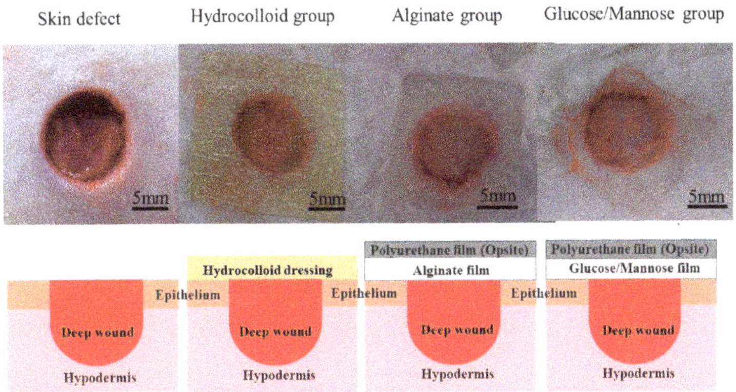

Figure 12. Images and illustrations of the application of hydrocolloid, alginate, and G/M dressing to skin defects.

3.5.2. Macroscopic Evaluation

The wound healing condition was recorded using a digital camera. The residual wound area of all wounds was identified using ImageJ Ver.1.51 (NIH, USA) software, and it was calculated using the following Equation (3):

$$Residual\ wound\ area\ (\%) = \frac{w_t}{w_o} \times 100 \tag{3}$$

where W_t and W_o represent the wound area at 1 and 2 weeks and initial wound area, respectively.

3.5.3. Histological Evaluation

The rats for each group were euthanized after 1 and 2 weeks post-surgery. Regenerated tissue including its surrounding healthy tissues was removed. The skin tissues were then fixed with a 5% of formaldehyde–phosphate buffered solution, followed by embedding in a paraffin block for tissue staining. The paraffin blocks were then sectioned into thin specimens of 6 μm thickness. The tissue specimens were then stained using Hematoxylin and eosin (HE), Masson's trichrome (MT), and picrosirius red (PSR) staining. All staining chemicals were procured from Muto Chemicals, Co. Ltd., Tokyo, Japan.

3.5.4. Angiogenesis Evaluation

The formation of new blood vessels for each treatment group was quantified from five random areas of the regenerated skin tissue. Images of the regenerated areas with HE staining were photographed with 20× magnification (2448 × 1980 pixels) using an optical microscope (BX53, OLYMPUS, Tokyo, Japan). The area of the image was converted from pixels to mm using ImageJ for further calculation. The formation of new blood vessels per mm^2 was determined with the following Formula (4):

$$New\ blood\ vessels\ count\ \left(\text{counts}/\text{mm}^2\right) = \frac{N}{A} \tag{4}$$

where N is the number of new blood vessels and A is the area of each image.

3.6. Statistical Analysis

All data were reported as mean ± standard deviation. All results were analyzed using one-way analysis of variance (ANOVA), with Tukey's post hoc test for multiple comparisons. Results were considered as significantly different with $p < 0.05$.

4. Conclusions

Crystalline glucose/mannose films (G/M) were prepared by solution casting method and possessed a structure resembling cellulose II polymorph. The crystalline films obtained were found to have adequate absorptivity, water permeability, and surface roughness for efficient wound healing. In the results of the wound-healing performance, the adhesion was observed in hydrocolloid and alginate groups at 1 week of healing. However, there was no adhesion in the G/M group. In the assessment at macroscopic and histological evaluation at 1 and 2 weeks post-surgery, it was found that the G/M group demonstrated faster wound healing than the alginate and hydrocolloid groups. Therefore, it was proven that the crystalline glucose/mannose dressing was a promising material for effective moist wound healing, which was a better dressing material than alginate and hydrocolloid dressings.

Author Contributions: Conceptualization, O.Y.; Validation, C.C.Q.W., K.T. and O.Y.; Formal analysis, C.C.Q.W., K.T. and O.Y.; Investigation, C.C.Q.W., K.T. and O.Y.; Writing—original draft, C.C.Q.W.; Writing—review & editing, O.Y.; Supervision, O.Y.; Project administration, O.Y.; Funding acquisition, O.Y. All authors have read and agreed to the published version of the manuscript.

Funding: This study was partly supported by Japan Science and Technology Agency (No. J23E000162).

Institutional Review Board Statement: The animal study protocol was approved by Yamagata University, approval code: R4035, approval date: 7 March 2022, and approval code: R5097, approval date: 6 March 2023.

Data Availability Statement: Data is contained within the article.

Conflicts of Interest: The authors declare no conflict of interest.

References

1. Dhivya, S.; Padma, V.V.; Santhini, E. Wound dressings—A review. *BioMedicine* **2015**, *5*, 22. [CrossRef] [PubMed]
2. Yan, J.; Ji, Y.; Huang, M.; Li, T.; Liu, Y.; Lü, S.; Liu, M. Nucleobase-Inspired Self-Adhesive and Inherently Antibacterial Hydrogel for Wound Dressing. *ACS Mater. Lett.* **2020**, *2*, 1375–1380. [CrossRef]
3. Lamke, L.O. Evaporative water loss from burns under different environmental conditions. *Scand. J. Plast. Reconstr. Surg.* **1971**, *5*, 77–81. [CrossRef] [PubMed]
4. Queen, D.; Gaylor, J.D.; Evans, J.H.; Courtney, J.M.; Reid, W.H. The preclinical evaluation of the water vapour transmission rate through burn wound dressings. *Biomaterials* **1987**, *8*, 367–371. [CrossRef] [PubMed]
5. Bajpai, M.; Bajpai, S.K.; Gautam, D. Investigation of Regenerated Cellulose/Poly(acrylic acid) Composite Films for Potential Wound Healing Applications: A Preliminary Study. *J. Appl. Chem.* **2014**, *2014*, 325627. [CrossRef]
6. Heyer, K.; Augustin, M.; Protz, K.; Herberger, K.; Spehr, C.; Rustenbach, S.J. Effectiveness of advanced versus conventional wound dressings on healing of chronic wounds: Systematic review and meta-analysis. *Dermatology* **2013**, *226*, 172–184. [CrossRef]
7. Rosique, R.G.; Rosique, M.J.; Farina Junior, J.A. Curbing Inflammation in Skin Wound Healing: A Review. *Int. J. Inflam.* **2015**, *2015*, 316235. [CrossRef]
8. Xu, R.; Xia, H.; He, W.; Li, Z.; Zhao, J.; Liu, B.; Wang, Y.; Lei, Q.; Kong, Y.; Bai, Y.; et al. Controlled water vapor transmission rate promotes wound-healing via wound re-epithelialization and contraction enhancement. *Sci. Rep.* **2016**, *6*, 24596. [CrossRef]
9. Nuutila, K.; Eriksson, E. Moist Wound Healing with Commonly Available Dressings. *Adv. Wound Care* **2021**, *10*, 685–698. [CrossRef]
10. Xue, M.; Jackson, C.J. Extracellular Matrix Reorganization During Wound Healing and Its Impact on Abnormal Scarring. *Adv. Wound Care* **2015**, *4*, 119–136. [CrossRef]
11. Takeuchi, T.; Ito, M.; Yamaguchi, S.; Watanabe, S.; Honda, M.; Imahashi, T.; Yamada, T.; Kokubo, T. Hydrocolloid dressing improves wound healing by increasing M2 macrophage polarization in mice with diabetes. *Nagoya J. Med. Sci.* **2020**, *82*, 487–498. [PubMed]
12. Barnes, H.R. Wound care: Fact and fiction about hydrocolloid dressings. *J. Gerontol. Nurs.* **1993**, *19*, 23–26. [CrossRef]
13. Aruan, N.M.; Sriyanti, I.; Edikresnha, D.; Suciati, T.; Munir, M.M.; Khairurrijal. Polyvinyl Alcohol/Soursop Leaves Extract Composite Nanofibers Synthesized Using Electrospinning Technique and their Potential as Antibacterial Wound Dressing. *Procedia Eng.* **2017**, *170*, 31–35. [CrossRef]
14. Bowling, F.L.; Rashid, S.T.; Boulton, A.J. Preventing and treating foot complications associated with diabetes mellitus. *Nat. Rev. Endocrinol.* **2015**, *11*, 606–616. [CrossRef] [PubMed]
15. Bharat, S.; Rucha, G.; Rahul, H. A Comprehensive Review on Wound Dressings and Their Comparative Effectiveness on Healing of Contaminated Wounds and Ulcers. *Arch. Anesthesiol. Crit. Care* **2022**, *8*. [CrossRef]

16. Bower, K.A.; Mulder, G.D.; Reineke, A.; Guide, S.V. Dermatologic Conditions and Symptom Control. In *Textbook of Interdisciplinary Pediatric Palliative Care*; Wolfe, J., Hinds, P.S., Sourkes, B.M., Eds.; W.B. Saunders: Philadelphia, PA, USA, 2011; pp. 350–367.
17. Lim, J.Z.; Ng, N.S.; Thomas, C. Prevention and treatment of diabetic foot ulcers. *J. R. Soc. Med.* **2017**, *110*, 104–109. [CrossRef]
18. Wietlisbach, C.M. 21—Wound Care. In *Fundamentals of Hand Therapy*, 2nd ed.; Cooper, C., Ed.; Mosby: Maryland Heights, MI, USA, 2014; pp. 206–218.
19. Zhao, Y.; Wang, X.; Qi, R.; Yuan, H. Recent Advances of Natural-Polymer-Based Hydrogels for Wound Antibacterial Therapeutics. *Polymers* **2023**, *15*, 3305. [CrossRef]
20. Sheokand, B.; Vats, M.; Kumar, A.; Srivastava, C.M.; Bahadur, I.; Pathak, S.R. Natural polymers used in the dressing materials for wound healing: Past, present and future. *J. Polym. Sci.* **2023**, *61*, 1389–1414. [CrossRef]
21. Hassan, M.A.; Tamer, T.M.; Valachová, K.; Omer, A.M.; El-Shafeey, M.; Mohy Eldin, M.S.; Šoltés, L. Antioxidant and antibacterial polyelectrolyte wound dressing based on chitosan/hyaluronan/phosphatidylcholine dihydroquercetin. *Int. J. Biol. Macromol.* **2021**, *166*, 18–31. [CrossRef]
22. Borbolla-Jiménez, F.V.; Peña-Corona, S.I.; Farah, S.J.; Jiménez-Valdés, M.T.; Pineda-Pérez, E.; Romero-Montero, A.; Del Prado-Audelo, M.L.; Bernal-Chávez, S.A.; Magaña, J.J.; Leyva-Gómez, G. Films for Wound Healing Fabricated Using a Solvent Casting Technique. *Pharmaceutics* **2023**, *15*, 1914. [CrossRef]
23. Weigelt, M.A.; Sanchez, D.P.; Lev-Tov, H. 20—Dressings and Wound Care Supplies for Hidradenitis Suppurativa. In *A Comprehensive Guide to Hidradenitis Suppurativa*; Shi, V.Y., Hsiao, J.L., Lowes, M.A., Hamzavi, I.H., Eds.; Elsevier: Amsterdam, The Netherlands, 2022; pp. 201–207.
24. Aderibigbe, B.A.; Buyana, B. Alginate in Wound Dressings. *Pharmaceutics* **2018**, *10*, 42. [CrossRef] [PubMed]
25. Agarwal, A.; McAnulty, J.F.; Schurr, M.J.; Murphy, C.J.; Abbott, N.L. Polymeric materials for chronic wound and burn dressings. In *Advanced Wound Repair Therapies*; Woodhead Publishing Limited: Sawston, UK, 2011; pp. 186–208.
26. Weller, C.; Weller, C.; Team, V. 4—Interactive dressings and their role in moist wound management. In *Advanced Textiles for Wound Care*, 2nd ed.; Rajendran, S., Ed.; Woodhead Publishing: Sawston, UK, 2019; pp. 105–134.
27. Huang, Y.-C.; Yang, C.-Y.; Chu, H.-W.; Wu, W.-C.; Tsai, J.-S. Effect of alkali on konjac glucomannan film and its application on wound healing. *Cellulose* **2015**, *22*, 737–747. [CrossRef]
28. Chen, H.; Lan, G.; Ran, L.; Xiao, Y.; Yu, K.; Lu, B.; Dai, F.; Wu, D.; Lu, F. A novel wound dressing based on a Konjac glucomannan/silver nanoparticle composite sponge effectively kills bacteria and accelerates wound healing. *Carbohydr. Polym.* **2018**, *183*, 70–80. [CrossRef] [PubMed]
29. Ganapathy, N.; Venkataraman, S.S.; Daniel, R.; Aravind, R.J.; Kumarakrishnan, V.B. Molecular biology of wound healing. *J. Pharm. Bioallied Sci.* **2012**, *4* (Suppl. S2), S334–S337. [CrossRef]
30. Wu, H.; Bu, N.; Chen, J.; Chen, Y.; Sun, R.; Wu, C.; Pang, J. Construction of Konjac Glucomannan/Oxidized Hyaluronic Acid Hydrogels for Controlled Drug Release. *Polymers* **2022**, *14*, 927. [CrossRef]
31. Nam, S.; French, A.D.; Condon, B.D.; Concha, M. Segal crystallinity index revisited by the simulation of X-ray diffraction patterns of cotton cellulose Iβ and cellulose II. *Carbohydr. Polym.* **2016**, *135*, 1–9. [CrossRef]
32. Albrecht, S.; van Muiswinkel, G.C.J.; Schols, H.A.; Voragen, A.G.J.; Gruppen, H. Introducing Capillary Electrophoresis with Laser-Induced Fluorescence Detection (CE-LIF) for the Characterization of Konjac Glucomannan Oligosaccharides and Their in Vitro Fermentation Behavior. *J. Agric. Food Chem.* **2009**, *57*, 3867–3876. [CrossRef]
33. Alves, A.; Miguel, S.P.; Araujo, A.; de Jesús Valle, M.J.; Sánchez Navarro, A.; Correia, I.J.; Ribeiro, M.P.; Coutinho, P. Xanthan Gum-Konjac Glucomannan Blend Hydrogel for Wound Healing. *Polymers* **2020**, *12*, 99. [CrossRef]
34. Zhou, L.; Xu, T.; Yan, J.; Li, X.; Xie, Y.; Chen, H. Fabrication and characterization of matrine-loaded konjac glucomannan/fish gelatin composite hydrogel as antimicrobial wound dressing. *Food Hydrocoll.* **2020**, *104*, 105702. [CrossRef]
35. Doloff, J.C.; Veiseh, O.; de Mezerville, R.; Sforza, M.; Perry, T.A.; Haupt, J.; Jamiel, M.; Chambers, C.; Nash, A.; Aghlara-Fotovat, S.; et al. The surface topography of silicone breast implants mediates the foreign body response in mice, rabbits and humans. *Nat. Biomed. Eng.* **2021**, *5*, 1115–1130. [CrossRef]
36. Nguyen, H.M.; Ngoc Le, T.T.; Nguyen, A.T.; Thien Le, H.N.; Pham, T.T. Biomedical materials for wound dressing: Recent advances and applications. *RSC Adv.* **2023**, *13*, 5509–5528. [CrossRef] [PubMed]
37. Qin, J.; Li, M.; Yuan, M.; Shi, X.; Song, J.; He, Y.; Mao, H.; Kong, D.; Gu, Z. Gallium(III)-Mediated Dual-Cross-Linked Alginate Hydrogels with Antibacterial Properties for Promoting Infected Wound Healing. *ACS Appl. Mater. Interfaces* **2022**, *14*, 22426–22442. [CrossRef] [PubMed]
38. Yang, L.; Zhao, Q.; Guo, Z.; Liu, Y.; Gao, W.; Pu, Y.; He, B. Konjac glucomannan hydrogel dressing and its combination with Chinese medicine for the wound treatment. *New J. Chem.* **2022**, *46*, 23077–23087. [CrossRef]
39. Wardhani, D.H.; Puspitosari, D.; Ashidiq, M.A.; Aryanti, N.; Prasetyaningrum, A. Effect of deacetylation on functional properties of glucomannan. *AIP Conf. Proc.* **2017**, *1855*, 030020.
40. Nunes, R.C.R. 13—Rubber nanocomposites with nanocellulose. In *Progress in Rubber Nanocomposites*; Thomas, S., Maria, H.J., Eds.; Woodhead Publishing: Sawston, UK, 2017; pp. 463–494.
41. Varshney, N.; Sahi, A.K.; Poddar, S.; Vishwakarma, N.K.; Kavimandan, G.; Prakash, A.; Mahto, S.K. Freeze–Thaw-Induced Physically Cross-linked Superabsorbent Polyvinyl Alcohol/Soy Protein Isolate Hydrogels for Skin Wound Dressing: In Vitro and In Vivo Characterization. *ACS Appl. Mater. Interfaces* **2022**, *14*, 14033–14048. [CrossRef]

42. Yamamoto, O.; Nagashima, M.; Nakata, Y.; Udagawa, E. The Significant Potential ofSimonkolleite Powder for Deep Wound Healing under a Moist Environment: In Vivo Histological Evaluation Using a Rat Model. *Bioengineering* **2023**, *10*, 375. [CrossRef]
43. Li, Y.; Wei, S.; Chu, H.; Jian, H.; Anand, A.; Nain, A.; Huang, Y.; Chang, H.; Huang, C.; Lai, J. Poly-quercetin-based nanoVelcro as a multifunctional wound dressing for effective treatment of chronic wound infections. *Chem. Eng. J.* **2022**, *437*, 135315. [CrossRef]
44. DiPietro, L.A. Angiogenesis and wound repair: When enough is enough. *J. Leukoc. Biol.* **2016**, *100*, 979–984. [CrossRef]

pharmaceuticals

MDPI

Article

Topical Biocomposites Based on Collagen, Hyaluronic Acid and Metronidazole as Periodontitis Treatment

Madalina Georgiana Albu Kaya [1], Alice Geanina Simonca [2], Ileana Rau [2], Alina Elena Coman [1,*], Minodora Maria Marin [2,*], Lacramioara Popa [3,4], Roxana Trusca [2], Cristina-Elena Dinu-Pirvu [3,4] and Mihaela Violeta Ghica [3,4]

1 Department of Collagen, National Research and Development Institute for Textiles and Leather—Division of Leather and Footwear Research Institute, 93 Ion Minulescu Str., 031215 Bucharest, Romania; albu_mada@yahoo.com

2 Faculty of Chemical Engineering and Biotechnology, National University of Science and Technology Politehnica Bucharest, 1-7 Gh. Polizu Street, 011061 Bucharest, Romania; simoncaalice@gmail.com (A.G.S.); ileana.rau@upb.ro (I.R.); roxana_doina.trusca@upb.ro (R.T.)

3 Department of Physical and Colloidal Chemistry, Faculty of Pharmacy, "Carol Davila" University of Medicine and Pharmacy, 6 Traian Vuia Str., 020956 Bucharest, Romania; lacramioara.popa@umfcd.ro (L.P.); cristina.dinu@umfcd.ro (C.-E.D.-P.); mihaela.ghica@umfcd.ro (M.V.G.)

4 Innovative Therapeutic Structures Research and Development Centre (InnoTher), "Carol Davila" University of Medicine and Pharmacy, 6 Traian Vuia Str., 020956 Bucharest, Romania

* Correspondence: coman.alina27@yahoo.com (A.E.C.); minodora.marin@ymail.com (M.M.M.); Tel.: +40-742535359 (A.E.C.); +40-764724044 (M.M.M.)

Abstract: Background: It is well known that periodontitis affects the gums and surrounding connective tissue. The chronic inflammatory response induced by bacteria in the gingival tissue leads to the loss of the collagen connection between the tooth and the bone and ultimately to bone loss. Methods: In this context, the aim of this research was the obtaining and characterization of a drug release supports in the form of sponges based on collagen, hyaluronic acid as a support and metronidazole as an antibiotic for the treatment of periodontitis. The sponges were characterized by FT-IR spectroscopy, water uptake, contact angle, SEM microscopy, in vitro metronidazole release analysis from sponges and data modeling. Results: The results showed that all the sponges had a porous structure with interconnected pores, the pore sizes being influenced by hyaluronic acid and metronidazole; the spongious structure became much more dense for samples with metronidazole content. All metronidazole-loaded sponges showed good surface wettability and an adequate swelling capacity for a suitable antimicrobial release at the periodontal pocket. The porous structures allow a controlled release, fast in the first hour, essential to control the initial microbial load at the periodontal level, which continues slowly in the following hours to ensure an effective treatment of periodontitis. Conclusions: Correlating all physical–chemical and bio-pharmaceutical results obtained, a promising solution for periodontitis treatment could be a met-ronidazole–collagen–hyaluronic system consisting of 1% collagen, 1.5% metronidazole and 0.8% hyaluronic acid, and in vitro and in vivo tests are recommended to continue studies.

Keywords: metronidazole; collagen sponges; hyaluronic acid; sustained drug release; periodontitis; freeze-drying

1. Introduction

Periodontitis affects the gingiva and surrounding connective tissue and represents a cellular inflammatory disease that destroys these tissues and bones that support teeth. The connective tissue, the periodontium, consists of four components: the cementum, the periodontal ligament (PDL), the alveolar bone, and the gingiva. Chronic adult periodontitis appears due to bacterial accumulations on teeth. The bacterially induced chronic inflammatory response in the gingival tissue leads to a loss in collagen connection between the tooth and the bone, and finally to bone losses [1–3].

The severe form of chronic periodontitis is a globally widespread pathology of the human oral cavity in the adult population, and affects almost 11% of the worldwide population, making it the sixth most prevalent disease of humanity [4–6]. Studies have shown that between 2011 and 2020, periodontitis impacted roughly 60% of the population, with about 24% of those suffering from the severe form. These studies demonstrate an extremely significant growth when compared to forecasts from 1990 to 2010 [7–9].

According to severity and progression, the present diagnostic classification of periodontitis is split into four phases and three grades. An appropriate periodontal therapy modality can be used once a patient's case has been properly classified.

Nowadays, non-surgical and surgical treatments, paired with pharmacological adjuncts are used in conventional periodontal therapies [10–12]. Scaling, root planning, and antibiotics are examples of treatments that may be used if the periodontitis is not advanced. Dental surgery, including flap surgery, soft tissue grafts, bone grafts, guided tissue regeneration, and tissue-stimulating proteins, could be necessary if the periodontitis is advanced [13–15].

Antibiotics treat infections by eradicating or stunting the growth of bacteria and other organisms, but they have many side effects, from minor allergic reactions to serious, incapacitating adverse outcomes, when ingested. Local treatments with antibiotics can be used in addition to oral therapy to prevent secondary effects of the latter [16–19].

Current antibacterial local therapy, commercially available, can be applied by the patient at home, or in a dental clinic. These local forms of antibacterial drug therapy can also be divided into non-sustained, sustained and controlled release systems. The active agent in the non-sustained systems is released immediately; supra and sub-gingival irrigation solutions are included here. On the other hand, sustained systems contain a high concentration of active agent released for an extended period. In order to provide a safe, efficient, long-lasting, and convenient drug delivery impact, sustained drug release systems, represent a prolonged and slow drug release. Biocomposites based on polymers are highly investigated for sustained release of an encapsulated active ingredient, especially hydrophilic and hydrophobic polymers [20,21], and core–shell structures [22].

The last category, controlled release systems, includes semi-solid systems (chips, films, strips), fibers, and nano or microparticle systems that incorporate the active ingredient in the delivery medium and are placed in the periodontal pocket by an expert in a dental office; these systems will gradually release adequate concentrations of the active ingredient over a period longer than 24 h [23–26].

According to scientific results obtained so far, this paper presents a new biomaterial, a sustained drug release system, with collagen, hyaluronic acid and metronidazole for periodontitis local treatment. The collagen we propose for this study is type I and of bovine origin, the most abundant type in the organism [27]. It is well known that the periodontium contains collagen and hyaluronic acid, leading to a better acceptance of this proposed composite by the organism.

Collagen represents the primary component and support for the periodontium. Collagen constitutes 60% of gingival tissues, 70–80% of the periodontal ligament, and 90% of the alveolar bone matrix [28–30]. Another important component that exists in all periodontal tissues is hyaluronic acid in different amounts. Gingiva and the periodontal ligament are more abundant in hyaluronic acid than cement and alveolar bone are [31]. The antibacterial and anti-inflammatory properties of hyaluronic acid lead to its use in periodontitis treatments [32].

The scientific literature presents many systems for locally applied periodontitis treatment, but none of them include collagen, hyaluronic acid and metronidazole in the same medical device. For example, for guided tissue regeneration (GTR), blended hydrogels composed of polyvinyl alcohol and fish collagen were prepared as GTR membranes [33] and for nanosystem treatment, metronidazole-loaded electrospun polylactide stereo complex nanofiber mats were successfully fabricated using the electrospinning process for treatment of periodontal disease [34]. Also, nanofibers with trilayer eccentric side-by-side structures, obtained through multiple-fluid electrospinning, represent a potential candidate to treat periodontitis [35].

According to our previous studies, the designed collagen hydrogels with metronidazole in different concentrations preserved the collagen triple helix structure, while the addition of strontium ranelate in the formulation led to a structural alteration. The kinetic parameters, the cumulative drug released percentage and the diffusion coefficient for the collagen hydrogels containing only metronidazole are influenced by the drug concentration, the best results being obtained for the sample containing 1.5% metronidazole-medium concentration level [36]. Also, other studies proved that an MTZ concentration higher than 2% induces an increase in the hydrogel viscosity, leading to a resistance of the drug diffusion through the polymeric network.

The aim of this research was to obtain and characterize some spongious collagen–hyaluronic acid supports with metronidazole in order to evaluate the physical–chemical, structural, and morphological properties as well as the drug deliverability in order to be used as a biomaterial for periodontitis.

2. Results and Discussion

The samples of collagen sponge with and without HA and MTZ were evaluated by morphology, structure and properties of support for drug delivery and the results are presented below.

2.1. FT-IR Spectroscopy for M1–M6 Sponges

The FT-IR for M1–M6 samples and for the main components of samples are presented in Figure 1.

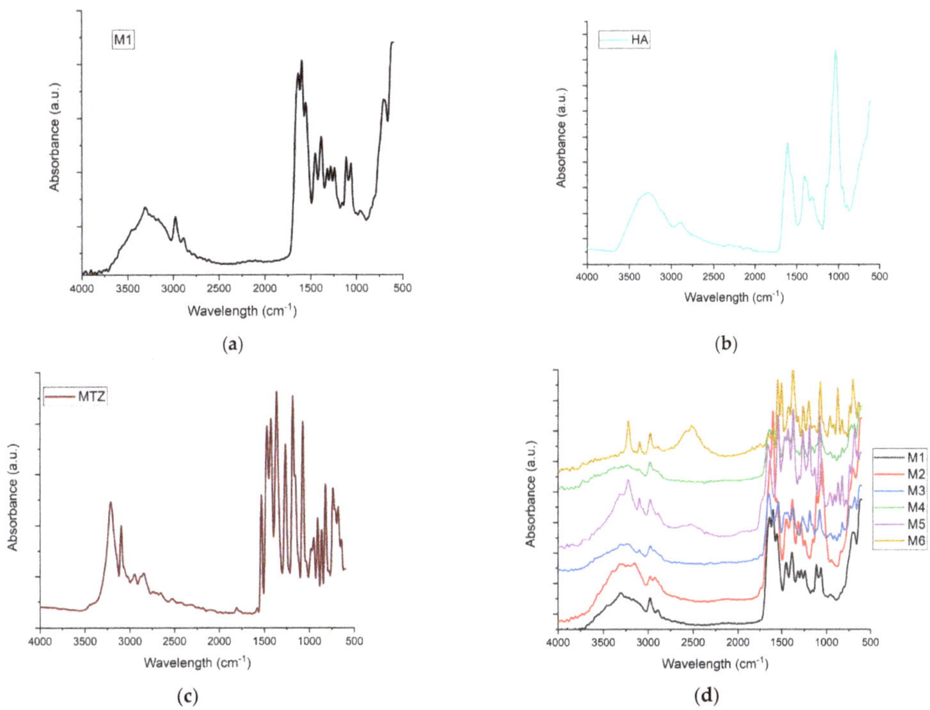

Figure 1. The FT-IR spectra for (**a**) M1 collagen; (**b**) HA-HA; (**c**) MTZ-MTZ; (**d**) the spongious matrices M1-M6.

The FT-IT spectra for collagen control (Figure 1a) show Amide A and B at 3309 and 2889 cm^{-1}, respectively, and Amide I, II and III at 1635, 1554 and 1451 cm^{-1} as our previous results showed for collagen. HA presents a broad band around 3272 cm^{-1} which is assigned to the O-H groups and a peak at 1606 cm^{-1} associated with C-O stretching of carboxylate anion [37]. The control sample of MTZ (MTZ) showed a characteristic vibrational peak for C-H stretching at 3211 cm^{-1}. The peaks at 1586 and 1530 cm^{-1} were assigned to C=C and C=N stretching, respectively. The N=O asymmetric stretching was assigned to peak at 1473 cm^{-1}, and the C-C stretching peak was assigned to peak at 1428 cm^{-1}. The absorption peaks at 1364 cm^{-1} were assigned to CH_3 bending and N=O asymmetric stretching, respectively. Further, absorption peaks at 1265, 1073 and 738 cm^{-1} were assigned to C-O stretching, C-N stretching, and =C-H bending, respectively. FT-IR data of control MTZ was well supported by the literature data [38]. The influence of MTZ on the samples is more evident in the samples which contain HA. The FT-IR proved that MTZ does not change the triple helical collagen structure as our previous results showed [36] but that there is a clear interaction between MTZ and HA, as the water absorption and contact angle showed. The characteristic vibrational peak for C-H stretching at 3223 cm^{-1} is very highlighted for samples M4 and M6, meanwhile for samples M3 and M5, which contain the same amount of MTZ, it is visible at the same intensity. Also of interest is the peak of 2400 cm^{-1}, which can be assigned to new crosslinking, more intense for the M6 than for the M4 sample and does not appear for the other sample. Comparing FT-IR spectra of M6 and M4, that peak is due to the higher presence of MTZ in sample M6.

2.2. *Scanning Electron Microscopy (SEM) of M1–M6 Sponges*

The SEM microscopy presents the spongious structure with interconnected pores for all the samples as Figure 2 shows. The control sponge, M1, showed a structure based on fibrils which form pores with sizes between 50 and 150 μm (Figure 2a). The addition of HA forms a structure with higher porosity and smaller pore sizes, the majority being about 100 μm (Figure 2b). Figure 2c proves the compact structure when the MTZ is added. At higher magnitudes (×2000 in Figure 2d and ×5000 in Figure 2e), the presence of MTZ on collagen fibrils is clearly visible. The M4 sponge looks like the most homogenous sample (Figure 2f); this can be due to the presence of hyaluronic acid. The pore sizes become smaller than the others without MTZ or HA and the MTZ is still visible on the fibrils of collagen.

The water absorption showed that the M5 and M6 samples became more compact, and less absorbent because of the higher amount of MTZ. This is visible by SEM in Figure 2h,i where the MTZ is in excess, the porous structure is very compact, and the size and form of pores are not so clear anymore.

2.3. *Water Uptake Ability of M1–M6 Sponges*

The water absorption results are presented in Figure 3 for all samples during 90 min, being at equilibrium after that period of time.

The controlled sample, M1, which contained only crosslinked collagen, uptook over 38 g/g water from the first moments and reached equilibrium at about 44 g/g, after one hour. The sample M2, which contained both collagen and HA, uptook about 37 g/g water in the first minutes, reached equilibrium in 10 min, and kept it for half an hour; then, the samples lost their weight in a slow degradation. A high statistical significance could be seen for samples that contained MTZ, all of which reduced their capacity of water absorption to less than half, uptaking about 18 g/g in the first minutes. The samples with a higher amount of MTZ uptook a smaller amount of water. This is because the MTZ is a lipophilic drug [39]. On the contrary, the samples with HA uptook a little bit more water than the ones without HA. Compared to the M1 matrix, it can be seen that the capacity to absorb the water of the M2 sample has a small variation in the first 45 min, followed by a significant decrease in the water uptake ability at 60 and 90 min. The samples with MTZ exhibit a highly significant decrease in the water absorption ability compared to the M1 sample, this behavior being related on the one hand to the presence of the drug and on the other hand to the presence in the same sample (M4 and M6) of the HA.

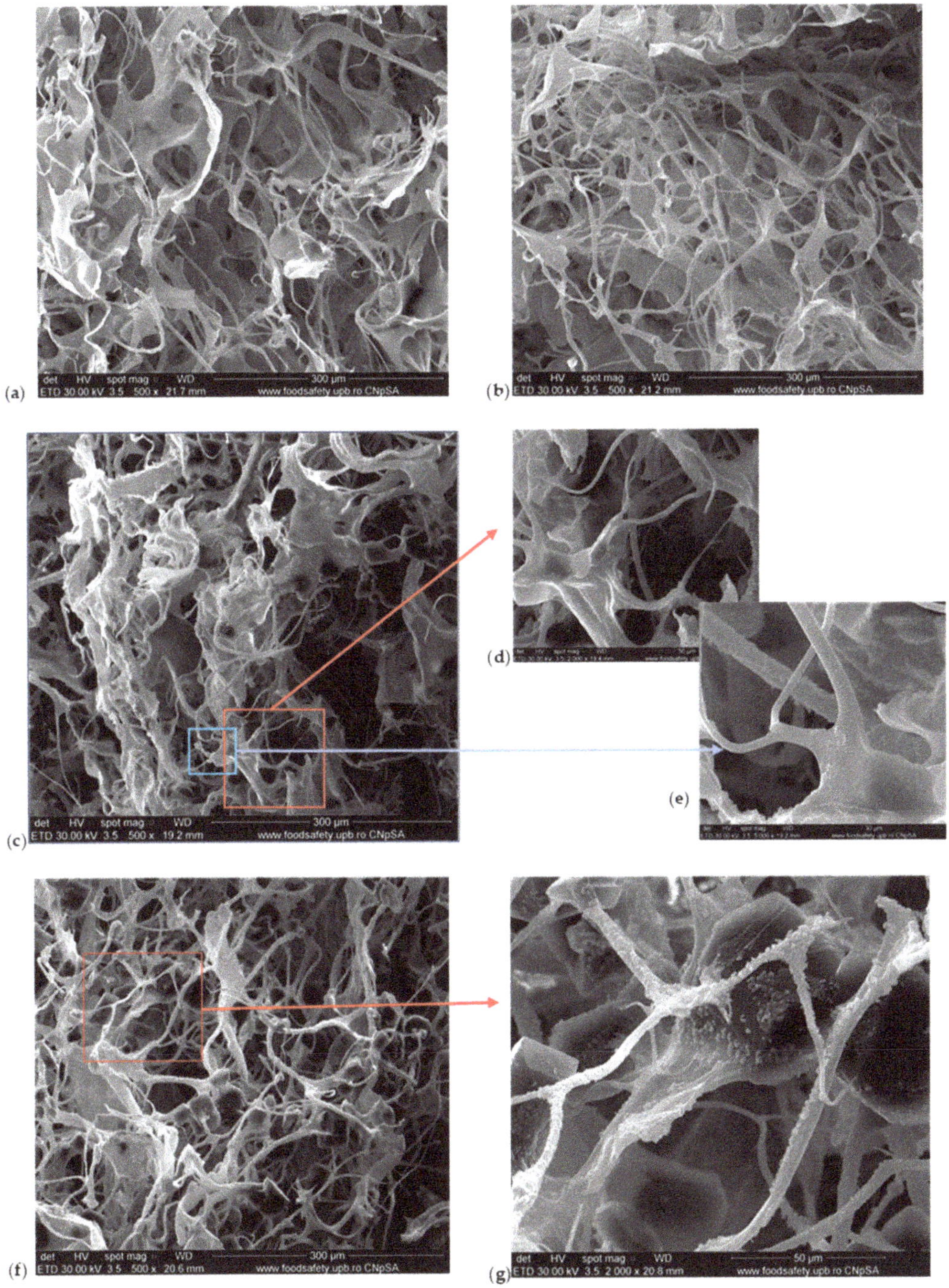

Figure 2. *Cont.*

(h) (i)

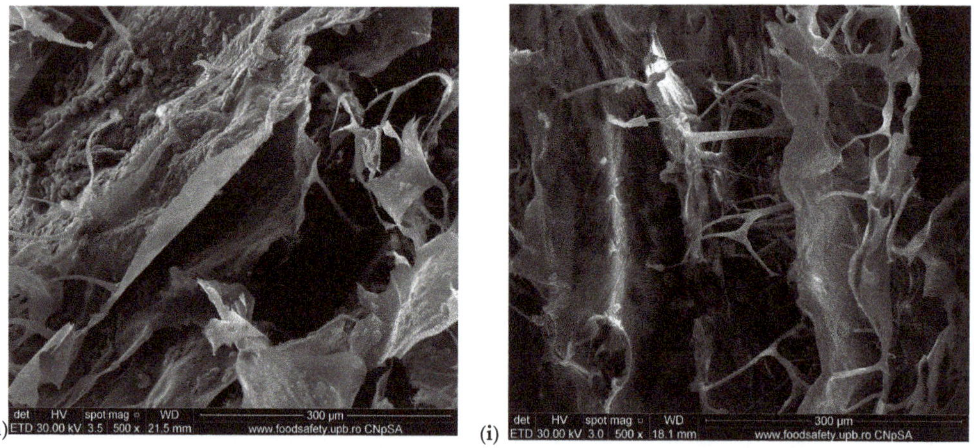

Figure 2. SEM images of M1–M6 sponges: (**a**) M1 (×500 magnification); (**b**) M2 (×500 magnification); (**c**) M3 (×500 magnification); (**d**) M3 (×2000 magnification); (**e**) M3 (×5000 magnification); (**f**) M4 (×500 magnification); (**g**) M4 (×2000 magnification); (**h**) M5 (×500 magnification); (**i**) M6 (×500 magnification).

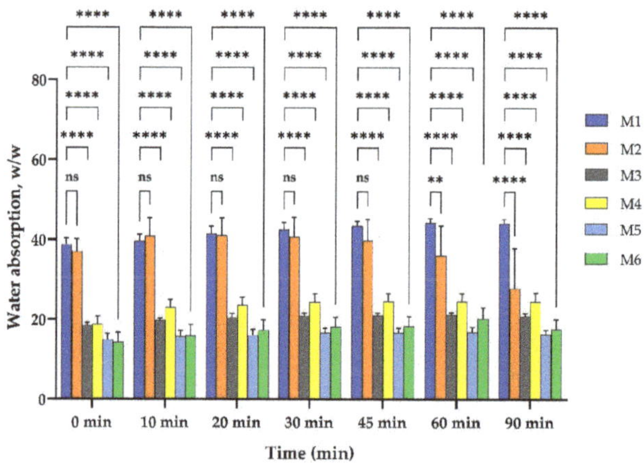

Figure 3. Water uptake ability of M1–M6 matrices. Results are not statistically significant (ns) for p-value > 0.05; results are statistically significant for p-value as follows: ** $p < 0.01$, **** $p < 0.0001$.

2.4. Contact Angle Evaluation of M1–M6 Sponges

The wetting behavior of the porous structure surface is important in different fields [40] including the medical one [41], and particularly for the design of spongious materials used as drug delivery supports [42]. The contact angle method was applied to determine the surface wetting ability of the sponges, with a lower contact angle value indicating a high hydrophilicity of the sponge surface [43]. The hydrophilicity is an important property facilitating the interaction between the sponge and biological environment [42], allowing both a rapid surface wetting and imbibition of the gingival crevicular fluid (GCF) within the drug release support. Due to the small values reported for the GCF, up to 8 μL under healthy conditions and up to 44 μL under inflammatory periodontal conditions [44,45], adequate sponge surface wetting is crucial for the penetration and diffusion of the dissolution liquid into the porous matrix structure, favoring the drug release from the supports.

In Figure 4 are illustrated examples of the drop shape images for the contact angle recorded for the tested sponges.

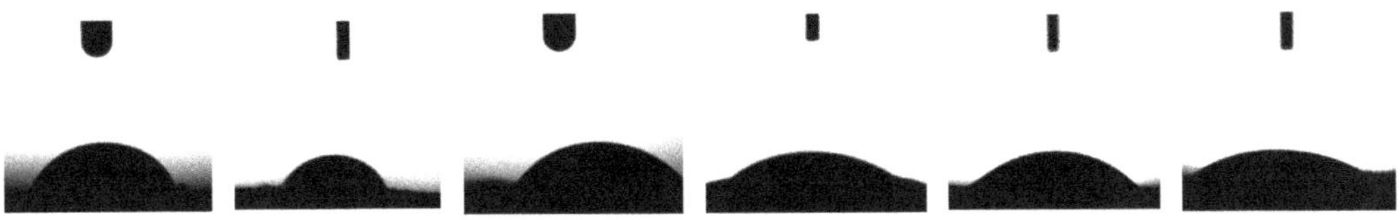

(a) 65.04 ± 2.42° (b) 55.59 ± 1.14° (c) 50.98 ± 1.09° (d) 38.51 ± 1.16° (e) 43.86 ± 1.36° (f) 28.71 ± 3.18°

Figure 4. Images of the drop shape and the corresponding contact angle mean values for the spongious matrices: (**a**) M1; (**b**) M2; (**c**) M3; (**d**) M4; (**e**) M5; (**f**) M6.

As can be seen from Figure 4, the sponge composition is reflected in the contact angle values obtained. The values recorded for the contact angles for all formulations were lower than 90°, ranging from 28.71 ± 3.18 (M6) to 65.04 ± 2.42° (M1). The highest value for the contact angle was noticed for the collagen sample without MTZ and HA, and the smallest one for the sample with a maximum concentration of drug and HA. The addition of HA (M2) in the formulation leads to a CA decrease of about 1.17 times reported in M1.

Analyzing the results obtained for the sponges M1, M3, and M5 based on collagen and MTZ, it can be seen that the presence of the drug at the inferior level in sample M3 leads to a CA decrease of about 1.27 times compared to M1, while the MTZ concentration of 2% generated a decrease of about 1.48 times. In the series M2, M4, and M6 with the presence of HA in the sponge formulation, a much higher decrease was observed, namely approximately 1.45 times for the M4 sponge (1.5% MTZ), and 1.94 times for the M6 sponge (2% MTZ), respectively, compared with the M2 sponge. One can remark that the presence of both MTZ and HA determined a higher hydrophilicity of the sponge surface, more obvious for a higher MTZ concentration. Comparing the samples M3 and M4 with 1.5% MTZ, and M5 and M6 with 2% MTZ, respectively, it can be observed that the CA value is more influenced by the presence of HA in the formulation (a decrease of about 1.34–1.2%), while evaluating sponges M3 and M5 and M4 and M6 ones, a higher drug concentration leads to a smaller CA decrease of approximately 1.16–1.32%. MTZ, a lipophylic drug, may not fully dominate the surface characteristics due to its dispersion within the collagen or HA matrix. Additionally, HA, which is known for its hydrophilic properties, likely offsets the hydrophobic tendencies of MTZ by enhancing the porosity and facilitating better surface wetting. This interplay results in the sponges showing improved wettability despite the presence of a hydrophobic drug.

On the other hand, it is known that the nature of porosity, such as pore size, distribution and interconnectivity, affects the contact angle. Smaller interconnected pores allow the liquid to imbibe more quickly, reducing the contact angle further. In contrast, larger or more isolated pores may slow down liquid penetration, resulting in higher initial contact angles [40,46]. Corroborating the results from the contact angle determination and the analysis of pore morphology using SEM analysis, it can be concluded that the inclusion of hyaluronic acid was found to increase the sponge's porosity, which corresponded to a significant decrease in contact angle values. This suggests that HA determined a more porous structure, and facilitated quicker liquid absorption, leading to a lower contact angle.

The obtained results showed a suitable hydrophilicity of all sponge surfaces. The combination of MTZ with other more hydrophilic materials, like HA, can overcome its hydrophobic nature, making the resulting material more suitable for biomedical applications. In the particular case of periodontal application, an adequate sponge surface wettability, as a critical key point for fluid absorption, facilitates the penetration of the gingival crevicular fluid into the porous structure and the subsequent diffusion of the drug through the polymer matrix architecture.

2.5. In Vitro Drug Release Analysis from Sponges and Data Modeling

An important aspect of the design and evaluation of antimicrobial-loaded topical biocomposite intended for periodontitis treatment is the investigation of the drug release characteristics.

Figure 5 illustrates the cumulative release profiles of the MTZ from the sponges in phosphate buffer pH 7.4 selected as in vitro release medium, compatible with the gingival fluid pH in periodontitis [47].

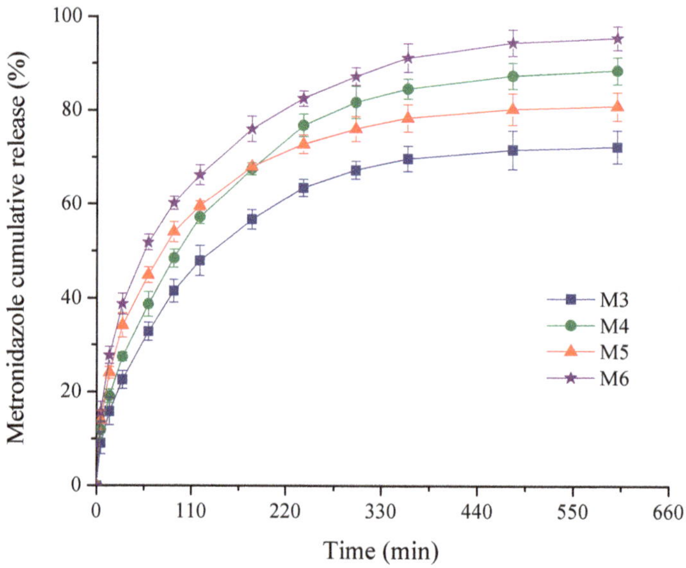

Figure 5. Plot of % cumulative drug release profiles from the sponges versus time.

As depicted in Figure 5, comparable kinetic patterns are obtained for the M3-M6 sponges with a variable composition in MTZ and HA. Thus, the drug delivery process was described by two different phases: an initial rapid release in the first 60 min, followed by the second stage of a slower and progressive release for the next 9 h.

For antimicrobial topical delivery, the biphasic kinetic profiles are targeted both for prophylactic and treatment of a periodontal infection [48–50]. The burst release effect is important to control the initial microbial load at the periodontal level, providing a rapid effect and attaining minimum inhibitory concentration (MIC) [50,51]. Among the pathogen bacteria incriminated in periodontitis, in accordance with the literature data, the least susceptibility was reported for the *Actinobacillus actinomycetemcomitans* (*Aggregatibacter actinomycetemcomitans*) [51]. This is the reason why, in the present work, we have chosen two higher MTZ concentrations to obtain a rapid burst release more than MIC of periodontal pathogenic bacteria. It is noticed that for the designed sponges with MTZ M3-M6, the released drug concentration after the first hour of the experiment was superior to the MIC reported [52] for the above periodontopathogen bacterium. The lowest burst release of 32.89% was obtained for the sponge M3 with lower MTZ concentration and without HA, while the highest value (51.91%) was recorded for the sponge M6 with higher MTZ concentration and HA.

The gradual and sustained MTZ release in the next hours further ensures the prevention of bacteria multiplication or invasion. With respect to the cumulative drug released percentage after 10 h of experiment, the sponges could be graded in the following order: M6 (95.57%) > M4 (88.59%) > M5 (80.98%) > M3 (72.36%). Comparing the results obtained for the samples M3 and M4, and M5 and M6, respectively, it seems that the drug released

(%) is affected by the presence of HA to a greater degree, an increase of about 1.20 times being recorded for the sponges M4 and M6, while the increase in the MTZ concentration in the sponge formulation has a smaller influence (Table 1).

Table 1. Correlation coefficients for different kinetic models; release kinetics parameters characteristics for the power law model and cumulative MTZ released percentage.

Sponges	Zero-Order Model			Higuchi Model			Power Law Model			Release Exponent	Kinetic Constant (1/min)	MTZ Released (%)
	R	Adj R^2	AIC_c	R	Adj R^2	AIC_c	R	Adj R^2	AIC_c			
M3	0.8701	0.7085	−46.18	0.9698	0.9290	−64.53	0.9841	0.9622	−72.74	0.37	0.077	72.36
M4	0.8796	0.7286	−42.07	0.9742	0.9390	−61.48	0.9862	0.9672	−69.55	0.37	0.089	88.59
M5	0.8295	0.6260	−41.27	0.9504	0.8842	−56.51	0.9845	0.9633	−71.47	0.30	0.131	80.98
M6	0.8511	0.6695	−38.97	0.9621	0.9109	−56.02	0.9897	0.9757	−72.90	0.31	0.141	95.57

Related to different reported studies, Kida et al. [52] performed an in vitro MTZ release from porous matrices, based on gelatin and two cellulose derivatives (carboxy methylcellulose and hydroxyethyl cellulose), over a period of 2 h. A burst release effect was noticed for all samples, more obvious in the first 20 min for the hydroxyethyl cellulose-based matrices. After an MTZ-loaded matrix single intra-pocket application, positive clinical results were obtained, indicating the local administration of the designed formulations as a promising alternative to the systemic one.

Panday et al. [53] described some MTZ microemulsion-loaded hydrogel for periodontitis prevention. The kinetic experiments were conducted over a period of 5 h, the released drug percentage varying from about 40 to 80%. The in vitro and ex vivo outcomes showed that the designed formulations could be effective in periodontitis treatment.

Hoang Nhan Ho et al. [54,55] reported that the MTZ release from different formulations (MTZ SLN-loaded HEC gel, MTZ SLNs and MTZ-loaded HEC gel) presented a considerable burst release effect, the amount of the drug delivered at 2 h varying from 61.41 to 91.05%. Moreover, the free drug (MTZ powder) was released more than 90% within 1 h. The MTZ incorporated free form in HEC gel was about 100% released after 3 h, while approximately 100% of the MTZ amount was released from the MTZ SLNs and MTZ SLN-loaded HEC gel at 24 h.

Besides the aforementioned works, different studies with MTZ-based formulations with a drug release extended more than 24 h were reported. Barat et al. [50] described chitosan inserts presenting an initial burst release of about 80% recorded at the end of 24 h (approximately 20% drug released in the first 4 h), independent of the formulation factors, followed by a sustained MTZ release in the next 6 days. In their paper, Jitrangsri et al. [55] developed an MTZ-loaded in situ forming matrix, using camphor as a matrix-forming agent. A variable burst release effect was noticed ranging from 20 to 80 in the first 6 h, followed by a sustained MTZ delivery reaching a maximum between 1.5 and 6 days, depending on the cosolvents. In another study, Khan et al. [56] developed biodegradable chitosan films based on MTZ and levofloxacin for periodontitis treatment. The cumulative MTZ release (%) was about 80% for the non-crosslinked films within 24 h, while for the crosslinked ones, it was less than 60%. After 24 h, the release was sustained and progressive up to 2–7 days depending on the crosslinking degree.

In this regard, it could be considered that our designed MTZ-loaded collagen sponges balanced well the effect of an initial rapid drug release with a gradual delivery for a longer period of time, essential for local antimicrobial therapy in periodontitis.

To predict the drug transport mechanism, different kinetic models were used, including the Higuchi, zero-order and power law models. The two primary metrics used to evaluate the goodness of fit of the kinetic models are the correlation coefficient (R) and adjusted R squared (R^2). Adjusted R^2 represents a relevant indicator when comparing the previous three models because, in addition to the evaluation of the goodness of fit, it also penalizes the kinetic models for their complexity. This aspect is essential when these three mathematical models are compared regarding their different complexities: the power law model involves more parameters (the release exponent n) than Higuchi and zero-order [57]. The R and adjusted R^2 values for all MTZ-loaded sponges according to the above model are listed in Table 1. The values obtained for the correlation coefficients showed that the drug release was best described by the power law model, with the R highest values ranging between 0.9841 and 0.9897, and the adjusted R^2 highest values varying from 0.9622 to 0.9757. The power law model presented the highest R and adjusted R^2 values compared to those of Higuchi and zero-order models, which means that this mathematical model is regarded to fit the experimental data better, considering the complexity of the model.

Moreover, we compared these kinetic models using a tool called Akaike Information Criterion (AIC) that is precisely designed to compare the models rather than a goodness of fit approach, which is best described by R and adjusted R^2. The AIC method generates numerical values which indicate both accuracy (goodness of fit) and precision (model variability) [58]. Considering the small number of experimental points, for kinetic analysis, the small-sample corrected AIC (AIC_c) was used. Thus, the model that best statistically represents the mechanism of the drug release is the one with the AIC_c lowest value [59]. As can be seen in Table 1, the smallest values of AIC_c are recorded for the power law model, which is regarded as a better fit for the data, taking into account the complexity of this model. Correlating all of these, the highest R and adjusted R^2 and the lowest AICc values were used to select the kinetic model with the best fit of the experimental data, which was the power law model.

The kinetic parameters specific to the power law model, namely release exponent and kinetic constant, are listed in Table 1. The release exponent values are smaller than 0.5 (varying from 0.31 to 0.37), indicating a deviation from the Higuchi model due to the complex processes that occur when the sponge comes into contact with the periodontal pocket. Initially, the drug retained onto or near the sponge surface (according to SEM images) is rapidly desorbed at contact with the crevicular gingival fluid, and then the absorption of the release medium in the porous structure takes place, followed by the polymer hydration and sponge swelling. This stage is associated with the burst release effect and is favored by an adequate sponge wetting ability, supported by the values of the contact angle smaller than 90° (varying between 28.71 and 50.98°), as well as by a suitable absorption in the first hour (Figure 1). Further, the diffusion-controlled release of the drug entrapped in the collagen fibrils (also concordant to images obtained from SEM analysis) takes place through the pores or channels within the polymer network, simultaneously with the gradual disintegration of the support [49,52]. This phase corresponds to the MTZ gradual and sustained release over the next 9 h of the experiment. We proposed for future investigations to use simulated crevicular gingival fluid in order to study the hydrophily, biodegradability and ability to release the drug.

3. Materials and Methods

3.1. Materials

Type I fibrillar collagen was extracted from calf hide using the technology currently available at the INCDTP-Division Leather and Footwear Research Institute—Collagen Department [60] with an initial concentration of 2.85% and acidic pH. Metronidazole (MTZ) was supplied from Hubei Hongyuan Pharmaceutical Technology Co., Ltd., Wuhan, China. Glutaraldehyde (GA) and hyaluronic acid (HA) were purchased from Sigma-Aldrich (Germany). All the experiments were carried out using ultra-pure water.

3.2. Methods

3.2.1. Preparation of Sponges by Freeze-Drying Hydrogels

The initial collagen gel (2.85%) was adjusted to a 1% (w/v) concentration and a pH of about 7.4 with 1 M sodium hydroxide solution and distilled water under mechanical stirring. Different proportions of MTZ and HA were added to the gel and then all the samples were crosslinked with 0.2% glutaraldehyde. The composition of hydrogels is presented below in Table 2.

Table 2. Composition of hydrogels (quantities of Coll, HA and MTZ are reported for 100 g gel).

Sample Code	Coll, %	MTZ, %	HA, %	GA, %
M1	1	0	0	0.2
M2	1	0	0.8	0.2
M3	1	1.5	0	0.2
M4	1	1.5	0.8	0.2
M5	1	2.0	0	0.2
M6	1	2.0	0.8	0.2

To obtain new sponges, the hydrogels presented in Table 2 were crosslinked, poured into glass Petri dishes with 5.2 cm diameter and left for 24 h at 4 °C and then the hydrogels were freeze-dried for 48 h using a Delta 2–24 LSC (Martin Christ, Osterode am Harz, Germany) as we previously described [61]. All the samples were used for further characterization, which is described below.

3.2.2. Fourier-Transform Infrared Spectrometry (FTIR) of Sponges

FTIR spectra were performed using a Vertex 70 Bruker FTIR spectrometer (Billerica, MA, USA) with an attenuated total reflectance (ATR) module. For the obtained samples, the FTIR spectra were recorded in the ATR-FTIR mode at a resolution of 4 cm^{-1} in 600–4000 cm^{-1} wave number region.

3.2.3. Scanning Electron Microscopy of Sponges

SEM analyses were performed on an FEI, Inspect F50 electron microscope equipped with a Schottky Field Emission source and an EDS detector, in the primary electron beam, on samples covered with a thin gold layer.

3.2.4. Water Uptake of Sponges

For the water absorption determination, the collagen samples were placed in water and maintained at a temperature of 37 °C. At fixed time intervals, the samples were withdrawn and weighed. The water absorption was determined using the equation (Equation (1)):

$$\%Water\ uptake = \frac{Wt - Wd}{Wd} \times 100(g/g) \quad (1)$$

where *Wd* represents the weight of the dry samples and *Wt* is the weight of the swollen samples at immersion time t. The experiments were conducted in triplicate.

3.2.5. Sponge Contact Angle Evaluation

The sponge surface properties were monitored through contact angle (CA) measurements, performed with a KSV Cam 101 Scientific Instrument, and the protocol was reported in our previous work [42,62]. Measurements were taken on smooth, representative areas to minimize the effects of porosity and surface irregularities. Young equation's (Equation (2)) was used for the contact angle evaluation:

$$\gamma_S = \gamma_{SL} + \gamma_L \cos\theta \quad (2)$$

where γ_S represents the surface tension of the solid, γ_{SL} is the solid/liquid interfacial tension, γ_L is the surface tension of the liquid, and θ is the contact angle made by the liquid drop with the solid porous surface. Contact angles were recorded immediately after droplet deposition to reduce liquid penetration. The initial contact angle was used for analysis. A high-speed camera (5 frames/16 ms) captured the droplet behavior, using the FAST method for precise evaluation. The experiments were carried out in triplicate.

3.2.6. In Vitro Drug Release Analysis from Sponges and Data Modeling

The drug release characteristics from the designed sponges were investigated using a sandwich device adapted to dissolution equipment in conjunction with paddle stirrers (Esadissolver), in accordance with the method previously detailed [48]. Aliquots withdrawn at defined time points (5, 15, 30, 60, 90, 120, 180, 240, 300, 360, 480, and 600 min) were collected from the release vessel, and the MTZ content in each sample was spectrophotometrically evaluated (Perkin Elmer UV-Vis Spectrophotometer) at its maximum absorbance associated with a wavelength of 319 nm [36]. Each release experiment was performed in triplicate.

The % cumulative release profiles as a function of time were built. To analyze the release mechanism, the experimental data were fitted to the general power law model (Equation (3)):

$$\frac{m_t}{m_\infty} = k \times t^n \tag{3}$$

where m_t/m_∞ represents the fraction of MTZ released at time t, k is the release kinetic constant (min^{-1}) considering the geometric and structural traits specific to the dosage form, and n is the release exponent (dimensionless) showing the drug delivery mechanism. Two particular cases of this kinetic model, zero-order (n = 1) and Higuchi time square root model (n = 0.5), respectively, were also applied. For the Higuchi model, the drug diffusion rate through the polymeric network is much lower than that of polymer relaxation, while for the zero-order, the release rate is independent of time, and the polymer relaxation rate becomes the determining factor of the overall drug transport. When n has different values than 0.5 and 1, both rates are comparable, and the drug release is related to other processes which happen simultaneously [63,64].

3.2.7. Statistical Analysis

Statistical analysis was carried out with GraphPad Prism 10.3.1, TableCurve 2D vs. 01, and Excel 2016 software. The experimental data were declared as means ± standard deviations (SDs). Multiple comparisons between the groups were realized employing two-way ANOVA (analysis of variance) with a 0.05 significance level Dunnett test. The obtained results were considered statistically significant for *p*-values less than 0.05.

4. Conclusions

Periodontitis has a lot of complications such as tooth and bone loss and many researchers are focused on developing new materials to prevent and treat it. In this context, collagen sponges with different metronidazole and hyaluronic acid concentrations intended for periodontitis treatment were designed and characterized. The sponges presented good surface wettability and an adequate swelling capacity for a suitable antimicrobial release at the periodontal pocket. The modulation of the MTZ and HA concentrations in the sponge formulation could balance the aforementioned characteristics well. FT-IR spectroscopy data show that the influence of metronidazole is more evident in samples containing hyaluronic acid. The recorded FTIR spectra demonstrated that the presence of metronidazole does not change the triple helical structure of collagen, as shown by previous results, but there is a clear interaction between metronidazole and hyaluronic acid, as shown by the results regarding water absorption capacity and hydrophilic–hydrophobic balance. SEM microscopy shows the spongious structure with interconnected pores for all samples. The presence of metronidazole is clearly visible on the collagen fibrils and forms a denser structure. The drug was fast released in the first hour, essential to control the initial microbial load at the periodontal level, followed by a gradual and sustained release of metronidazole over the next hours ensuring further prevention of bacterial multiplication or invasion. The designed spongious forms could be a viable alternative for periodontitis treatment and a starting point for new metronidazole-based formulations. Correlating all physical–chemical and biopharmaceutical results obtained, a promising solution for periodontitis treatment could be a metronidazole–collagen–hyaluronic system consisting of 1% collagen, 1.5%

metronidazole and 0.8% hyaluronic acid, and in vitro and in vivo tests are recommended to continue studies.

Author Contributions: Conceptualization, I.R., A.E.C., M.M.M., M.G.A.K. and M.V.G.; Methodology, L.P., M.G.A.K. and M.V.G.; Formal analysis A.G.S., A.E.C., M.M.M., R.T., M.G.A.K. and M.V.G.; Investigation, A.G.S., A.E.C., M.M.M., L.P., R.T., C.-E.D.-P., M.G.A.K. and M.V.G.; Resources, C.-E.D.-P. and M.G.A.K.; Writing—original draft preparation, A.E.C., M.M.M. and M.G.A.K.; Writing—review and editing, I.R., A.E.C., M.G.A.K. and M.V.G.; Visualization, I.R., A.E.C., M.M.M., R.T., C.-E.D.-P., M.G.A.K. and M.V.G.; Supervision, I.R., A.E.C., M.M.M., L.P., R.T., C.-E.D.-P., M.G.A.K. and M.V.G.; and Project administration, C.-E.D.-P. and M.G.A.K.; All authors have read and agreed to the published version of the manuscript.

Funding: This research received no external funding.

Institutional Review Board Statement: Not applicable.

Informed Consent Statement: Not applicable.

Data Availability Statement: Data is contained within the article.

Acknowledgments: This paper was financially supported by Carol Davila University of Medicine and Pharmacy Bucharest, Romania, through Contract No. CNFIS-FDI-2024-F-0570, and by a grant of the Ministry of Research, Innovation and Digitalization, project number PN 23 26 01 01/2023.

Conflicts of Interest: The authors declare no conflicts of interest.

References

1. Loesche, W. Dental Caries and Periodontitis: Contrasting Two Infections That Have Medical Implications. *Infect. Dis. Clin. N. Am.* **2007**, *21*, 471–502. [CrossRef] [PubMed]
2. Tatakis, D.N.; Kumar, P.S. Etiology and Pathogenesis of Periodontal Diseases. *Dent. Clin. N. Am.* **2005**, *49*, 491–516. [CrossRef] [PubMed]
3. Offenbacher, S.; Barros, S.P.; Singer, R.E.; Moss, K.; Williams, R.C.; Beck, J.D. Periodontal Disease at the Biofilm–Gingival Interface. *J. Periodontol.* **2007**, *78*, 1911–1925. [CrossRef] [PubMed]
4. Dubey, P.; Mittal, N. Periodontal Diseases—A Brief Review. *Int. J. Oral Health Dent.* **2020**, *6*, 177–187. [CrossRef]
5. Sanz, M.; D'Aiuto, F.; Deanfield, J.; Fernandez-Aviles, F. European Workshop in Periodontal Health and Cardiovascular Disease—Scientific Evidence on the Association between Periodontal and Cardiovascular Diseases: A Review of the Literature. *Eur. Heart J. Suppl.* **2010**, *12*, B3–B12. [CrossRef]
6. Kassebaum, N.J.; Bernabé, E.; Dahiya, M.; Bhandari, B.; Murray, C.J.L.; Marcenes, W. Global Burden of Severe Periodontitis in 1990–2010. *J. Dent. Res.* **2014**, *93*, 1045–1053. [CrossRef]
7. Marcenes, W.; Kassebaum, N.J.; Bernabé, E.; Flaxman, A.; Naghavi, M.; Lopez, A.; Murray, C.J.L. Global Burden of Oral Conditions in 1990–2010. *J. Dent. Res.* **2013**, *92*, 592–597. [CrossRef]
8. Kassebaum, N.J.; Smith, A.G.C.; Bernabé, E.; Fleming, T.D.; Reynolds, A.E.; Vos, T.; Murray, C.J.L.; Marcenes, W.; Abyu, G.Y.; Alsharif, U.; et al. Global, Regional, and National Prevalence, Incidence, and Disability-Adjusted Life Years for Oral Conditions for 195 Countries, 1990–2015: A Systematic Analysis for the Global Burden of Diseases, Injuries, and Risk Factors. *J. Dent. Res.* **2017**, *96*, 380–387. [CrossRef]
9. Trindade, D.; Carvalho, R.; Machado, V.; Chambrone, L.; Mendes, J.J.; Botelho, J. Prevalence of Periodontitis in Dentate People between 2011 and 2020: A Systematic Review and Meta-analysis of Epidemiological Studies. *J. Clin. Periodontol.* **2023**, *50*, 604–626. [CrossRef]
10. Caton, J.G.; Armitage, G.; Berglundh, T.; Chapple, I.L.C.; Jepsen, S.; Kornman, K.S.; Mealey, B.L.; Papapanou, P.N.; Sanz, M.; Tonetti, M.S. A New Classification Scheme for Periodontal and Peri-implant Diseases and Conditions—Introduction and Key Changes from the 1999 Classification. *J. Periodontol.* **2018**, *89*, S1–S8. [CrossRef]
11. Deas, D.E.; Moritz, A.J.; Sagun, R.S.; Gruwell, S.F.; Powell, C.A. Scaling and Root Planing vs. Conservative Surgery in the Treatment of Chronic Periodontitis. *Periodontol. 2000* **2016**, *71*, 128–139. [CrossRef] [PubMed]
12. Sheridan, R.A.; Wang, H.L.; Eber, R.; Oh, T.J. Systemic Chemotherapeutic Agents as Adjunctive Periodontal Therapy: A Narrative Review and Suggested Clinical Recommendations. *J. Int. Acad. Periodontol.* **2015**, *17*, 123–134. [PubMed]
13. Kwon, T.; Lamster, I.B.; Levin, L. Current Concepts in the Management of Periodontitis. *Int. Dent. J.* **2021**, *71*, 462–476. [CrossRef] [PubMed]
14. Kao, R.T.; Nares, S.; Reynolds, M.A. Periodontal Regeneration—Intrabony Defects: A Systematic Review From the AAP Regeneration Workshop. *J. Periodontol.* **2015**, *86*, S77–S104. [CrossRef]
15. Hämmerle, C.H.F.; Jung, R.E.; Feloutzis, A. A Systematic Review of the Survival of Implants in Bone Sites Augmented with Barrier Membranes (Guided Bone Regeneration) in Partially Edentulous Patients. *J. Clin. Periodontol.* **2002**, *29*, 226–231. [CrossRef]

16. Jain, N.; Jain, G.K.; Javed, S.; Iqbal, Z.; Talegaonkar, S.; Ahmad, F.J.; Khar, R.K. Recent Approaches for the Treatment of Periodontitis. *Drug Discov. Today* **2008**, *13*, 932–943. [CrossRef]
17. Mura, S.; Nicolas, J.; Couvreur, P. Stimuli-Responsive Nanocarriers for Drug Delivery. *Nat. Mater.* **2013**, *12*, 991–1003. [CrossRef]
18. Wei, Y.; Deng, Y.; Ma, S.; Ran, M.; Jia, Y.; Meng, J.; Han, F.; Gou, J.; Yin, T.; He, H.; et al. Local Drug Delivery Systems as Therapeutic Strategies against Periodontitis: A Systematic Review. *J. Control. Release* **2021**, *333*, 269–282. [CrossRef]
19. Fenton, O.S.; Olafson, K.N.; Pillai, P.S.; Mitchell, M.J.; Langer, R. Advances in Biomaterials for Drug Delivery. *Adv. Mater.* **2018**, *30*, 1705328. [CrossRef]
20. Zhang, Z.; Liu, H.; Yu, D.-G.; Bligh, S.-W.A. Alginate-Based Electrospun Nanofibers and the Enabled Drug Controlled Release Profiles: A Review. *Biomolecules* **2024**, *14*, 789. [CrossRef]
21. Dong, R.; Gong, W.; Guo, Q.; Liu, H.; Yu, D.-G. Synergistic Effects of Radical Distributions of Soluble and Insoluble Polymers within Electrospun Nanofibers for an Extending Release of Ferulic Acid. *Polymers* **2024**, *16*, 2614. [CrossRef] [PubMed]
22. Chen, Y.; Gong, W.; Zhang, Z.; Zhou, J.; Yu, D.-G.; Yi, T. Reverse Gradient Distributions of Drug and Polymer Molecules within Electrospun Core–Shell Nanofibers for Sustained Release. *Int. J. Mol. Sci.* **2024**, *25*, 9524. [CrossRef]
23. Rajeshwari, H.R.; Dhamecha, D.; Jagwani, S.; Rao, M.; Jadhav, K.; Shaikh, S.; Puzhankara, L.; Jalalpure, S. Local Drug Delivery Systems in the Management of Periodontitis: A Scientific Review. *J. Control. Release* **2019**, *307*, 393–409. [CrossRef]
24. Mandlik, V.; Jha, A. Periochip. *Med. J. Armed Forces India* **2007**, *63*, 368–369. [CrossRef]
25. John, P. Adjunctive Effects of A Piscean Collagen-Based Controlled-Release Chlorhexidine Chip in the Treatment of Chronic Periodontitis: A Clinical and Microbiological Study. *J. Clin. Diagn. Res.* **2015**, *9*, ZC70–ZC74. [CrossRef] [PubMed]
26. Paolantonio, M.; D'Angelo, M.; Grassi, R.F.; Perinetti, G.; Piccolomini, R.; Pizzo, G.; Annunziata, M.; D'Archivio, D.; D'Ercole, S.; Nardi, G.; et al. Clinical and Microbiologic Effects of Subgingival Controlled-Release Delivery of Chlorhexidine Chip in the Treatment of Periodontitis: A Multicenter Study. *J. Periodontol.* **2008**, *79*, 271–282. [CrossRef] [PubMed]
27. Vancea, C.-V.; Grosu-Bularda, A.; Cretu, A.; Hodea, F.-V.; Al-Falah, K.; Stoian, A.; Chiotoriu, A.L.; Mihai, C.; Hariga, C.S.; Lascar, I.; et al. Therapeutic Strategies for Nerve Injuries: Current Findings and Future Perspectives. Are Textile Technologies a Potential Solution? *Ind. Textila* **2022**, *73*, 704–712. [CrossRef]
28. Melcher, A.H. On the Repair Potential of Periodontal Tissues. *J. Periodontol.* **1976**, *47*, 256–260. [CrossRef]
29. Ali, M.; Yang, F.; Plachokova, A.S.; Jansen, J.A.; Walboomers, X.F. Application of Specialized Pro-resolving Mediators in Periodontitis and Peri-implantitis: A Review. *Eur. J. Oral Sci.* **2021**, *129*, e12759. [CrossRef]
30. Binlateh, T.; Thammanichanon, P.; Rittipakorn, P.; Thinsathid, N.; Jitprasertwong, P. Collagen-Based Biomaterials in Periodontal Regeneration: Current Applications and Future Perspectives of Plant-Based Collagen. *Biomimetics* **2022**, *7*, 34. [CrossRef]
31. Embery, G.; Waddington, R.J.; Hall, R.C.; Last, K.S. Connective Tissue Elements as Diagnostic Aids in Periodontology. *Periodontol 2000* **2000**, *24*, 193–214. [CrossRef] [PubMed]
32. Gontiya, G.; Galgali, S. Effect of Hyaluronan on Periodontitis: A Clinical and Histological Study. *J. Indian Soc. Periodontol.* **2012**, *16*, 184. [CrossRef] [PubMed]
33. Zhou, T.; Zheng, K.; Sui, B.; Boccaccini, A.R.; Sun, J. In Vitro Evaluation of Poly (Vinyl Alcohol)/Collagen Blended Hydrogels for Regulating Human Periodontal Ligament Fibroblasts and Gingival Fibroblasts. *Int. J. Biol. Macromol.* **2020**, *163*, 1938–1946. [CrossRef] [PubMed]
34. Srithep, Y.; Akkaprasa, T.; Pholharn, D.; Morris, J.; Liu, S.-J.; Patrojanasophon, P.; Ngawhirunpat, T. Metronidazole-Loaded Polylactide Stereocomplex Electrospun Nanofiber Mats for Treatment of Periodontal Disease. *J. Drug Deliv. Sci. Technol.* **2021**, *64*, 102582. [CrossRef]
35. Zhao, P.; Zhou, K.; Xia, Y.; Qian, C.; Yu, D.-G.; Xie, Y.; Liao, Y. Electrospun Trilayer Eccentric Janus Nanofibers for a Combined Treatment of Periodontitis. *Adv. Fiber Mater.* **2024**, *6*, 1053–1073. [CrossRef]
36. Simonca, A.G.; Kaya, M.G.A.; Rău, I.; Marin, M.M.; Dinu-Pîrvu, C.-E.; Ghica, M.V. The Influence of the Formula-Tion Factors on the Design and Characterization of Some Collagen-Based Hydrogels with Metronidazole. *Sci. Bull. -Univ. Politeh. Buchar. Ser. B* **2023**, *85*, 43–52.
37. Manju, S.; Sreenivasan, K. Conjugation of Curcumin onto Hyaluronic Acid Enhances Its Aqueous Solubility and Stability. *J. Colloid. Interface Sci.* **2011**, *359*, 318–325. [CrossRef]
38. Kumar Trivedi, M. Spectroscopic Characterization of Biofield Treated Metronidazole and Tinidazole. *Med. Chem.* **2015**, *5*, 7. [CrossRef]
39. Bahman, M.; Jalili, H.; Etesam, M.; Amrane, A. Investigation of Pharmaceutical Compounds (Metronidazole, Rosuvastatin and Codeine Phosphate) Removal by Synechocystis Sp. PCC6803 Microalga. *J. Water Process Eng.* **2022**, *47*, 102820. [CrossRef]
40. Krainer, S.; Hirn, U. Contact Angle Measurement on Porous Substrates: Effect of Liquid Absorption and Drop Size. *Colloids Surf. A Physicochem. Eng. Asp.* **2021**, *619*, 126503. [CrossRef]
41. Menzies, K.L.; Jones, L. The Impact of Contact Angle on the Biocompatibility of Biomaterials. *Optom. Vis. Sci.* **2010**, *87*, 387–399. [CrossRef] [PubMed]
42. Ghica, M.V.; Albu, M.G.; Popa, L.; Moisescu, S. Response Surface Methodology and Taguchi Approach to Assess the Combined Effect of Formulation Factors on Minocycline Delivery from Collagen Sponges. *Die Pharm. Int. J. Pharm. Sci.* **2013**, *68*, 340–348.
43. Xia, G.; Zhai, D.; Sun, Y.; Hou, L.; Guo, X.; Wang, L.; Li, Z.; Wang, F. Preparation of a Novel Asymmetric Wettable Chitosan-Based Sponge and Its Role in Promoting Chronic Wound Healing. *Carbohydr. Polym.* **2020**, *227*, 115296. [CrossRef] [PubMed]

44. Bergamo, A.Z.; Nelson-Filho, P.; Romano, F.L.; da Silva, R.A.; Saraiva, M.C.; da Silva, L.A.; Matsumoto, M.A. Gingival Crevicular Fluid Volume and Periodontal Parameters Alterations after Use of Conventional and Self-Ligating Brackets. *J. Orthod.* **2016**, *43*, 260–267. [CrossRef]
45. Drummond, S.; Canavarro, C.; Perinetti, G.; Teles, R.; Capelli, J. The Monitoring of Gingival Crevicular Fluid Volume during Orthodontic Treatment: A Longitudinal Randomized Split-Mouth Study. *Eur. J. Orthod.* **2012**, *34*, 109–113. [CrossRef]
46. Holm, R.; Borkenfelt, S.; Allesø, M.; Andersen, J.E.T.; Beato, S.; Holm, P. Investigation of Surface Porosity Measurements and Compaction Pressure as Means to Ensure Consistent Contact Angle Determinations. *Int. J. Pharm.* **2016**, *498*, 355–361. [CrossRef] [PubMed]
47. Zhao, J.; Wei, Y.; Xiong, J.; Liu, H.; Lv, G.; Zhao, J.; He, H.; Gou, J.; Yin, T.; Tang, X.; et al. A Multiple Controlled-Release Hydrophilicity Minocycline Hydrochloride Delivery System for the Efficient Treatment of Periodontitis. *Int. J. Pharm.* **2023**, *636*, 122802. [CrossRef]
48. Tihan, G.T.; Rău, I.; Zgârian, R.G.; Ungureanu, C.; Barbaresso, R.C.; Kaya, M.G.A.; Dinu-Pîrvu, C.; Ghica, M.V. Oxytetracycline versus Doxycycline Collagen Sponges Designed as Potential Carrier Supports in Biomedical Applications. *Pharmaceutics* **2019**, *11*, 363. [CrossRef]
49. Ioan, D.-C.; Rău, I.; Albu Kaya, M.G.; Radu, N.; Bostan, M.; Zgârian, R.G.; Tihan, G.T.; Dinu-Pîrvu, C.-E.; Lupuliasa, A.; Ghica, M.V. Ciprofloxacin-Collagen-Based Materials with Potential Oral Surgical Applications. *Polymers* **2020**, *12*, 1915. [CrossRef]
50. Barat, R.; Srinatha, A.; Pandit, J.; Anupurba, S.; Mittal, N. Chitosan Inserts for Periodontitis: Influence of Drug Loading, Plasticizer and Crosslinking on in Vitro Metronidazole Release. *Acta Pharm.* **2007**, *57*, 469–477. [CrossRef]
51. Ghavami-Lahiji, M.; Shafiei, F.; Najafi, F.; Erfan, M. Drug-Loaded Polymeric Films as a Promising Tool for the Treatment of Periodontitis. *J. Drug Deliv. Sci. Technol.* **2019**, *52*, 122–129. [CrossRef]
52. Kida, D.; Karolewicz, B.; Junka, A.; Sender-Janeczek, A.; Duś, I.; Marciniak, D.; Szulc, M. Metronidazole-Loaded Porous Matrices for Local Periodontitis Treatment: In Vitro Evaluation and In Vivo Pilot Study. *Appl. Sci.* **2019**, *9*, 4545. [CrossRef]
53. Pandey, S.; Das, U.; Patil, A. Formulation and Ex-Vivo Evaluation of Metronidazole Microemulsion Loaded Hydrogel for Prevention of Periodontitis. *J. Pharm. Investig.* **2014**, *44*, 225–236. [CrossRef]
54. Ho, H.N.; Le, H.H.; Le, T.G.; Duong, T.H.A.; Ngo, V.Q.T.; Dang, C.T.; Nguyen, V.M.; Tran, T.H.; Nguyen, C.N. Formulation and Characterization of Hydroxyethyl Cellulose-Based Gel Containing Metronidazole-Loaded Solid Lipid Nanoparticles for Buccal Mucosal Drug Delivery. *Int. J. Biol. Macromol.* **2022**, *194*, 1010–1018. [CrossRef]
55. Jitrangsri, K.; Lertsuphotvanit, N.; Kabthong, N.; Phaechamud, T. Metronidazole-Loaded Camphor-Based In Situ Forming Matrix for Periodontitis Treatment. *AAPS PharmSciTech* **2023**, *24*, 185. [CrossRef]
56. Khan, G.; Yadav, S.K.; Patel, R.R.; Nath, G.; Bansal, M.; Mishra, B. Development and Evaluation of Biodegradable Chitosan Films of Metronidazole and Levofloxacin for the Management of Periodontitis. *AAPS PharmSciTech* **2016**, *17*, 1312–1325. [CrossRef] [PubMed]
57. Kan, H.J.; Kharrazi, H.; Chang, H.-Y.; Bodycombe, D.; Lemke, K.; Weiner, J.P. Exploring the Use of Machine Learning for Risk Adjustment: A Comparison of Standard and Penalized Linear Regression Models in Predicting Health Care Costs in Older Adults. *PLoS ONE* **2019**, *14*, e0213258. [CrossRef]
58. Saffron, C.M.; Park, J.-H.; Dale, B.E.; Voice, T.C. Kinetics of Contaminant Desorption from Soil: Comparison of Model Formulations Using the Akaike Information Criterion. *Environ. Sci. Technol.* **2006**, *40*, 7662–7667. [CrossRef]
59. Romero, A.I.; Villegas, M.; Cid, A.G.; Parentis, M.L.; Gonzo, E.E.; Bermúdez, J.M. Validation of Kinetic Modeling of Progesterone Release from Polymeric Membranes. *Asian J. Pharm. Sci.* **2018**, *13*, 54–62. [CrossRef]
60. Albu, M.G. *Collagen Gels and Matrices for Biomedical Applications*; Lambert Academic Publishing: Saarbrücken, Germany, 2011.
61. Sleiman, L.; Lazăr (Popa), A.-D.; Albu-Kaya, M.; Marin, M.M.; Kaya, D.A.; Vasile, O.-R.; Dinescu, S. Development and Investigation of an Innovative 3D Biohybrid Based on Collagen and Silk Sericin Enriched with Flavonoids for Potential Wound Healing Applications. *Polymers* **2024**, *16*, 1627. [CrossRef]
62. Popa, L.; Ghica, M.V.; Albu, M.G.; Ortan, A.; Dinu-Pîrvu, C.E. Hysteresis of contact angle. Dynamic wettability studies of collagen and doxycycline porous matrices crosslinked with tannic acid. *Dig. J. Nanomater. Biostruct.* **2013**, *8*, 937–943.
63. Askarizadeh, M.; Esfandiari, N.; Honarvar, B.; Sajadian, S.A.; Azdarpour, A. Kinetic Modeling to Explain the Release of Medicine from Drug Delivery Systems. *ChemBioEng Rev.* **2023**, *10*, 1006–1049. [CrossRef]
64. Ștefania, M.; Albu Kaya, M.G.; Ghica, M.V.; Dinu-Pîrvu, C.; Popa, L.; Udeanu, D.I.; Mihai, G.; Enachescu, M. Collagen-Polyvinyl Alcohol-Indomethacin Biohybrid Matrices as Wound Dressings. *Pharmaceutics* **2018**, *10*, 224. [CrossRef] [PubMed]

pharmaceuticals

MDPI

Article

Development of Smart pH-Sensitive Collagen-Hydroxyethylcellulose Films with Naproxen for Burn Wound Healing

Elena-Emilia Tudoroiu [1,2], Mădălina Georgiana Albu Kaya [3,*], Cristina Elena Dinu-Pîrvu [1,2,*], Lăcrămioara Popa [1,2], Valentina Anuța [1,2], Mădălina Ignat [4], Emilia Visileanu [5], Durmuș Alpaslan Kaya [6], Răzvan Mihai Prisada [1,2] and Mihaela Violeta Ghica [1,2]

[1] Department of Physical and Colloidal Chemistry, Faculty of Pharmacy, "Carol Davila" University of Medicine and Pharmacy, 6 Traian Vuia Str., 020956 Bucharest, Romania; elena-emilia.tudoroiu@drd.umfcd.ro (E.-E.T.); lacramioara.popa@umfcd.ro (L.P.); valentina.anuta@umfcd.ro (V.A.); razvan.prisada@umfcd.ro (R.M.P.); mihaela.ghica@umfcd.ro (M.V.G.)

[2] Innovative Therapeutic Structures Research and Development Center (InnoTher), "Carol Davila" University of Medicine and Pharmacy, 6 Traian Vuia Str., 020956 Bucharest, Romania

[3] Department of Collagen, Division of Leather and Footwear Research Institute, National Research and Development Institute for Textiles and Leather, 93 Ion Minulescu Str., 031215 Bucharest, Romania

[4] Department of Testing and Quality Control, Division of Leather and Footwear Research Institute, National Research and Development Institute for Textiles and Leather, 93 Ion Minulescu Str., 031215 Bucharest, Romania; madalina.fleancu@yahoo.com

[5] National Research and Development Institute for Textiles and Leather, 16 Lucrețiu Pătrășcanu Str., 030508 Bucharest, Romania; e.visileanu@incdtp.ro

[6] Department of Field Crops, Faculty of Agriculture, Hatay Mustafa Kemal University, 31034 Antakya-Hatay, Turkey; dak1976@msn.com

* Correspondence: albu_mada@yahoo.com (M.G.A.K.); cristina.dinu@umfcd.ro (C.E.D.-P.); Tel.: +40-72-339-5108 (M.G.A.K.); +40-72-230-4894 (C.E.D.-P.)

Abstract: Background: Developing versatile dressings that offer wound protection, maintain a moist environment, and facilitate healing represents an important therapeutic approach for burn patients. **Objectives**: This study presents the development of new smart pH-sensitive collagen-hydroxyethylcellulose films, incorporating naproxen and phenol red, designed to provide controlled drug release while enabling real-time pH monitoring for burn care. **Methods**: Biopolymeric films were prepared by the solvent-casting method using ethanol and glycerol as plasticizers. **Results**: Orange-colored films were thin, flexible, and easily peelable, with uniform, smooth, and nonporous morphology. Tensile strength varied from 0.61 N/mm^2 to 3.33 N/mm^2, indicating improved mechanical properties with increasing collagen content, while wetting analysis indicated a hydrophilic surface with contact angle values between 17.61° and 75.51°. Maximum swelling occurred at pH 7.4, ranging from 5.65 g/g to 9.20 g/g and pH 8.5, with values from 4.74 g/g to 7.92 g/g, suggesting effective exudate absorption. In vitro degradation proved structural stability maintenance for at least one day, with more than 40% weight loss. Films presented a biphasic naproxen release profile with more than 75% of the drug released after 24 h, properly managing inflammation and pain on the first-day post-burn. The pH variation mimicking the stages of the healing process demonstrated the color transition from yellow (pH 5.5) to orange (pH 7.4) and finally to bright fuchsia (pH 8.5), enabling easy visual evaluation of the wound environment. **Conclusions**: New multifunctional films combine diagnostic and therapeutic functions, providing a promising platform for monitoring wound healing, making them suitable for real-time wound assessment.

Keywords: smart polymeric dressing; pH-sensitive films; phenol red indicator; colorimetric pH detection; drug release; burn wound healing

1. Introduction

Wound healing is a highly intricate regenerative process that relies on the coordinated actions of various tissues and cell types [1]. The pH level within the wound environment plays a crucial role in therapeutic wound care, as it not only indicates but also affects key physiological and biochemical processes involved in tissue remodeling [2]. Under normal conditions, the skin's surface maintains an acidic pH ranging from 4 to 6, which contributes to its protective barrier function and helps prevent microbial colonization [3]. However, this acidic environment can be easily disrupted by wounds, as they lead to the mixing of external skin fluids with the body's internal fluids, which have a pH of 7.4 [4].

Clinical studies have shown that initially, burns typically exhibit a more alkaline pH compared to unburned skin, with an average pH value between 8.1 and 8.5, due to cellular impairment, exudate accumulation, and bacterial colonization. This alkaline phase promotes bacterial growth and persistent inflammation, which can delay the healing process and increase the risk of infection [5–7]. Burn wounds that progress successfully toward healing shift back to a neutral pH and finally to an acidic environment. This acidic medium during the later stages of healing is associated with keratinocyte migration, fibroblast activity, angiogenesis, and epithelialization. Furthermore, an acidic pH promotes the release of oxygen, encourages the enzymatic activity necessary for skin tissue remodeling, and impedes bacterial proliferation [8,9]. These affirmations suggest that pH can serve as a reliable indicator of wound healing [10]. Given its significance, real-time monitoring of wound surface pH could play a crucial role in guiding clinical management and optimizing treatment strategies for improved healing outcomes [11].

Recent studies have explored colorimetric pH sensors for wound monitoring using various pH indicators. Kiti et al. [12] and Petkowska et al. [13] developed colorimetric pH-sensitive wound dressings based on biopolymers and pH indicators (anthocyanins from *Clitoria ternatea* flower and grape, respectively). However, while their systems successfully achieved visual wound pH monitoring, they did not incorporate active drug delivery functionalities. Additionally, neither study comprehensively addressed critical parameters for a wound dressing, such as wetting and swelling capacity, mechanical properties, enzymatic degradation behavior, or drug release kinetics. Liu et al. [14] described a pH-sensitive alginate/polyacrylamide hydrogel wound dressing, loaded with phenol red, achieving rapid color changes, yet lacking wetting behavior, degradation study, and drug delivery functionality to promote wound healing. In contrast, we developed a collagen-hydroxyethylcellulose-based biocomposite with dual function: (1) diagnostic—real-time pH wound monitoring through color change using phenol red and (2) therapeutic—localized controlled release of naproxen (NPX) to actively reduce inflammation and pain, providing a multifunctional platform for burn wound care. We performed a detailed characterization, including swelling tests at different pH levels, enzymatic degradation studies, and drug release profiles, offering a comprehensive physicochemical and biopharmaceutical evaluation not always present in the previously mentioned studies. Finally, we specifically targeted the clinically relevant pH range (5.5–8.5) for burn injuries, linking the dressing color changes with actual healing stages, thereby enhancing the clinical applicability of our system.

This study belongs to a complex research. Collagen-based materials have been widely acknowledged for their outstanding biocompatibility, biodegradability, and ability to promote wound healing [15,16]. As a key component of the extracellular matrix (ECM), collagen plays an essential role in tissue repair and regeneration [17,18]. However, despite its beneficial properties, collagen alone often lacks the necessary mechanical strength and stability for long-term wound coverage. To address these limitations, combining collagen with other polymers can improve its properties [19]. Considering all of the above, in the first stage of our research, we presented an extensive literature screening of cellulose derivative applications as wound dressings addressed for many types of wounds [20]. Starting with the major findings from this previous study, we selected two cellulose derivatives, methylcellulose (MC) and hydroxyethylcellulose (HEC), to combine them with collagen.

The development of polymer-based wound dressings is being studied continuously. The polymeric support has a fundamental role because it directly comes into contact with the wound exudates, which it can properly absorb to maintain a suitable moist environment to promote the healing process [21]. In the last years, multiple polymeric dressings have been developed based on various polymer combinations with clinical applications: human-like collagen, hyaluronic acid, and carboxylated chitosan hydrogels designed as burn wound dressing [22], collagen and gellan gum hydrogels for full-thickness burn injury therapy [23], chitosan nanocomposites for chronic tissue repair [24], hyaluronic acid hydrogels loaded with silver nanoparticles designed to prevent infection, facilitating burn healing [25], and collagen with basic fibroblast growth factor hydrogel, designed as a delivery system for second-degree burn treatment [26].

Considering all the literature research, in the second stage of our research, we designed some spongious matrices by mixing the collagen gel with MC/HEC gels in different ratios. The results showed that collagen and both cellulose derivatives were biocompatible and preserved the collagen native triple helix structure for a maximum content of 30% MC/HEC gels. Moreover, newly designed scaffolds exhibited suitable swelling and wettability capacity to absorb the wound exudates; these findings make these systems optimal supports for drug delivery and wound dressing applications [27].

In the third stage of our extensive research, based on the underexplored potential of HEC and our previous studies' results, we designed and optimized some spongious drug delivery systems, loaded with naproxen, using a 3-factor, 3-level Box-Behnken design, coupled with response surface methodology. Naproxen, a non-selective non-steroidal anti-inflammatory drug (NSAID), was selected as an anti-inflammatory drug model due to its well-known pharmacological action in managing inflammation and pain, both symptoms being critical in the acute phase (24–48 h) of the healing process of a burn injury [28]. Commonly, NSAIDs, including NPX and their selective cyclooxygenase-2 (COX-2) inhibitors, are described as active substances that inhibit prostaglandin production, reduce inflammation, and act as efficient painkillers [29,30]. Compared to COX-2 selective inhibitors, NPX is more frequently used in topical and localized delivery systems as a result of its suitable permeability and cutaneous tissue retention [31]. Previous studies have strongly formulated this anti-inflammatory drug in hydrogels [32–36], films [37,38], and nanofibers [39] for localized therapy. Accordingly, when NPX is applied topically, it has low toxicity, with limited systemic absorption, which means reduced side effects on the gastrointestinal and cardiovascular levels [32,33]. The use of selective COX-2 inhibitors in topical wound care is limited. Furthermore, regarding the beneficial therapeutic effect on wound healing of selective COX-2 inhibitors, there are few reported studies where some of these drugs (celecoxib and meloxicam) had severe side effects (hepatic toxicity, exaggerated inflammatory processes) on wounded mice [40], a negative impact on wound healing (delaying the reepithelialization and the wound closure) [30,41]. Based on these findings, NPX was incorporated into these collagen-HEC spongious delivery systems to have a localized drug release that can provide targeted therapeutic action while minimizing systemic side effects [42]. That study continued with the optimization process using the Taguchi technique, and four optimal formulations were selected. Their regenerating effect on burn healing was in vivo demonstrated by applying them to experimentally induced burns on Wistar rats (manuscript under review).

Based on the previous results regarding the beneficial anti-inflammatory and epithelializing effects on animals of the optimal formulations, in this study, we developed some smart pH-sensitive films according to the optimal compositions to monitor the pH variation, which can provide important information for burn status and care. The pH indicator dye was phenol red, whose changes in color vary with pH: in acidic pH, it is yellow, in neutral pH it is orange, and in alkaline pH, it is bright fuchsia [43,44]. These novel smart dressings focus on both monitoring burn healing with color transition depending on the pH wound and controlling the inflammation by delivering the anti-inflammatory drug in a controlled manner.

2. Results and Discussion

2.1. Physical Evaluation of pH-Sensitive Films

The resulting pH-sensitive film dressings were found to be orange-colored because the final pH of the collagen-HEC hydrogels before drying was between 7.2 and 7.4, the physiological pH, where the color of the phenol red indicator is orange. Films were flexible, odorless, without air bubbles, being easily peelable from Petri dishes. One important property of biopolymeric films is their transparency, which is essential for an optimal wound dressing because it allows the physician to monitor the evolution of the healing process [45]. The main physical characteristics of film dressings are presented in Table 1.

Table 1. Physical evaluation of pH-sensitive film dressings.

Film Code	Transparency	Air Bubbles	Flexibility	Peelability
F1	✓	×	✓	✓
F2	✓	×	✓	✓
F3	✓	×	✓	✓
F4	✓	×	✓	✓

The pH-sensitive films developed for burn wound healing and tissue regeneration should have a uniform thickness to ensure consistent mechanical properties [45]. The thickness of the prepared films is primarily influenced by an appropriate homogenization of polymer gels and plasticizers and by a homogeneous distribution of the drug in the film structure. Moreover, the thickness is also controlled by the quantity of hydrogels that are poured into the Petri dishes and by the flatness of the used molds. To ensure a regular distribution of all components, the prepared gels were vigorously mixed before pouring them into the Petri dishes. For every sample, an equal amount of hydrogels was used to cast the pH-sensitive films, and the hydrogels were dried on a flat surface. The results are presented in Table 2. Film thickness values were quite close, ranging from 0.12 mm for F3 to 0.19 mm for F1.

Table 2. Thickness and mechanical characterization of pH-sensitive film dressings.

Film Code	Thickness (mm)	Tensile Strength (N/mm^2)
F1	0.19	0.61
F2	0.16	3.33
F3	0.12	1.56
F4	0.16	0.62

2.2. Mechanical Characterization

Mechanical properties of film dressings play a substantial role in establishing the film's structural integrity during its application at the lesion site, which is a predominant factor in regulating the target wound [46,47]. Film dressings must be able to endure the applied stress on the injury area and must present large resistance to swelling or motion-caused deformation to avoid damage by exudate absorption and by the movement of the patient. The ductility behavior was quantified through the determination of tensile strength [14].

The results obtained from the mechanical testing are shown in Table 2. The values of tensile strength ranged from 0.61 for F1 to 3.33 for F2. The F2 sample with maximum collagen gel and crosslinking agent concentrations presented the highest tensile strength value. The absence of HEC gel and the presence of 100% collagen gel provided a dense and structurally strong membrane, which significantly improved the mechanical strength. This behavior can be assigned to the unique structural characteristics of collagen. Its specific triple-helix configuration, stabilized by extensive hydrogen bonding and covalent crosslinks, contributed to higher tensile strength and structural rigidity [48–50]. Moreover, the crosslinking reaction of collagen with glutaraldehyde (GA) strengthened the polymer network by inserting more covalent bonds, which improved the mechanical durability [51]. These molecular interactions demonstrated the higher tensile strength of films based on 100% collagen gel compared to the samples that also contain HEC gel. Glutaraldehyde was used in very low concentrations (0.005 and 0.010%), which completely reacted with the amine groups of collagen, with the formation of new covalent crosslinks. With the entire consumption of glutaraldehyde during the crosslinking reaction, we did not have an excess of the crosslinking agent in the final formulations, so no residuals were predicted to remain. Accordingly, the quantification of glutaraldehyde residuals was not performed. This approach encourages the safety of the newly designed pH-sensitive films for burn wound application, with the maintenance of their structural integrity when they come in contact with the injury exudates.

For F1, F3, and F4 formulations, the mechanical properties are lower than those of F2, this behavior is due to the presence of 15–30% HEC gel. This polymer is more soluble in water and mechanically weaker than collagen, thus reducing the mechanical properties of films compared to F2. Although F1 and F3 had the same polymer composition, F3 had a tensile strength 2.55 times higher than F1. It would be expected that the presence of GA in F1 could increase the tensile strength compared to F3. However, F3 was more resistant to breakage, suggesting that the low GA (0.005%) from F1 was not sufficient to crosslink the collagen molecule in the presence of a high quantity of HEC gel. This phenomenon could be attributed to the possible physical and chemical interactions of HEC with GA crosslinking sites, as presented in previous studies [52–54]. Even though F4 had more collagen gel than F1 and the same GA concentration, the tensile strength value of F4 was similar to F1, indicating that the decrease in HEC gel content did not improve the tensile strength.

Taking into account all the findings, it can be concluded that F2 was the strongest film, with the best mechanical properties, being ideal for wound applications where structural stability and mechanical durability are desired. F3 exhibited moderate mechanical traits, with higher elasticity, representing an adequate alternative for flexible wound dressings if some stretchability is required. The least mechanically strong were F1 and F4, but they still can be an option for highly flexible wound dressings, where the structural support is not as necessary.

2.3. Scanning Electron Microscopy (SEM)

The surface morphology represents a fundamental feature of wound dressings. Accordingly, the surface morphology and the microstructure of the biopolymeric films were examined by scanning electron microscopy. SEM analysis produced high-resolution images that revealed intricate details about the fiber and drug distribution, porosity, and surface topography [55]. This analysis also offered information about the distribution of the drug through the polymeric network, which is important for the drug release performance in the healing process. The micrographs of the designed pH-sensitive film dressings are shown in Figure 1.

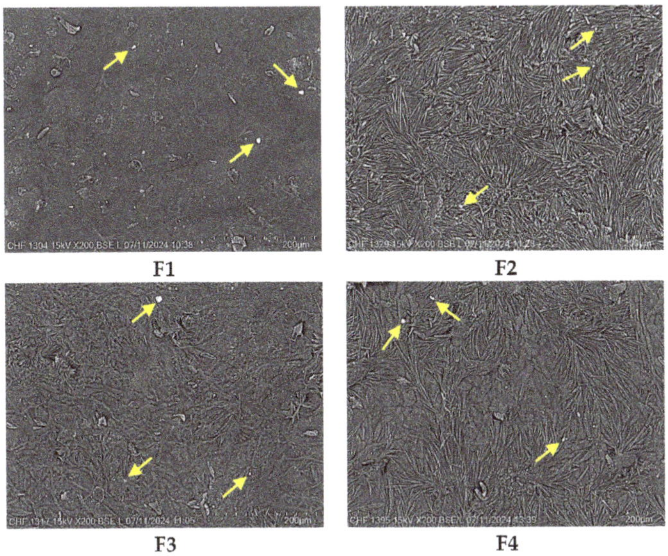

Figure 1. SEM micrographs of pH-sensitive film dressings at 200× magnification, scale bar of 200 μm. Yellow arrows indicated the presence of the drug particles on the surface of the film.

Commonly, the morphology of the film dressings should seem homogeneous and regular to establish uniform distribution of the drug into the biopolymeric blend (Figure 1). All formulations appeared to have a quite smooth, compact, nonporous, and continuous surface, suggesting a regular molecular network. The micrographs of the blended films illustrated a homogeneous morphology without cracks, voids, friable areas, agglomerations, or phase separation between the components. The smooth appearance of the films could be attributed to the use of an oven without a vacuum for the samples' drying [56].

However, small parts of the surface of the films seemed to be slightly rough because, during the drying process, intermolecular and convective forces occurred [57]. This aspect was more obvious when the drug was added, with the presence of its particles on the surface (white spots), which were highlighted through the yellow arrows in the SEM images (Figure 1). The roughness of films could also be influenced by the polymeric composition. Thus, the F2 sample with 100% collagen gel was slightly rougher than the other samples containing 15–30% HEC gel. The appearance of surface roughness could also be assigned to the interaction between the collagen and GA for F1, F2, and F4. GA crosslinking happens principally through the reaction with the free amine groups present in the amino acid residues of collagen [58]. This interaction can lead to microstructural rearrangements and heterogeneity in the film network due to localized differences in crosslinking density, resulting in slight surface roughness [52]. The rough surface of film dressings can have a helpful role in the healing process because it promotes the differentiation, migration, and adhesion of the cells [59]. The rough surface promotes cell adhesion through the formation of more binding sites that enhance the attachment of keratinocytes, fibroblasts, and other cells involved in the restoration process of the skin. Film surface roughness also creates topographical keys that manage cell migration, promoting rapid coverage of the lesion area. Moreover, the rough surface can activate the differentiation of fibroblasts into myofibroblasts, accelerating the injury contraction and consequently its healing [60–62].

These findings suggested a high miscibility and mixture homogeneity between collagen and HEC gels, plasticizers, and NPX. Thus, pH-sensitive films seem to fulfill the content uniformity criteria.

2.4. Wettability Analysis

Wettability is a crucial factor that influences the interaction of wound dressings with biological tissues and the drug release profile [63]. For an ideal dressing, hydrophilic behavior is essential, facilitating the absorption of injury exudates and stimulating the healing process [64]. To investigate the wettability (hydrophilicity or hydrophobicity) of pH-sensitive films, contact angle (CA) is proposed as a valuable evaluation index [65]. When its value is less than 90°, a material has a hydrophilic nature, while a material is considered hydrophobic when the CA value is higher than 90° [51]. Moreover, very low (less than 50°) or very high (higher than 150°) CA values can characterize a material as superhydrophilic or superhydrophobic, respectively [66]. The wetting behavior of pH-sensitive film dressings is illustrated in Figure 2.

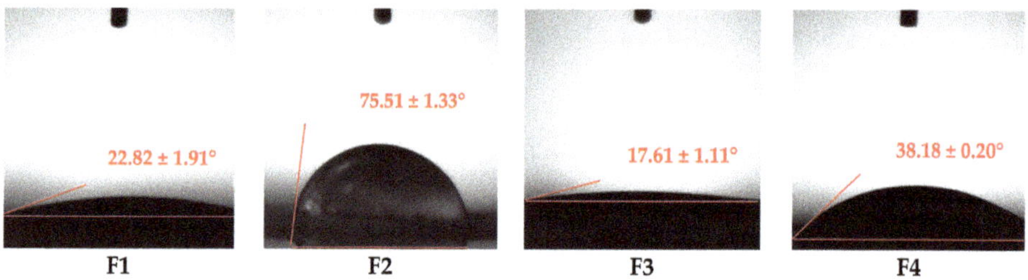

Figure 2. Water droplet contact angles registered on the surface of pH-sensitive film dressings. Values are mean ± SD (n = 3).

According to Figure 2, all films exhibited CA values lower than 90°, confirming their hydrophilic nature. CA values varied from 17.61 ± 1.11° for F3 to 75.51 ± 1.33° for F2.

The combination of two different polymers, collagen (natural) and HEC (semisynthetic), is advantageous because it increases the hydrophilicity of the developed films, as can be seen from the CA values obtained. This behavior can be explained through the following specific features: collagen is a highly hydrophilic polymer due to the presence of multiple polar amino acids in its molecule, which allow it to rapidly swell and retain water, maintaining its structural stability, without dissolving [67]. On the other hand, HEC, a cellulose derivative, also has a hydrophilic nature due to the many hydroxyethyl groups in its molecule, but compared to collagen, HEC is highly water soluble [68]. These findings are also well correlated with the swelling behavior regarding the high swelling capacity and the preservation of the structural integrity of the film dressings.

Considering the previously mentioned, the highest CA was registered for F2 due to the presence of maximum collagen gel and GA concentration, without HEC, and the lowest CA was noticed for F3, the formulation with the maximum content of HEC and without crosslinking agent. The cross-linking of F2 formed a more rigid and durable structure due to the formation of crosslinks between the collagen fibers. This chemical reaction explained the highest CA from all formulations.

The formulations with the maximum quantity of HEC gel (30%), F1 and F3, showed the smallest CA values, having a superhydrophilic nature. F1 had a slightly higher CA than F3 because F1 was crosslinked with GA, enhancing the mechanical strength [69]. The influence of polymer concentration is easily visible when comparing F1 with F4, which had the same concentration of NPX and GA but different concentrations of HEC gel; thus, F4 had a higher CA due to the smaller content of HEC gel (15%) compared to F1 (30%). Even if F4 had a higher CA than F1, it also exhibited superhydrophilic behavior.

Wettability analysis illustrated that the designed film dressings had high hydrophilicity, which is a desired property for the novel designed formulations.

2.5. Swelling Behavior

Swelling behavior represents a significant aspect of evaluating modern wound dressings because it indicates their capacity to interact with lesions' exudates under the influence of some external stimuli (pH, temperature, and ionic strength) [59]. An optimal swelling profile ensures the maintenance of a moist environment, prevents dehydration and inflammation, and facilitates painless dressing removal without destroying the newly formed epithelial tissue [70]. Furthermore, swelling behavior directly influences drug release rates and the structural integrity of the films in biological environments [21]. The swelling behavior in three different pH media—acidic for healthy skin (pH 5.5), neutral for the early-stage wound (pH 7.4), and alkaline for the post-burn wound (pH 8.5) [7]—was conducted to observe the pH response of films. The swelling behavior of pH-sensitive films performed for 72 h is shown in Figure 3.

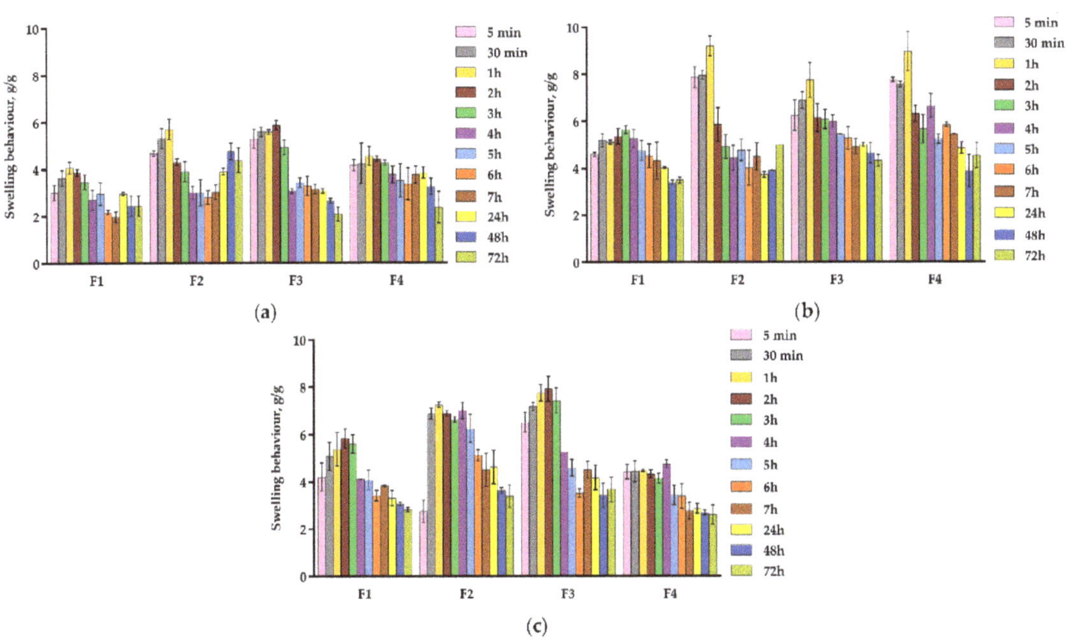

Figure 3. Swelling behavior of pH-sensitive film dressings in different pH media at room temperature for 72 h: (**a**) 5.5; (**b**) 7.4; (**c**) 8.5. Values are mean ± SD (n = 3).

As can be seen in Figure 3, all formulations remained intact even after 72 h in all three phosphate buffer solutions, meaning that the frequency of their removal at the lesion site can be reduced, thus enhancing the patients' life quality. When a film membrane is immersed in various pH media, it absorbs the solutions and swells. This process is representative of the healing process because wound dressing with an optimal swelling behavior will absorb the lesion exudate when it is applied to the wounded skin. This mechanism facilitates the drug release from the film structure, reducing inflammation and pain, and the collagen-HEC support that remains in the wound area stimulates the healing process [71].

The swelling analysis of all formulations showed distinct behavior due to the various structural and physico-chemical properties, as we explained in the wettability analysis. The combination of collagen with HEC enhanced the hydrophilic nature and the structural integrity of the prepared films [19]. The diffusion process is managed by the attraction between the solvent and the polymer chains [56]. The swelling behavior varied depending on pH, with prominent differences in peak swelling times, with higher swelling at pH 7.4 and 8.5 compared to pH 5.5 due to the differences in the electrostatic interactions between the chemical groups of the polymers and solvent. Generally, all formulations presented the highest swelling at neutral pH, followed by the alkaline and then the acidic ones. These findings confirm their application as wound dressings.

In the neutral medium, carboxylic acid and amide groups from the collagen molecule, respectively, and the hydroxyl groups from the HEC molecule exist in both forms, ionized and non-ionized. Negatively charged carboxylic acid and hydroxyl groups can form hydrogen linkages with both protonated amide groups or molecules of water, increasing the electrostatic repulsion, which causes the highest swelling behavior [72]. According to Figure 3, the highest swelling was recorded for F2 (9.20 g/g), F4 (8.96 g/g), and F3 (7.74 g/g) after 1h, followed by F1 (5.65 g/g) after 3 h.

On the other hand, at pH 8.5, the swelling values were slightly lower than those registered at pH 7.4; this behavior could be due to the deprotonation of functional groups [59]. Thus, the highest swelling was noticed for F3 (7.92 g/g) after 2 h, followed by F2 (7.25 g/g) after 1 h, F1 (5.84 g/g) after 2 h, and F4 (4.74 g/g) after 4 h.

The lowest swelling values were recorded at pH 5.5, where the protonation of the carboxylic acid and hydroxyl groups decreased the swelling behavior because of the stronger intermolecular interactions [59]. All samples showed the maximum swelling after 1 h as follows: F3 (6.07 g/g), F2 (5.70 g/g), F4 (4.54 g/g), and F1 (4.08 g/g).

At each pH level, after these maximum absorption points, each sample registered a consecutive slow decrease, reaching the equilibrium state, which indicated the stabilization of the film structure. These fast maximum absorptions, recorded for the three pH values in a short time interval between one and four hours, are beneficial to managing the burn exudates in the early stages of the wound, thus promoting the healing process.

At all pH values, F1 exhibited lower swelling than F3 (formulations with the same polymer and drug concentration but different GA amounts) due to the crosslinking effect of GA, generating a denser, more compact formulation, impeding the rapid penetration of the solutions through its structure [73]. When F1 is compared with F4 (samples with the same concentration of NPX and GA but different polymer ratios), the influence on swelling behavior of both hydrophilic polymers, but also of the pH media, is noticed. At pH 5.5 and 7.4, from Figure 3, it can be seen that F4 had a slightly higher swelling than F1, but F1 had a higher swelling at pH 8. At every pH, the highest swelling capacity was registered for F3 because it was the only uncrosslinked sample and had the maximum concentration of HEC gel (30%), conferring higher hydrophilicity. Due to the hydroxyl groups from the HEC molecule, the swelling behavior of F3 was the most significant due to the hydrogen bonds that formed with the aqueous solutions of phosphate buffer.

The highest swelling values at pH 7.4 and 8.5 indicate that the obtained formulations could be used as potential dressings for post-burn wounds.

2.6. In Vitro Enzymatic Biodegradation

In vitro enzymatic biodegradation is fundamental for evaluating wound dressings, ensuring their degradation rate aligns with the wound healing process [74]. Collagenase, a key enzyme present at the lesion site, degrades the collagen triple helix structure during the inflammatory phase, thereby stimulating tissue remodeling [75]. Moreover, this investigation provides insight into the structural integrity of the pH-sensitive films, a critical factor in determining the appropriate replacement rate of the dressing at the wound site. Figure 4 shows the variation of weight loss (%) over time for polymeric films.

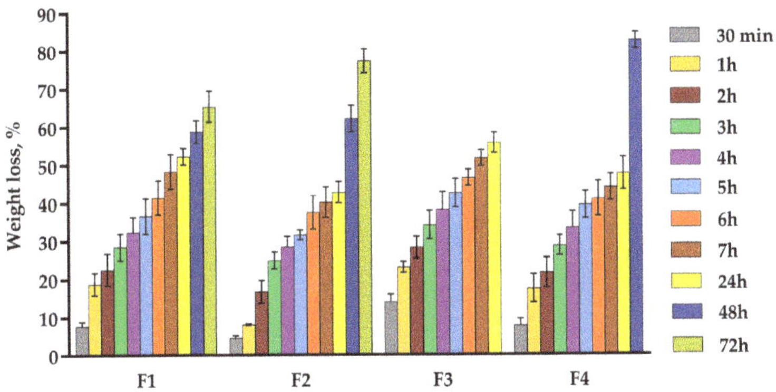

Figure 4. Weight loss of pH-sensitive film dressings in collagenase solution at 37 °C for 72 h. Values are mean ± SD (n = 3).

This analysis investigated the residual amount of film dressings after three days of incubation in collagenase solution. According to Figure 4, all samples registered a gradual increase in weight loss, with two of four formulations maintaining their structural stability after three days (F1 and F2), while F3 degraded after 24 h and F4 after 48 h.

The degradation rate of wound dressing has a meaningful effect on the drug release from the polymeric support and also on the replacement frequency of the wounded skin. After 24 h, F1 and F3 degraded more than 50%: 52.23% for F1 and 55.70% for F3. This behavior can be explained by the highest content of HEC gel in their composition, which is a very water-soluble polymer due to the multiple hydroxyl groups that are contained in its structure, being a cellulose derivative. Moreover, higher percentages of disintegration are also due to the small concentration of the crosslinking agent or its absence; thus, the samples are more exposed to degradation by the collagenase. F2 and F4 registered lower weight loss after one day: 42.78% for F2 and 47.64% for F4. The smallest weight loss of the F2 film can be explained by the 100% collagen gel content and the highest amount of GA, which formed a denser structure [73], impeding the accelerated disintegration. F4 had a slightly higher degradation because it had a lower concentration of collagen gel (85%) and of GA (0.005%) compared to F2.

The only uncrosslinked formulation (F2) suffered considerable changes in its structural stability because it presented the highest degradation rate: after 24 h, more than 50% of the total mass was degraded, with a total degradation after 48 h. F2 was followed by F4, which was almost completely digested after 48 h (82.60%), with a total degradation after three days. This comportment can be explained by the small concentration of crosslinking agent (0.005%), but also by the higher amount of collagen. The total disintegration of F3 and the maintenance of structural stability of the other three formulations after 24 h can be explained by the presence of the crosslinking agent, which enhanced the mechanical properties of the films.

2.7. In Vitro Drug Release Assay

Inflammation and pain are major challenges during burn healing, causing significant physical and psychological discomfort that negatively impacts the patients' life quality. Therefore, an appropriate option to reduce these symptoms is NSAIDs like NPX [35].

The drug release from the pH-sensitive films varied from fast to slow and prolonged trends depending on the film nature and characteristics (polymeric composition, thickness) and also on the dissolution media [76]. The drug release profile is presented in terms of cumulative percentage for 24 h in Figure 5.

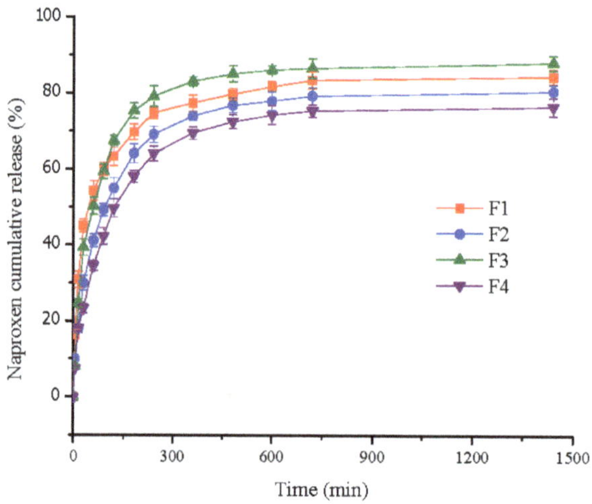

Figure 5. Release profile of NPX from pH-sensitive films for 24 h. Values are mean ± SD (n = 3).

The pH-sensitive films exhibited a biphasic drug release profile over 24 h (Figure 5). Initially, a burst release occurred within the first hour due to loosely interacting or weakly bound NPX on the film surface, as confirmed by SEM analysis. This fast release was succeeded by a slower and sustained release phase for the next 24 h [57]. This behavior is explained by the remaining drug fraction incorporated within the polymeric film. Thus, NPX is slightly released when the hydrated polymeric support begins to swell and the drug diffuses through the loose swollen membrane [70]. A complex is formed between the polymeric matrix and drug molecules ("host-guest complex"), leading to a delay in the drug delivery [21].

According to Figure 5, in the first hour, the highest burst release (54.39%) was registered for F1, closely followed by F3 (50.29%). The highest burst release values for both samples were due to the maximum content of HEC gel (30%), a very hydrophilic polymer. A lower level of HEC gel and an increase in collagen gel in the formulations led to a decrease in burst release values for F2 (41.24%) with 100% collagen gel and, respectively, F4 (34.54%) with 15% collagen gel. After the first hour, a slower and sustained drug release was recorded for over 24 h. After this period, the cumulative NPX release percentages varied from 76.60% for F4 to 88.19% for F3. As we explained above, at the burst release effect, the values recorded after 24 h are also strongly influenced by the composition of the film. Thus, the highest values were obtained for F3 and F1 due to the highest concentration of HEC gel (30%). Moreover, F1 had a slower NPX release than F3 because it was crosslinked with GA, resulting in a more compact network that slowly delivers the drug in the medium. F2 and F4 registered lower values than F1 and F3, with the lowest value for F4; this behavior is explained by the reduction in the concentration of HEC gel: 0% for F2 and 15% for F4.

An immediate release of NPX is beneficial for quickly reducing the acute symptoms of inflammation and pain that occur immediately after the skin is burned. Moreover, equally significant is the slower and more controlled release of the anti-inflammatory drug in the later hours after the initial injury because the first 24–48 h correspond to the inflammatory period of the burn healing process [77]. Such combined effects substantially promote the patient's quality of life and induce a reduction of the wound dressing exchange and consequently a reduction of treatment costs [78].

Several studies have explored the NSAIDs release behavior from biopolymeric films intended for wound healing. Thu et al. [79] developed an alginate-bilayer hydrocolloid film, releasing ibuprofen slowly over 8 h due to a swelling-controlled mechanism. Maver et al. [78] reported some cellulose-based films with a fast burst release of diclofenac in the first 5 min, followed by a stationary phase for 4 h. Jantrawut et al. [57] evaluated low-methoxyl pectin-based films with different plasticizers for indomethacin release and found that over 50% of the drug was released in the first 120 min, with no significant differences between formulations regardless of the plasticizer used. Mishra et al. [38] demonstrated that chitosan-based films exhibited a burst release in the first 120 min, with 20–60% NPX released. Moreover, the addition of polyethylene glycol led to a sustained release of NPX for over 24 h. Bernardo et al. [37] achieved a delayed NPX release from alginate-hydroxyapatite-based films for over 48 h. Compared to these systems, our collagen-HEC films offer a biphasic release profile that can properly handle the burn treatment: an initial burst release to control acute inflammation and pain, followed by a prolonged drug delivery for over 24 h, which ensures an optimal anti-inflammatory effect for this period, corresponding to the inflammatory phase of the healing process.

To set up the release mechanism of NPX from the pH-sensitive films, the experimental data were fitted with two kinetic models: Higuchi and Power Law. To evaluate the goodness of fit for every previous kinetic model, two fundamental metrics are used: correlation coefficient (R) and adjusted R squared (R^2). The last indicator is important when the kinetic models are compared because, besides goodness of fit assessment, adjusted R squared also penalizes the mathematical models for their complexity. This metric is fundamental when kinetic release models are compared regarding the number of predictors: the Power Law model has more parameters (diffusional exponent, n) than Higuchi [80]. Table 3 indicates the values of the correlation coefficient and adjusted R squared.

Table 3. Kinetic parameters registered for different kinetic mathematical models; cumulative NPX released percentages.

Films Code	Higuchi Model			Power Law Model			Kinetic Constant, k ($1/min^n$)	Diffusional Exponent, n	Drug Released (%)
	R	Adj R^2	AIC_c	R	Adj R^2	AIC_c			
F1	0.8502	0.6999	81.30	0.9675	0.9310	60.73	0.228	0.22	84.59
F2	0.8870	0.7692	78.79	0.9601	0.9154	64.74	0.147	0.26	80.68
F3	0.8527	0.7050	84.82	0.9508	0.8915	70.81	0.196	0.23	88.19
F4	0.9028	0.7998	75.83	0.9616	0.9186	63.23	0.120	0.28	76.60

According to Table 3, the highest R and adjusted R^2 values were recorded for the Power Law model, which means that the experimental release data were best fitted by this mathematical model. R values ranged between 0.9508 and 0.9675, while the adjusted R^2 values varied from 0.8915 to 0.9310. Compared to the other kinetic model, the Higuchi, Power Law model had the highest values of both important metrics (R and adjusted R^2), indicating that this kinetic model is considered the best model to fit the experimental data, considering the Power Law model complexity.

The kinetic model ranking based only on accuracy, including the comparison of correlation coefficient values, is not sufficient because the model variability is not described. Therefore, the kinetic model comparison and evaluation were performed using the Akaike Information Criterion (AIC) metric. This tool also indicates the model variability (precision), in addition to the goodness of fit (accuracy) [81]. For this study, we used the AIC_c (small-sample corrected AIC) values, taking into account the small number of experimental points. The kinetic mathematical model that best represents statistically the NPX release is the model that presents the lowest AIC_c values [82].

Table 3 shows that the lowest AIC_c values were registered for the Power Law model, being lower than the AICc values registered for the Higuchi model. This aspect means that the Power Law model is considered the best model to fit the experimental release data, considering the model's complexity. Considering all mentioned, the highest values of R and adjusted R^2 and the smallest values of AIC_c were used to choose the kinetic mathematical model that best fit the experimental data. The kinetic model that fulfilled these characteristics was the Power Law model, which properly explained the NPX release mechanism from the pH-sensitive films.

As can be seen in Table 3, the diffusional exponent values varied from 0.22 to 0.28, which indicates a non-Fickian drug transport [83], which includes three various mechanisms: firstly, the NPX release from pH-sensitive film surface; secondly, the drug diffusion from the swollen films; thirdly, the NPX release due to the polymeric scaffold erosion [84].

2.8. Colorimetric Analysis

In the development of pH-sensitive materials for wound pH monitoring, it is essential to ensure that the color change can be distinguished by the naked eye [3]. Collagen-HEC films loaded with phenol red as a pH indicator were analyzed in different pH buffer solutions to simulate the clinical environment [72]. Their color modifications were captured by a camera, as can be seen in Figure 6.

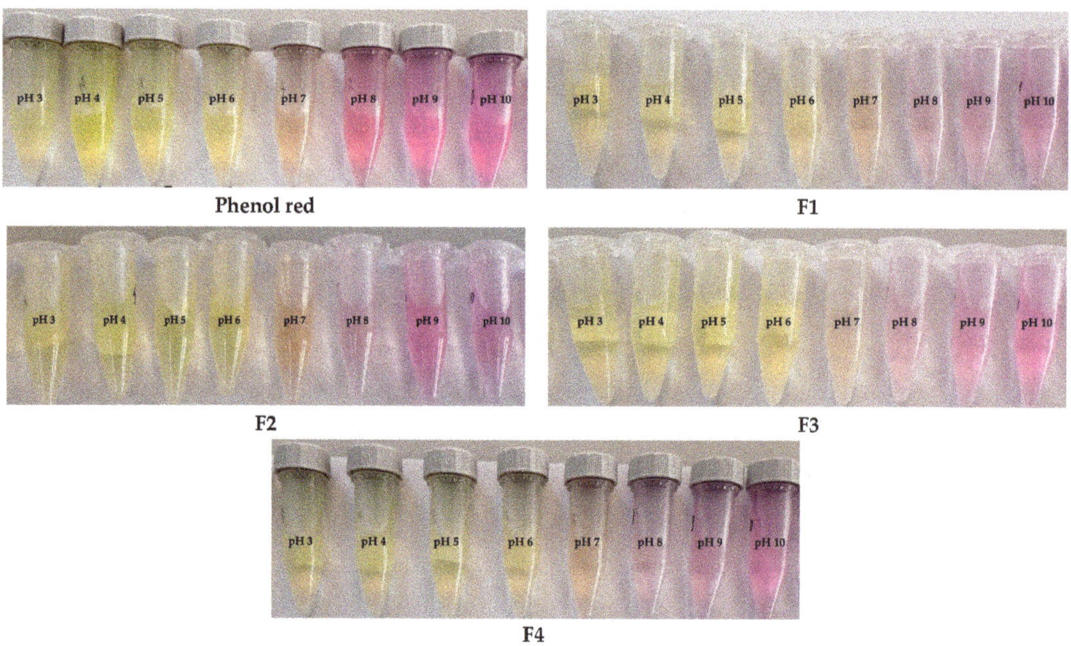

Figure 6. Image of pH-sensitive film dressings in buffer solutions with pH 3 to pH 10.

As can be seen in Figure 6, as the pH shifted from 3 to 10, the film dressings transitioned from yellow (pH lower than 6.8) to orange (pH 6.8–7.5) and finally to fuchsia (pH higher than 7.5), clearly visible to the naked eye. The color modifications furnished valuable insights. Thus, the pH interval of the color changes matches the pH window, which is required to indicate the status of a burn wound. As the injury heals, its environment progresses from an alkaline form to a neutral one and later to an acidic status [14]. Table 4 presents the color parameters of the pH-sensitive films in pH 3–10 buffer solutions.

Table 4. Color parameters of pH-sensitive films immersed in different pH buffer solutions.

	F1				F2				F3				F4			
pH	L*	a*	b*	ΔE	L*	a*	b*	ΔE	L*	a*	b*	ΔE	L*	a*	b*	ΔE
3	92.03	0.15	−8.20	1.60	92.52	−0.31	−7.93	2.82	91.92	−0.32	−7.39	0.55	92.47	−0.72	−7.12	1.42
4	92.04	1.91	−11.29	4.41	91.80	1.32	−9.83	3.09	91.63	1.64	−10.45	3.82	92.16	1.13	−9.59	2.95
5	91.82	2.05	−11.14	3.25	91.83	1.71	−10.20	3.13	91.65	1.97	−10.74	3.35	92.42	1.65	−10.35	3.33
6	91.76	2.39	−12.11	2.31	92.34	2.25	−10.90	1.83	91.81	2.37	−11.19	1.55	91.62	1.78	−8.61	1.42
7	91.96	2.64	−12.46	2.18	92.24	2.64	−10.71	0.92	91.84	3.04	−11.66	1.18	91.95	2.29	−9.79	1.19
8	92.60	3.07	−12.89	2.68	91.75	3.26	−13.17	1.97	91.56	3.38	−12.07	2.68	91.57	3.12	−12.67	2.56
9	91.54	3.53	−13.92	2.02	91.56	4.16	−14.18	2.34	91.72	3.96	−13.24	2.90	91.67	3.30	−14.02	2.08
10	91.42	3.94	−14.40	2.41	90.71	3.70	−14.19	1.68	90.73	4.44	−14.75	1.24	91.54	4.09	−14.05	1.54

According to Table 4, for all formulations, a* values increased with the increase in pH: from 0.15 at pH 3 to 3.94 at pH 10 for F1, from −0.31 at pH 3 to 3.70 at pH 10 for F2, from −0.32 at pH 3 to 4.44 at pH 10 for F3, and from −0.72 at pH 3 to 4.09 at pH 10 for F4. This aspect indicated that the films' color gradually turned redder at higher pH, consistent with phenol red behavior. On the other hand, b* became more negative with the increase in pH: for F1 from −8.20 at pH 3 to −14.40 at pH 10, for F2 from −7.93 at pH 3 to −14.19 at pH 10, for F3 from −7.39 at pH 3 to −14.75 at pH 10, and for F4 from −7.12 at pH 3 to −14.05 at pH 10, suggesting that the color progressively turned to blue/purple tones [85]. For F1, ΔE registered a visible increase from 1.60 (pH 3) to 4.41 (pH 4), showing early sensitivity. Then, the ΔE value slowly decreased with the increase in pH but also remained visible to the naked eye. F2 exhibited an increase in ΔE at pH 4–5, followed by a decrease at the next pH levels, while F3 registered a sharp jump from pH 3 to pH 4 and 5, where the ΔE value was about 3.5, meaning the sample is quite responsive in the acidic medium. The same trend was observed for the F4 sample, with a visible increase in ΔE from 1.42 (pH 3) to 3.33 (pH 5). Larger ΔE values signify that the pH-sensitive films can have proper color variation according to the pH value, which suggests adequate visual color variability [86]. The color changes of biopolymeric films were perceptible to the naked eye in multiple pH solutions, indicating that the designed films have a sensitive response to pH modification. Taking into account that the pH-sensitive films will be handled as wound dressings and the average pH of an injury is around 7, the color of the wound dressing will turn orange. When the skin is burned, the local pH will increase to around 8–8.5, and the color of the film dressing will change to fuchsia. If the burn injury heals, the film color will progressively change to yellow because normal skin has a pH value close to 5.5 [87].

These color transitions of the films, when applied at the lesion site, represent an excellent indicator of wound status, guiding the physicians to properly choose the treatment for rapid and effective healing.

3. Materials and Methods

3.1. Materials

Calf skin was used as the primary source to extract type I fibrillar collagen in gel form using the method that was set up by the Collagen Research Department of the Leather and Footwear Research Institute Division from the National Research & Development Institute for Textiles and Leather, Bucharest, Romania [88]. The initial collagen gel had a 2.43% concentration (*w/w*), and the pH was acidic. Hydroxyethylcellulose (analytical grade) was acquired from Sigma-Aldrich, Steinheim, Germany, and had a viscosity of 4000 cPs. Naproxen ((S)-(+)-2-(6-Methoxy-2-naphtyl)propionic acid, 99% purity) was obtained from Thermo Fisher, Kandel, Germany, and type I collagenase (*Clostridium histolyticum*, analytical grade) was purchased from Sigma-Aldrich, St. Louis, MO, USA. Orthophosphoric acid (85% analytical grade), phenol red (analytical grade), glutaraldehyde (25% aqueous solution, ≥98% purity), and sodium hydroxide (analytical grade) were provided by Merck, Darmstadt, Germany. Disodium hydrogen phosphate, potassium dihydrogen phosphate, ethanol absolute, and glycerol (analytical grades) were supplied by Chemical Company S.A., Iași, Romania. The distilled water was used for sample preparation and different analyses.

3.2. Methods

3.2.1. Preparation of Biopolymeric Films

The collagen gel used for the preparation of the film dressings had a concentration of 1.1% (*w/v*) and a neutral pH (7.2–7.4), being obtained from the initial acid collagen gel of 2.43% concentration with distilled water and 1 M sodium hydroxide under continuous mixing with a mechanical stirrer. To prepare a 3% HEC hydrogel, the HEC powder was dispersed in distilled water at room temperature under continuous stirring until the hydrogel was obtained. Consequently, collagen and HEC hydrogels were mixed in different ratios; then, NPX was added in various concentrations according to Table 5.

Table 5. Composition of the different dried films.

Film Code	Coll/HEC [1,2], (g%/g%)	NPX [2] (g%)	GA [2] (g%)
F1	70:30	1.00	0.005
F2	100:0	0.50	0.010
F3	70:30	1.00	0.000
F4	85:15	1.00	0.005

[1] The ratio between collagen and HEC gels. [2] Quantities of Coll/HEC, NPX, and GA are reported to 100 g gel.

To these formulations, a mixture of two plasticizers, ethanol absolute (3 mL) and glycerol (0.3 mL), was added under mechanical stirring to obtain a homogenized mixture. The pH of the samples was adjusted to the physiological one, varying between 7.2 and 7.4 using sodium hydroxide solution (1M). After this important step of pH regulation, a small volume (1.5 mL) of 0.02% phenol red aqueous solution was added, resulting in orange-colored hydrogels (color of the phenol red at neutral pH). The final stage of the preparation process was the crosslinking of three hydrogels with 0.005% or 0.010% glutaraldehyde, one sample remaining uncrosslinked. Hydrogels were then poured into 5 cm Petri dishes and maintained in the oven at 33 °C to obtain the dried films. When completely dry, the films were removed from the Petri dishes very carefully and placed in plastic bags individually for further analysis. The compositions were named F1, F2, F3, and F4. The biopolymeric films obtained were characterized by multiple analyses: physical characterization, mechanical properties, scanning electron microscopy, water contact angle test, swelling behavior, in vitro enzymatic degradation, drug release kinetics, and colorimetric analysis.

3.2.2. Physical Evaluation of pH-Sensitive Films

The designed pH-sensitive film dressings were physically investigated by visual inspection for their color, odor, air bubbles, transparency, flexibility, ease of difficulty regarding their peelability from Petri dishes, and thickness. Transparency was investigated by putting the films over a printed text and evaluating if the text remained readable without compelling blurring. We considered the films to be transparent because the text was readable [45]. To evaluate the presence of air bubbles, we placed them in an ambient light. The films did not present any form of air bubbles. Flexibility was assessed by performing the folding endurance test. Accordingly, this analysis was performed by manually folding every formulation repetitively in the same place until it cracked. Films that can be folded more than 300 times without cracking were presumed to pass the folding test [70]. Our formulations successfully passed this test, indicating proper flexibility to be attached to the wounded skin without cracking. All our formulations were considered peelable because they were easily removed from the Petri dishes without fracturing and adhering to the casting molds [89].

3.2.3. Mechanical Characterization

To evaluate the mechanical properties of pH-sensitive film dressings (film thickness and tensile strength), the samples were analyzed according to an actual standard, SR EN ISO 3376:2020 *Determination of tensile strength and percentage elongation* [90]. Tests were conducted in the Leather and Footwear Research Institute (ICPI) accredited laboratory, using the traction test machine "Tinius Olsen" (India).

3.2.4. Scanning Electron Microscopy (SEM)

The morphology of the film's surface was analyzed by a Tabletop TM 4000 Plus (Hitachi, Japan) scanning electron microscope using small pieces of dried films, at 15 kV accelerating voltage, in a low vacuum mode, and a backscattered electron detector. Microstructural characteristics of dried formulations were studied without the coverage of the samples with a conductive layer. Micrographs were captured at 200× magnification, with a scale bar of 200 μm.

3.2.5. Wettability Analysis

The water static contact angle of the biopolymeric films was measured at room temperature using a CAM 101 goniometer (KSV Instruments Ltd., Espoo, Finland). Briefly, the film was placed on a glass slide, and the distilled water was cautiously dropped from a Hamilton syringe onto the dried film surface. The moment when the water droplet came into contact with the film surface was captured with a digital video camera. Contact angles were measured three times on different zones of each surface and averaged.

3.2.6. Swelling Behavior

The gravimetric method [91] was used to investigate the swelling behavior of the dried films at different pH levels of phosphate buffer solutions: acidic, neutral, and alkaline (pH 5.5, 7.4, and 8.5). The films were cut into a square shape (0.25 cm^2), and the initial weight was accurately measured (W_0). The small pieces were subsequently soaked in 3 mL of pH media at room temperature. Then, swollen film pieces were removed from the different media after specific time intervals (30 min, 1, 2, 3, 4, 5, 6, 7, 24, 48, and 72 h) and weighed again at room temperature on a digital balance (W_s). The experiment was conducted three times to obtain precise results. The swelling behavior of the dried films was calculated using Equation (1) [72]. For every formulation, the mean and standard deviation were estimated.

$$\text{Swelling behaviour (g/g)} = \frac{W_s - W_0}{W_0} \quad (1)$$

3.2.7. In Vitro Enzymatic Biodegradation

The in vitro enzymatic degradation of films was assessed by measuring weight loss over time in a collagenase solution. Identically shaped film samples with similar initial weight were first immersed in a solution of phosphate buffer (pH 7.4) for 24 h to reach equilibrium. Once fully hydrated, the swollen samples were weighed (W_0). Subsequently, they were transferred into a 3 mL solution of phosphate buffer (pH 7.4) containing collagenase (10^{-6} μg/mL) and incubated at 37 °C (simulation of physiological conditions) for various time intervals: 30 min, 1, 2, 3, 4, 5, 6, 7, 24, 48, and 72 h. After each incubation period, the film pieces were pulled out and weighed (W_t). Each measurement was performed in triplicate, and the average value was determined. The percentage weight loss of the polymeric films was then calculated following Equation (2):

$$\text{Weight loss } (\%) = \frac{W_0 - W_t}{W_0} \times 100 \quad (2)$$

3.2.8. In Vitro Drug Release Assay

The in vitro drug delivery was performed using the paddle dissolution apparatus (Vision G2 Classic 6 Dissolution Tester, Hanson Research, Chatsworth, CA, USA) and the corresponding disks for testing topical membranes (d = 35 mm, mesh 40, Sotax, Orléans, France). NPX-loaded pH-sensitive films with a 5 cm diameter were placed onto the disk. The resulting excess was removed, and the obtained films were weighed and assembled in the disk. The pH of wound fluid is similar to a physiological buffer solution (pH 7.4), considering the ion content and pH value [92]. Accordingly, the release characteristics of NPX from collagen-HEC films were studied in phosphate buffer solution (PBS, pH 7.4, heated at 37 ± 0.5 °C), simulating the physiological conditions of a real wound and plasmatic environment at 50 rpm [51]. When the medium temperature reached 37 °C, the disks were placed into the vessels of the tester. At specific time intervals (5, 15, 30, 60, 90, 120, 180, 240, 360, 480, 600, 1440 min), 5 mL of each sample was taken with a syringe and replaced with 5 mL of fresh PBS (37 °C) to maintain the volume of release medium in the vessels. The standard calibration curve (R^2 = 0.9996) was used to calculate the NPX concentration in the release medium at an absorbance of λ = 262 nm, using a UV–Vis spectrophotometer (Jasco, Tokyo, Japan). The drug release assay was performed in triplicate for 24 h.

Analyzing the NPX release using adequate mathematical models facilitates a better understanding of the underlying release mechanisms. To identify the mechanism governing the NPX release from the pH-sensitive film dressings, the cumulative release data were fitted with two models: the Power Law model (Equation (3)) and its specific case—Higuchi model (n = 0.5):

$$\frac{M_t}{M_\infty} = kt^n \quad (3)$$

where: M_t and M_∞ are described as the released amount of NPX at t time and equilibrium, M_t/M_∞ is the fractional release of NPX in t time, "k" is the release rate constant characteristic to collagen-HEC-NPX system (expressed in $1/\text{min}^n$), and "n" is defined as the diffusional exponent specific to the drug release process (dimensionless).

3.2.9. Colorimetric Analysis

Color changes of pH-sensitive films were analyzed in the pH range of 3 to 10. Films were immersed in the buffer solutions and stirred for 1 min. To determine their colorimetric response, soft cotton materials were submerged in the previously obtained colored solutions. Materials were left for a few minutes in the solutions, then were taken out and left at room temperature to dry. The color of the impregnated cotton materials was investigated by a UltraScan® PRO spectrophotometer (Hunter Associates Laboratory Inc., Reston, VA, USA). To correlate the color changes, CIE (International Commission Illumination) color space coordinates were measured. Mention that L* indicates lightness (+) and darkness (−), a* corresponds to redder (+) and greener (−), and b* suggests yellower (+) and bluer (−) [93]. For each film dressing, the total color difference (ΔE) was calculated according to Equation (4) [44].

$$\Delta E = \sqrt{(\Delta L)^2 + (\Delta a)^2 + (\Delta b)^2} \quad (4)$$

4. Conclusions

This study was focused on the development of some pH-sensitive film dressings based on collagen, hydroxyethylcellulose, and naproxen, loaded with a pH indicator, phenol red, to be used for the pH detection of a wound and to indicate the healing status. The films demonstrated desirable physicochemical and functional properties, including optimal flexibility, peelability, and hydrophilicity to support their use for burn wound application. The films exhibited proper mechanical and swelling properties, with variations dependent on the polymeric composition, supporting their capacity to absorb the exudates that form at the lesion site while maintaining their structural integrity for more than 24 h. The high capacity to absorb lesion exudates favors the drug release from the polymeric membrane and rapid local effect at the beginning of the burn when the inflammation is very high. The naproxen release from the pH-sensitive films showed a biphasic profile: the burst release effect in the first hour with an immediate drug release, followed by a sustained and prolonged release for the next 24 h, ensuring a suitable control of acute inflammation and pain. Moreover, the pH-sensitive color changes from yellow (acidic pH) to fuchsia (alkaline pH) across a pH interval of 3–10 furnished a visually perceptible indicator of environmental pH, a meaningful characteristic for real-time monitoring of injury status.

While these outcomes are promising for burn wound healing, one limitation of this study is the lack of evaluation of the films' biological safety. Future studies will include in vitro cytotoxic assessment, in vivo validation using murine burn models, and process scalability of newly pH-sensitive films to support their clinical application. Concluding, the dual function of the designed films positions them as strong options with considerable potential for real-time wound control and therapeutic applications.

Author Contributions: Conceptualization, E.-E.T., M.G.A.K., M.I., E.V. and M.V.G.; methodology, E.-E.T., M.G.A.K., L.P., V.A., M.I., E.V. and M.V.G.; software, E.-E.T., M.G.A.K., M.I., E.V. and M.V.G.; validation, M.G.A.K., C.E.D.-P., L.P., V.A., M.I., E.V. and M.V.G.; formal analysis, E.-E.T., M.G.A.K., M.I., E.V., D.A.K., R.M.P. and M.V.G.; investigation, E.-E.T., M.G.A.K., C.E.D.-P., L.P., V.A., D.A.K., R.M.P. and M.V.G.; resources, C.E.D.-P.; data curation, E.-E.T., M.G.A.K., M.I., E.V. and M.V.G.; writing—original draft preparation, E.-E.T.; writing—review and editing, M.G.A.K. and M.V.G.; visualization, E.-E.T., M.G.A.K., M.I., E.V., D.A.K., R.M.P. and M.V.G.; supervision, M.G.A.K., C.E.D.-P., L.P., V.A. and M.V.G.; project administration, C.E.D.-P.; funding acquisition, C.E.D.-P. All authors have read and agreed to the published version of the manuscript.

Funding: This work was financially supported by "Carol Davila" University of Medicine and Pharmacy Bucharest, Romania through Contract No. CNFIS-FDI-2025-F-0646.

Institutional Review Board Statement: Not applicable.

Informed Consent Statement: Not applicable.

Data Availability Statement: The data presented in this research are available in the article.

Conflicts of Interest: The authors declare no conflicts of interest.

References

1. Eskilson, O.; Zattarin, E.; Berglund, L.; Oksman, K.; Hanna, K.; Rakar, J.; Sivlér, P.; Skog, M.; Rinklake, I.; Shamasha, R.; et al. Nanocellulose composite wound dressings for real-time pH wound monitoring. *Mater. Today Bio* **2023**, *19*, 100574. [CrossRef] [PubMed]
2. Metcalf, D.G.; Haalboom, M.; Bowler, P.G.; Gamerith, C.; Sigl, E.; Heinzle, A.; Burnet, M.W.M. Elevated wound fluid pH correlates with increased risk of wound infection. *Wound Med.* **2019**, *26*, 100166. [CrossRef]
3. Gamerith, C.; Luschnig, D.; Ortner, A.; Pietrzik, N.; Guse, J.-H.; Burnet, M.; Haalboom, M.; van der Palen, J.; Heinzle, A.; Sigl, E.; et al. pH-responsive materials for optical monitoring of wound status. *Sens. Actuators B Chem.* **2019**, *301*, 126966. [CrossRef]
4. Kuo, S.-H.; Shen, C.-J.; Shen, C.-F.; Cheng, C.-M. Role of pH Value in Clinically Relevant Diagnosis. *Diagnostics* **2020**, *10*, 107. [CrossRef]
5. Richards, H.; Falder, S. pH of a burn wound. *Burns* **2018**, *44*, 2104–2105. [CrossRef] [PubMed]
6. Ono, S.; Imai, R.; Ida, Y.; Shibata, D.; Komiya, T.; Matsumura, H. Increased wound pH as an indicator of local wound infection in second degree burns. *Burns* **2015**, *41*, 820–824. [CrossRef]
7. Osti, E. Skin ph variations from the acute phase to re-epithelialization in burn patients treated with new materials (burnshield®, semipermeable adhesive film, dermasilk®, and hyalomatrix®). Non-invasive preliminary experimental clinical trial. *Ann. Burn. Fire Disasters* **2008**, *21*, 73–77.
8. Schneider, L.A.; Korber, A.; Grabbe, S.; Dissemond, J. Influence of pH on wound-healing: A new perspective for wound-therapy? *Arch. Dermatol. Res.* **2007**, *298*, 413–420. [CrossRef]
9. Sim, P.; Song, Y.; Yang, G.N.; Cowin, A.J.; Garg, S. In Vitro Wound Healing Properties of Novel Acidic Treatment Regimen in Enhancing Metabolic Activity and Migration of Skin Cells. *Int. J. Mol. Sci.* **2022**, *23*, 7188. [CrossRef]
10. Pourali, P.; Razavianzadeh, N.; Khojasteh, L.; Yahyaei, B. Assessment of the cutaneous wound healing efficiency of acidic, neutral and alkaline bacterial cellulose membrane in rat. *J. Mater. Sci. Mater. Med.* **2018**, *29*, 90. [CrossRef]
11. Bazbouz, M.B.; Tronci, G. Two-layer Electrospun System Enabling Wound Exudate Management and Visual Infection Response. *Sensors* **2019**, *19*, 991. [CrossRef] [PubMed]
12. Kiti, K.; Thanomsilp, C.; Suwantong, O. The potential use of colorimetric pH sensor from Clitoria ternatea flower for indicating bacterial infection in wound dressing application. *Microchem. J.* **2022**, *177*, 107277. [CrossRef]
13. Petkovska, J.; Geskovski, N.; Marković, D.; Dimova, V.; Mirakovski, D.; Radetić, M.; Jordanov, I. Chitosan-pectin multilayer coating with anthocyanin grape dye as pH indicating wound dressing: Synthesis and characterization. *Carbohydr. Polym. Technol. Appl.* **2024**, *7*, 100438. [CrossRef]
14. Liu, L.; Li, X.; Nagao, M.; Elias, A.L.; Narain, R.; Chung, H.-J. A pH-Indicating Colorimetric Tough Hydrogel Patch towards Applications in a Substrate for Smart Wound Dressings. *Polymers* **2017**, *9*, 558. [CrossRef]
15. Ghica, M.V.; Albu, M.G.; Popa, L.; Moisescu, S. Response surface methodology and Taguchi approach to assess the combined effect of formulation factors on minocycline delivery from collagen sponges. *Die Pharm. Int. J. Pharm. Sci.* **2013**, *68*, 340–348. [CrossRef]
16. Tihan, G.T.; Rău, I.; Zgârian, R.G.; Ghica, M.V. Collagen-based biomaterials for ibuprofen delivery. *Comptes Rendus. Chim.* **2016**, *19*, 390–394. [CrossRef]
17. Li, Y.; Liu, Y.; Li, R.; Bai, H.; Zhu, Z.; Zhu, L.; Zhu, C.; Che, Z.; Liu, H.; Wang, J.; et al. Collagen-based biomaterials for bone tissue engineering. *Mater. Des.* **2021**, *210*, 110049. [CrossRef]
18. Marin, Ș.; Albu Kaya, M.G.; Ghica, M.V.; Dinu-Pîrvu, C.; Popa, L.; Udeanu, D.I.; Mihai, G.; Enachescu, M. Collagen-Polyvinyl Alcohol-Indomethacin Biohybrid Matrices as Wound Dressings. *Pharmaceutics* **2018**, *10*, 224. [CrossRef]
19. Sionkowska, A. Collagen blended with natural polymers: Recent advances and trends. *Prog. Polym. Sci.* **2021**, *122*, 101452. [CrossRef]
20. Tudoroiu, E.-E.; Dinu-Pîrvu, C.-E.; Albu Kaya, M.G.; Popa, L.; Anuța, V.; Prisada, R.M.; Ghica, M.V. An Overview of Cellulose Derivatives-Based Dressings for Wound-Healing Management. *Pharmaceuticals* **2021**, *14*, 1215. [CrossRef]
21. Silva, C.N.S.; Cruz, M.V.; Fernandes, K.F.; Batista, K.A. Production of anti-inflammatory films based on cashew gum polysaccharide and polyvinyl alcohol for wound dressing applications. *3 Biotech* **2023**, *13*, 299. [CrossRef] [PubMed]
22. Lei, H.; Zhu, C.; Fan, D. Optimization of human-like collagen composite polysaccharide hydrogel dressing preparation using response surface for burn repair. *Carbohydr. Polym.* **2020**, *239*, 116249. [CrossRef] [PubMed]
23. Ng, J.Y.; Zhu, X.; Mukherjee, D.; Zhang, C.; Hong, S.; Kumar, Y.; Gokhale, R.; Ee, P.L.R. Pristine Gellan Gum–Collagen Interpenetrating Network Hydrogels as Mechanically Enhanced Anti-inflammatory Biologic Wound Dressings for Burn Wound Therapy. *ACS Appl. Bio Mater.* **2021**, *4*, 1470–1482. [CrossRef]
24. Halarnekar, D.; Ayyanar, M.; Gangapriya, P.; Kalaskar, M.; Redasani, V.; Gurav, N.; Nadaf, S.; Saoji, S.; Rarokar, N.; Gurav, S. Eco synthesized chitosan/zinc oxide nanocomposites as the next generation of nano-delivery for antibacterial, antioxidant, antidiabetic potential, and chronic wound repair. *Int. J. Biol. Macromol.* **2023**, *242*, 124764. [CrossRef] [PubMed]

25. Chen, J.; Zhao, X.; Qiao, L.; Huang, Y.; Yang, Y.; Chu, D.; Guo, B. Multifunctional On-Demand Removability Hydrogel Dressing Based on in Situ Formed AgNPs, Silk Microfibers and Hydrazide Hyaluronic Acid for Burn Wound Healing. *Adv. Healthc. Mater.* **2024**, *13*, 2303157. [CrossRef]
26. Chakrabarti, S.; Mazumder, B.; Rajkonwar, J.; Pathak, M.P.; Patowary, P.; Chattopadhyay, P. bFGF and collagen matrix hydrogel attenuates burn wound inflammation through activation of ERK and TRK pathway. *Sci. Rep.* **2021**, *11*, 3357. [CrossRef]
27. Tudoroiu, E.-E.; Albu Kaya, M.G.; Titorencu, I.; Dinu-Pîrvu, C.E.; Marin, M.M.; Roșca, A.-M.; Popa, L.; Anuța, V.; Antoniac, A.; Chelaru, C.; et al. Design and evaluation of new wound dressings based on collagen-cellulose derivatives. *Mater. Des.* **2023**, *236*, 112469. [CrossRef]
28. Al-Khoury, H.; Espinosa-Cano, E.; Aguilar, M.R.; Román, J.S.; Syrowatka, F.; Schmidt, G.; Groth, T. Anti-inflammatory Surface Coatings Based on Polyelectrolyte Multilayers of Heparin and Polycationic Nanoparticles of Naproxen-Bearing Polymeric Drugs. *Biomacromolecules* **2019**, *20*, 4015–4025. [CrossRef]
29. Wong, R.S.Y. Role of Nonsteroidal Anti-Inflammatory Drugs (NSAIDs) in Cancer Prevention and Cancer Promotion. *Adv. Pharmacol. Pharm. Sci.* **2019**, *2019*, 3418975. [CrossRef]
30. Su, W.-H.; Cheng, M.-H.; Lee, W.-L.; Tsou, T.-S.; Chang, W.-H.; Chen, C.-S.; Wang, P.-H. Nonsteroidal Anti-Inflammatory Drugs for Wounds: Pain Relief or Excessive Scar Formation? *Mediat. Inflamm.* **2010**, *2010*, 413238. [CrossRef]
31. Shah, H.; Nair, A.B.; Shah, J.; Jacob, S.; Bharadia, P.; Haroun, M. Proniosomal vesicles as an effective strategy to optimize naproxen transdermal delivery. *J. Drug Deliv. Sci. Technol.* **2021**, *63*, 102479. [CrossRef]
32. Van den Ouweland, F.A.; Eenhoorn, P.C.; Tan, Y.; Gribnau, F.W.J. Transcutaneous absorption of naproxen gel. *Eur. J. Clin. Pharmacol.* **1989**, *36*, 209–211. [CrossRef] [PubMed]
33. Barakat, N.S. Evaluation of Glycofurol-Based Gel as a New Vehicle for Topical Application of Naproxen. *AAPS PharmSciTech* **2010**, *11*, 1138–1146. [CrossRef]
34. Yurdasiper, A.; Ertan, G.; Heard, C.M. Enhanced delivery of naproxen to the viable epidermis from an activated poly N-isopropylacrylamide (PNIPAM) Nanogel: Skin penetration, modulation of COX-2 expression and rat paw oedema. *Nanomed. Nanotechnol. Biol. Med.* **2018**, *14*, 2051–2059. [CrossRef] [PubMed]
35. Wang, Y.; Pang, X.; Luo, J.; Wen, Q.; Wu, Z.; Ding, Q.; Zhao, L.; Yang, L.; Wang, B.; Fu, S. Naproxen Nanoparticle-Loaded Thermosensitive Chitosan Hydrogel for Prevention of Postoperative Adhesions. *ACS Biomater. Sci. Eng.* **2019**, *5*, 1580–1588. [CrossRef] [PubMed]
36. Eslamian, L.; Kianipour, A.; Mortazavi, S.A.R. The Analgesic Efficacy of 5% Naproxen Gel for Pain Associated with Orthodontic Separator Placement: A Randomized Double-Blind Controlled Trial. *Anesthesiol. Pain Med.* **2017**, *7*, e42708. [CrossRef]
37. Bernardo, M.P.; Pasquini, D.; Mattoso, L.H.C. Enhanced antibacterial activity of wound dressings based on alginate/hydroxyapatite modified with copper and naproxen. *J. Mater. Res.* **2024**, *39*, 762–773. [CrossRef]
38. Mishra, S.K.; Mary, D.S.; Kannan, S. Copper incorporated microporous chitosan-polyethylene glycol hydrogels loaded with naproxen for effective drug release and anti-infection wound dressing. *Int. J. Biol. Macromol.* **2017**, *95*, 928–937. [CrossRef]
39. Purnamasari, W.; Budiastanti, T.A.; Aminatun, A.; Rahmah, U.; Sumarsih, S.; Chang, J.-Y.; Fahmi, M.Z. Naproxen release behaviour from graphene oxide/cellulose acetate composite nanofibers. *RSC Adv.* **2022**, *12*, 8019–8029. [CrossRef]
40. Jiao, W.; Kiang, J.G.; Cary, L.; Elliott, T.B.; Pellmar, T.C.; Ledney, G.D. COX-2 Inhibitors Are Contraindicated for Treatment of Combined Injury. *Radiat. Res.* **2009**, *172*, 686–697. [CrossRef]
41. Fairweather, M.; Heit, Y.I.; Buie, J.; Rosenberg, L.M.; Briggs, A.; Orgill, D.P.; Bertagnolli, M.M. Celecoxib inhibits early cutaneous wound healing. *J. Surg. Res.* **2015**, *194*, 717–724. [CrossRef]
42. Goder, D.; Eshkol-Yogev, I.; Matsliah, L.; Lemberger, M.; Harlev, M.; Furer, A.; Zilberman, M.; Egozi, D. In vivo study of the efficacy of bupivacaine-eluting novel soy protein wound dressings in a rat burn model. *Burns* **2022**, *48*, 623–632. [CrossRef]
43. Morgan, A.; Babu, D.; Reiz, B.; Whittal, R.; Suh, L.Y.K.; Siraki, A.G. Caution for the routine use of phenol red—It is more than just a pH indicator. *Chem. Biol. Interact.* **2019**, *310*, 108739. [CrossRef] [PubMed]
44. Chalitangkoon, J.; Ronte, A.; Sintoppun, T.; Manapradit, N.; Monvisade, P. Dual Cross-Linked Chitosan-Based Films with pH-Sensitive Coloration and Drug Release Kinetics for Smart Wound Dressings. *ACS Omega* **2025**, *10*, 7770–7782. [CrossRef]
45. Ahmad, N.; Tayyeb, D.; Ali, I.; K. Alruwaili, N.; Ahmad, W.; ur Rehman, A.; Khan, A.H.; Iqbal, M.S. Development and Characterization of Hemicellulose-Based Films for Antibacterial Wound-Dressing Application. *Polymers* **2020**, *12*, 548. [CrossRef] [PubMed]
46. Arafa, A.A.; Nada, A.A.; Ibrahim, A.Y.; Sajkiewicz, P.; Zahran, M.K.; Hakeim, O.A. Preparation and characterization of smart therapeutic pH-sensitive wound dressing from red cabbage extract and chitosan hydrogel. *Int. J. Biol. Macromol.* **2021**, *182*, 1820–1831. [CrossRef]
47. Aycan, D.; Selmi, B.; Kelel, E.; Yildirim, T.; Alemdar, N. Conductive polymeric film loaded with ibuprofen as a wound dressing material. *Eur. Polym. J.* **2019**, *121*, 109308. [CrossRef]
48. Shoulders, M.D.; Raines, R.T. Collagen Structure and Stability. *Annu. Rev. Biochem.* **2009**, *78*, 929–958. [CrossRef]

49. Kirkness, M.W.H.; Lehmann, K.; Forde, N.R. Mechanics and structural stability of the collagen triple helix. *Curr. Opin. Chem. Biol.* **2019**, *53*, 98–105. [CrossRef]
50. Fratzl, P. Collagen: Structure and Mechanics, an Introduction. In *Collagen: Structure and Mechanics*; Fratzl, P., Ed.; Springer: Boston, MA, USA, 2008; pp. 1–13.
51. Ahmed, M.; Bhat, A.R.; Verma, A.K.; Patel, R. Collagen–PVA Films Plasticized with Choline Acetate Ionic Liquid for Sustained Drug Release: UV Shielding, Mechanical, Antioxidant, and Antibacterial Properties. *ACS Appl. Bio Mater.* **2023**, *6*, 663–673. [CrossRef]
52. Sionkowska, A. Current research on the blends of natural and synthetic polymers as new biomaterials: Review. *Prog. Polym. Sci.* **2011**, *36*, 1254–1276. [CrossRef]
53. Ferreira, A.M.; Gentile, P.; Chiono, V.; Ciardelli, G. Collagen for bone tissue regeneration. *Acta Biomater.* **2012**, *8*, 3191–3200. [CrossRef] [PubMed]
54. Yu, Z.; Wu, J.; Zhang, T.; Chen, C.; Ma, Y.; Liu, H.; Chiou, B.-S.; Liu, F.; Li, J. Improving the crosslinking of collagen casing and glutaraldehyde by facilitating the formation of conjugate structure via pH. *Collagen Leather* **2024**, *6*, 29. [CrossRef]
55. Ning, F.; Zhang, J.; Kang, M.X.; Ma, C.P.; Li, H.; Qiu, Z.M. Hydroxyethyl cellulose hydrogel modified with tannic acid as methylene blue adsorbent. *J. Appl. Polym. Sci.* **2021**, *138*, 17. [CrossRef]
56. Khan, M.U.A.; Iqbal, I.; Ansari, M.N.M.; Razak, S.I.A.; Raza, M.A.; Sajjad, A.; Jabeen, F.; Riduan Mohamad, M.; Jusoh, N. Development of antibacterial, degradable and ph-responsive chitosan/guar gum/polyvinyl alcohol blended hydrogels for wound dressing. *Molecules* **2021**, *26*, 5937. [CrossRef] [PubMed]
57. Jantrawut, P.; Chaiwarit, T.; Jantanasakulwong, K.; Brachais, C.H.; Chambin, O. Effect of Plasticizer Type on Tensile Property and In Vitro Indomethacin Release of Thin Films Based on Low-Methoxyl Pectin. *Polymers* **2017**, *9*, 289. [CrossRef]
58. Adamiak, K.; Sionkowska, A. Current methods of collagen cross-linking: Review. *Int. J. Biol. Macromol.* **2020**, *161*, 550–560. [CrossRef]
59. Khan, M.U.; Razaq, S.I.; Mehboob, H.; Rehman, S.; Al-Arjan, W.S.; Amin, R. Antibacterial and Hemocompatible pH-Responsive Hydrogel for Skin Wound Healing Application: In Vitro Drug Release. *Polymers* **2021**, *13*, 3703. [CrossRef]
60. Zeugolis, D.I.; Khew, S.T.; Yew, E.S.Y.; Ekaputra, A.K.; Tong, Y.W.; Yung, L.-Y.L.; Hutmacher, D.W.; Sheppard, C.; Raghunath, M. Electro-spinning of pure collagen nano-fibres—Just an expensive way to make gelatin? *Biomaterials* **2008**, *29*, 2293–2305. [CrossRef]
61. Zhang, Y.; Wang, Y.; Li, Y.; Yang, Y.; Jin, M.; Lin, X.; Zhuang, Z.; Guo, K.; Zhang, T.; Tan, W. Application of Collagen-Based Hydrogel in Skin Wound Healing. *Gels* **2023**, *9*, 185. [CrossRef]
62. Tu, C.-X.; Gao, C.-Y. Recent Advances on Surface-modified Biomaterials Promoting Selective Adhesion and Directional Migration of Cells. *Chin. J. Polym. Sci.* **2021**, *39*, 815–823. [CrossRef]
63. Singh, D.; Dilip Saoji, S. The Role of Surface Energy and Wettability in Polymer-Based Drug Delivery Systems: Enhancing Bioadhesion and Drug Release Efficiency. *J. Macromol. Sci. Part B* **2024**, 1–8. [CrossRef]
64. Liu, T.; Dan, W.; Dan, N.; Liu, X.; Liu, X.; Peng, X. A novel grapheme oxide-modified collagen-chitosan bio-film for controlled growth factor release in wound healing applications. *Mater. Sci. Eng. C* **2017**, *77*, 202–211. [CrossRef]
65. Sun, L.; Guo, J.; Chen, H.; Zhang, D.; Shang, L.; Zhang, B.; Zhao, Y. Tailoring Materials with Specific Wettability in Biomedical Engineering. *Adv. Sci.* **2021**, *8*, 2100126. [CrossRef]
66. Li, B.; Liu, X.; Zhang, X.; Zou, J.; Chai, W.; Lou, Y. Rapid adsorption for oil using superhydrophobic and superoleophilic polyurethane sponge. *J. Chem. Technol. Biotechnol.* **2015**, *90*, 2106–2112. [CrossRef]
67. Rodrigues, A.P.H.; Pereira, I.M.; de Souza, S.D.; Gil, C.S.B.; Machado, G.; Carvalho, S.M.; Pereira, F.V.; Paiva, P.R.P.; de Oliveira, L.C.A.; de O. Patricio, P.S. Control of properties of nanocomposites bio-based collagen and cellulose nanocrystals. *Cellulose* **2017**, *24*, 1731–1744. [CrossRef]
68. Sun, N.; Wang, T.; Yan, X. Self-assembled supermolecular hydrogel based on hydroxyethyl cellulose: Formation, *in vitro* release and bacteriostasis application. *Carbohydr. Polym.* **2017**, *172*, 49–59. [CrossRef] [PubMed]
69. Perez-Puyana, V.; Romero, A.; Guerrero, A. Influence of collagen concentration and glutaraldehyde on collagen-based scaffold properties. *J. Biomed. Mater. Res. Part A* **2016**, *104*, 1462–1468. [CrossRef]
70. Ghataty, D.S.; Amer, R.I.; Wasfi, R.; Shamma, R.N. Novel linezolid loaded bio-composite films as dressings for effective wound healing: Experimental design, development, optimization, and antimicrobial activity. *Drug Deliv.* **2022**, *29*, 3168–3185. [CrossRef]
71. Rizwan, M.; Yahya, R.; Hassan, A.; Yar, M.; Azzahari, A.D.; Selvanathan, V.; Sonsudin, F.; Abouloula, C.N. pH Sensitive Hydrogels in Drug Delivery: Brief History, Properties, Swelling, and Release Mechanism, Material Selection and Applications. *Polymers* **2017**, *9*, 137. [CrossRef]
72. Arafa, A.A.; Nada, A.A.; Ibrahim, A.Y.; Zahran, M.K.; Hakeim, O.A. Greener therapeutic pH-sensing wound dressing based on Curcuma Longa and cellulose hydrogel. *Eur. Polym. J.* **2021**, *159*, 110744. [CrossRef]
73. Zhang, T.; Yu, Z.; Ma, Y.; Chiou, B.-S.; Liu, F.; Zhong, F. Modulating physicochemical properties of collagen films by cross-linking with glutaraldehyde at varied pH values. *Food Hydrocoll.* **2022**, *124*, 107270. [CrossRef]

74. Marin, M.M.; Ianchis, R.; Leu Alexa, R.; Gifu, I.C.; Kaya, M.G.; Savu, D.I.; Popescu, R.C.; Alexandrescu, E.; Ninciuleanu, C.M.; Preda, S.; et al. Development of New Collagen/Clay Composite Biomaterials. *Int. J. Mol. Sci.* **2022**, *23*, 401. [CrossRef]
75. Neacsu, I.A.; Leau, S.-A.; Marin, S.; Holban, A.M.; Vasile, B.-S.; Nicoara, A.-I.; Ene, V.L.; Bleotu, C.; Albu Kaya, M.G.; Ficai, A. Collagen-Carboxymethylcellulose Biocomposite Wound-Dressings with Antimicrobial Activity. *Materials* **2021**, *14*, 1153. [CrossRef] [PubMed]
76. Di Martino, A.; Drannikov, A.; Surgutskaia, N.S.; Ozaltin, K.; Postnikov, P.S.; Marina, T.E.; Sedlarik, V. Chitosan-collagen based film for controlled delivery of a combination of short life anesthetics. *Int. J. Biol. Macromol.* **2019**, *140*, 1183–1193. [CrossRef] [PubMed]
77. Pawar, H.V.; Tetteh, J.; Boateng, J.S. Preparation, optimisation and characterisation of novel wound healing film dressings loaded with streptomycin and diclofenac. *Colloids Surf. B Biointerfaces* **2013**, *102*, 102–110. [CrossRef]
78. Maver, T.; Maver, U.; Mostegel, F.; Griesser, T.; Spirk, S.; Smrke, D.M.; Stana-Kleinschek, K. Cellulose based thin films as a platform for drug release studies to mimick wound dressing materials. *Cellulose* **2015**, *22*, 749–761. [CrossRef]
79. Thu, H.-E.; Zulfakar, M.H.; Ng, S.-F. Alginate based bilayer hydrocolloid films as potential slow-release modern wound dressing. *Int. J. Pharm.* **2012**, *434*, 375–383. [CrossRef] [PubMed]
80. Kan, H.J.; Kharrazi, H.; Chang, H.-Y.; Bodycombe, D.; Lemke, K.; Weiner, J.P. Exploring the use of machine learning for risk adjustment: A comparison of standard and penalized linear regression models in predicting health care costs in older adults. *PLoS ONE* **2019**, *14*, e0213258. [CrossRef]
81. Saffron, C.M.; Park, J.-H.; Dale, B.E.; Voice, T.C. Kinetics of Contaminant Desorption from Soil: Comparison of Model Formulations Using the Akaike Information Criterion. *Environ. Sci. Technol.* **2006**, *40*, 7662–7667. [CrossRef]
82. Romero, A.I.; Villegas, M.; Cid, A.G.; Parentis, M.L.; Gonzo, E.E.; Bermúdez, J.M. Validation of kinetic modeling of progesterone release from polymeric membranes. *Asian J. Pharm. Sci.* **2018**, *13*, 54–62. [CrossRef] [PubMed]
83. Dash, S.; Murthy, P.N.; Nath, L.; Chowdhury, P. Kinetic modeling on drug release from controlled drug delivery systems. *Acta Pol. Pharm.* **2010**, *67*, 217–223.
84. Unagolla, J.M.; Jayasuriya, A.C. Drug transport mechanisms and in vitro release kinetics of vancomycin encapsulated chitosan-alginate polyelectrolyte microparticles as a controlled drug delivery system. *Eur. J. Pharm. Sci. Off. J. Eur. Fed. Pharm. Sci.* **2018**, *114*, 199–209. [CrossRef] [PubMed]
85. Chen, S.; Wu, M.; Lu, P.; Gao, L.; Yan, S.; Wang, S. Development of pH indicator and antimicrobial cellulose nanofibre packaging film based on purple sweet potato anthocyanin and oregano essential oil. *Int. J. Biol. Macromol.* **2020**, *149*, 271–280. [CrossRef]
86. Choi, I.; Lee, J.Y.; Lacroix, M.; Han, J. Intelligent pH indicator film composed of agar/potato starch and anthocyanin extracts from purple sweet potato. *Food Chem.* **2017**, *218*, 122–128. [CrossRef]
87. Arafat, M.T.; Mahmud, M.M.; Wong, S.Y.; Li, X. PVA/PAA based electrospun nanofibers with pH-responsive color change using bromothymol blue and on-demand ciprofloxacin release properties. *J. Drug Deliv. Sci. Technol.* **2021**, *61*, 102297. [CrossRef]
88. Albu, M.G. *Collagen Gels and Matrices for Biomedical Applications*; Lap Lambert Academic Publishing: Saarbrücken, Germany, 2011; pp. 23–24.
89. Boateng, J.S.; Matthews, K.H.; Stevens, H.N.E.; Eccleston, G.M. Wound Healing Dressings and Drug Delivery Systems: A Review. *J. Pharm. Sci.* **2008**, *97*, 2892–2923. [CrossRef] [PubMed]
90. *SR EN ISO 3376:2020*; Leather—Physical and Mechanical Tests—Determination of Tensile Strength and Percentage Elongation. International Organization for Standardization. ASRO: Bucharest, Romania, 2020.
91. Güngör, Z.; Ozay, H. Ultra-fast pH determination with a new colorimetric pH-sensing hydrogel for biomedical and environmental applications. *React. Funct. Polym.* **2022**, *180*, 105398. [CrossRef]
92. Vinklárková, L.; Masteiková, R.; Vetchý, D.; Doležel, P.; Bernatonienė, J. Formulation of Novel Layered Sodium Carboxymethylcellulose Film Wound Dressings with Ibuprofen for Alleviating Wound Pain. *BioMed Res. Int.* **2015**, *2015*, 892671. [CrossRef]
93. Pourjavaher, S.; Almasi, H.; Meshkini, S.; Pirsa, S.; Parandi, E. Development of a colorimetric pH indicator based on bacterial cellulose nanofibers and red cabbage (*Brassica oleraceae*) extract. *Carbohydr. Polym.* **2017**, *156*, 193–201. [CrossRef]

pharmaceuticals

MDPI

Article

Wound-Healing Potential of *Myristica fragrans* Essential Oil: A Multi-Targeted Approach Involving Inflammation, Oxidative Stress, and Apoptosis Regulation

Yahya I. Asiri and Krishnaraju Venkatesan *

Department of Pharmacology, College of Pharmacy, King Khalid University, Abha 62529, Saudi Arabia; yialmuawad@kku.edu.sa
* Correspondence: kvenkatesan@kku.edu.sa

Abstract: Background: Essential oils are widely studied for their therapeutic potential, including their role in wound healing. *Myristica fragrans* essential oil (MEO) has been previously investigated for various pharmacological activities, including anti-inflammatory and antimicrobial effects. However, its mechanistic role in accelerating wound healing and modulating critical pathways, such as oxidative stress, inflammation, and apoptosis, remains poorly characterized. MEO contains a rich profile of monoterpene esters, sesquiterpenoids, and phenolic acids, which may contribute to its bioactivity through unique multi-targeted mechanisms. **Objective:** This research aims to investigate the curative properties of MEO on wound repair, specifically its capacity to regulate inflammation, oxidative stress, and apoptosis in an excision wound model using Wistar rats. **Methods:** Chemical characterization via GC-MS analysis identified Nitrobenzoate Esters (12.85%), Terpenoid/Cineole (6.99%), and Gamma-Terpinene (4.67%) as the dominant constituents. This study utilized a full-thickness excision wound model, and wound contraction, inflammatory cytokines (IL-1β and TNF-α), a macrophage cell surface marker (CD68), oxidative stress markers (ROS MDA, SOD, GSH), and apoptotic regulation (Caspase-3) was evaluated using macroscopic, histopathological, and immunohistochemical analyses. **Result:** MEO treatment significantly reduced pro-inflammatory cytokines IL-1β (658.3 ± 32.7 pg/mg, *** $p < 0.005$) and TNF-α (266.7 ± 33.3 pg/mg, *** $p < 0.005$), compared to the control group (983.3 ± 60.1 and 650 ± 42.8 ** $p < 0.05$, respectively). CD68 expression was also markedly decreased (12.67 ± 0.71 ng/mL, *** $p < 0.005$). Furthermore, MEO effectively attenuated oxidative stress by reducing ROS and MDA levels while restoring antioxidant enzymes GSH and SOD. **Conclusions:** This study demonstrates that Mace Essential Oil (MEO) effectively promotes wound healing by modulating inflammation, oxidative stress, and apoptosis in a preclinical rat model. Its unique bioactive components suggest significant therapeutic potential as a botanical agent for skin repair. Further research is warranted to explore its application in advanced wound-care formulations.

Keywords: mace oil; essential oil; wound healing; *Myristica fragrans*

1. Introduction

Wound healing is a complex and tightly regulated biological process essential for restoring skin integrity following trauma. It involves a cascade of molecular, biochemical, and cellular events, including hemostasis, inflammation, proliferation, and tissue remodelling that work in concert to repair damaged tissue. However, this process often faces complications such as infection, chronic inflammation, and impaired regeneration, making effective wound management a persistent clinical challenge [1].

Current therapeutic strategies include topical antimicrobials (e.g., silver sulfadiazine and mupirocin) [2], advanced wound dressings (e.g., hydrocolloid, alginate, and bioactive matrices) [3], and, in more severe cases, autologous or allogeneic skin grafts [4]. Despite their widespread use, these interventions often exhibit limitations, including prolonged healing times [5], high costs [6], and the growing threat of antibiotic resistance [7]. This underscores the urgent need for safer, cost-effective, and biologically active alternatives that can accelerate healing and reduce complications.

In this context, the use of natural agents, particularly essential oils, has garnered increasing attention due to their broad spectrum of pharmacological properties. Essential oils have been reported to exhibit anti-inflammatory, antimicrobial, antioxidant, and wound-contracting activities, which are crucial for effective tissue repair [8,9]. Studies have shown that essential oils such as lavender, tea tree, and eucalyptus can enhance fibroblast proliferation, promote collagen deposition, and accelerate re-epithelialization, ultimately contributing to improved wound closure [10]. These beneficial effects are attributed to their diverse bioactive constituents, including monoterpenes, sesquiterpenes, and phenolic compounds, which exert synergistic effects on the wound-healing process [11,12].

Although a previous study has reported the wound-healing potential of *Myristica fragrans* essential oil (MEO) [13], its mechanistic role remains underexplored. MEO is characterized by a unique chemical composition, including high levels of monoterpene esters (e.g., terpinyl acetate, geranyl formate), sesquiterpenoids, and phenolic compounds, which have been associated with antioxidant, anti-inflammatory, and antimicrobial activities [14–16]. However, how these constituents collectively influence the wound-healing cascade, particularly oxidative stress modulation and apoptosis regulation, remains to be elucidated.

While previous studies have primarily focused on fibroblast activity and angiogenesis, recent evidence suggests that modulating oxidative stress and apoptosis also play critical roles in wound repair. Excessive oxidative stress impairs healing, while regulated antioxidant activity supports tissue regeneration [17]. Similarly, the inappropriate activation of apoptosis, especially via caspase-3, can hinder epithelial restoration by depleting viable fibroblasts. Therefore, understanding how MEO influences oxidative and apoptotic pathways may reveal important therapeutic mechanisms [18].

Although *Myristica fragrans* essential oil (MEO) has demonstrated anti-inflammatory, antioxidant, and antimicrobial activities in prior studies [13–16], there is limited mechanistic insight into how it contributes to wound healing beyond basic endpoints. Given the increasing demand for plant-based wound therapeutics with scientifically validated mechanisms, a deeper understanding of MEO's biological effects on wound repair is both timely and essential. In particular, its influence on apoptotic regulation and oxidative stress modulation, two pivotal processes in tissue regeneration, remains poorly defined [17,18]. Therefore, this study investigates the wound-healing potential of MEO in a full-thickness excision wound model in Wistar rats, focusing on its ability to modulate key inflammatory cytokines (IL-1β and TNF-α), CD68, oxidative stress markers (ROS, MDA, GSH, SOD), and apoptotic activity (Caspase-3). By integrating biochemical, histopathological, and immunohistochemical analyses, this study aims to fill a critical knowledge gap and provide a scientific basis for MEO's application in regenerative wound therapy.

2. Results

Our findings indicate a significant difference in wound-healing duration among the groups. Wounds in the reference and control groups demonstrated a significantly prolonged recovery time. In contrast, wounds treated with MEO exhibited a markedly accelerated healing period ($p < 0.05$), highlighting the efficacy of this oil in wound healing.

2.1. Chemical Characterization of Essential Oil

The GC-MS analysis (Table 1, Figure 1) of MEO identified various volatile compounds, predominantly constituted by monoterpenes, sesquiterpenes, esters, and phenolic acids. The primary components, determined by peak area percentage, were Nitrobenzoate Esters (12.85%), Terpenoid/Cineole (6.99%), and Gamma-Terpinene (4.67%), followed by Caryophyllane sesquiterpenoids (3.77%), Monolignols/Myristicin (3.69%), and phenolic acids/Shikimic acid derivatives (3.73%). Moreover, geranyl formate (3.04%), terpinyl acetate (3.03%), and Alpha-Terpineol (1.56%) were identified as minor constituents. The chemical profile reveals that MEO comprises a complex amalgamation of bioactive compounds, indicating its potential for biological activity.

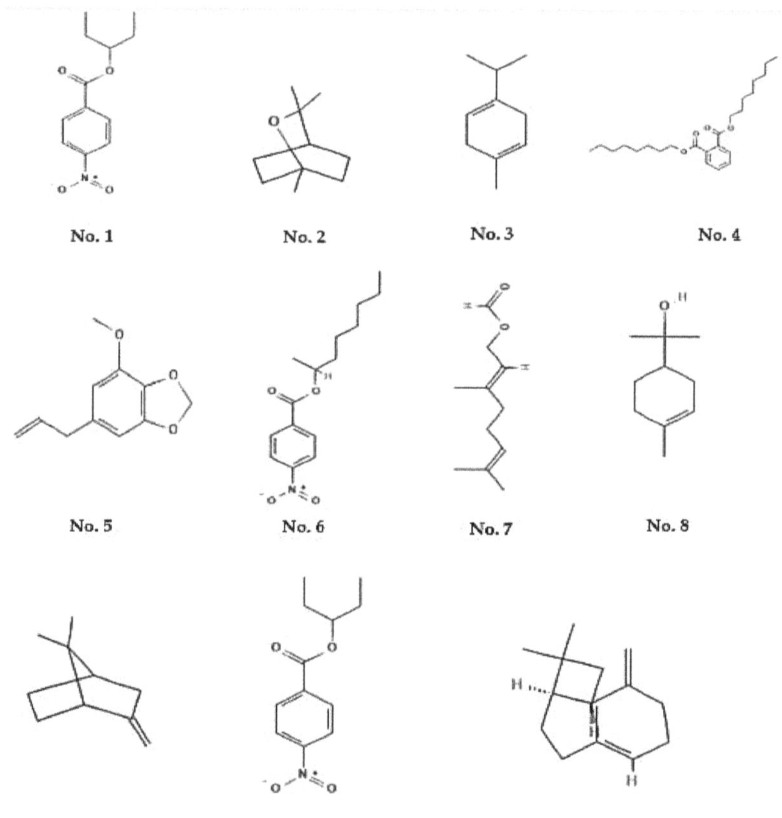

Figure 1. Structure of major compounds identified in an MEO. (**No. 1**) 4-Nitrobenzoic acid, 3-pentyl ester, (**No. 2**) Eucalyptol, (**No. 3**) 1,4-cyclohexadiene, 1-methyl-4-(1-methylethyl), (**No. 4**) Di-n-octyl phthalate, (**No. 5**) 1,3-Benzodioxole, 4-methoxy-6-(2-propenyl), (**No. 6**) 4-Nitro-benzoic acid, 1-methyl-heptyl ester, (**No. 7**) 2,6-octadien-1-ol, 3,7-dimethyl-, formate, (e)-, (**No. 8**) 3-cyclohexene-1-methanol, .alpha.,.alpha.,4-trimethyl, (**No. 9**) Bicyclo[2.2.1]heptane, 7,7-dimethyl-2-methylene-, (**No. 10**) 4-Nitrobenzoic acid, 3-pentyl ester, and (**No. 11**) Caryophyllene.

Table 1. Compounds have a peak area percentage greater than 1.0%, according to the GCMS data on frankincense oil.

Retention Duration (Min)	Name of the Compound	Peak Area (%)	Molecular Formula	Chemical Class
29.996	4-nitrobenzoic acid, 3-pentyl ester	12.85	$C_{12}H_{15}NO_4$	Nitrobenzoate Esters
7.416	Eucalyptol	6.99	$C_{10}H_{18}O$	Terpenoid/Cineole
5.627	1,4-cyclohexadiene,1-methyl-4-(1-methylethyl)-	4.67	$C_{10}H_{16}$	Gamma-Terpinene
17.468	-)-5-oxatricyclo[8.2.0.0(4,6)]dodecane,,12-trimethyl-9-	3.77	$C_{15}H_{24}O$	Caryophyllene Sesquiterpenoids
29.293	Di-N-octyl phthalate	3.73	$C_{24}H_{38}O_4$	Phenolic Acids/Shikimic Acids And Derivatives
16.423	1,3-benzodioxole, 4-methoxy-6-(2-propenyl)-	3.69	$C_{11}H_{12}O_3$	Monolignols/ Myristicin
30.293	4-nitro-benzoic acid, 1-methyl-heptyl ester	3.51	$C_{15}H_{21}NO_4$	Nitrobenzoate Esters
6.433	2,6-octadien-1-ol, 3,7-dimethyl-, formate, (e)-	3.04	$C_{11}H_{18}O_2$	Geranyl Formate
13.429	3-cyclohexene-1-methanol, .alpha.,.alpha.,4-trimethyl-,	3.03	$C_{12}H_{20}O_2$	Terpinyl Acetate
6.322	Bicyclo[2.2.1]heptane, 7,7-dimethyl-2-methylene-	2.51	$C_{10}H_{16}$	Monoterpene/ Alpha-Fenchene
30.133	4-nitrobenzoic acid, 3-pentyl ester	2.44	$C_{12}H_{15}NO_4$	Nitrobenzoate Esters
14.722	Caryophyllene	2.17	$C_{15}H_{24}$	Polycyclic Sesquiterpenes
30.354	1,2-benzene dicarboxylic acid, dioctyl ester	2.02	$C_{24}H_{38}O_4$	Phthalic Acids-Diethylhexyl Phthalate
17.164	8-acetoxycarvotanacetone	1.96	$C_{12}H_{18}O_3$	Terpinenes
10.538	3-cyclohexene-1-methanol, .alpha.,.alpha.,4-trimethyl-	1.56	$C_{10}H_{18}O$	Alpha-Terpineol
18.161	2,6,6-trimethylbicyclo[3.1.1]heptane-2,3-diol	1.72	$C_{10}H_{18}O_2$	Monoterpenoids-Pinane Monoterpenoids
14.901	2-((1r,4r)-4-Hydroxy-4-Methylcyclohex-2-Enyl)Propan-2-Yl Acetate	1.48	$C_{12}H_{20}O_3$	Cannabidiol
11.621	1,5-dimethyl-1-vinyl-4-hexenyl 2-aminobenzoate	1.41	$C_{17}H_{23}NO_2$	Arene-Linalyl Anthranilate
13.608	Eugenol	1.37	$C_{10}H_{12}O_2$	Caffeic Acids–Eugenol
15.362	2-((1r,4r)-4-Hydroxy-4-Methylcyclohex-2-Enyl)Propan-2-Yl Acetate	1.21	$C_{12}H_{20}O_3$	Cannabidiol
8.687	1,6-octadien-3-ol, 3,7-dimethyl-	1.21	$C_{10}H_{18}O$	Monoterpenoid-Linalool

Table 1. *Cont.*

Retention Duration (Min)	Name of the Compound	Peak Area (%)	Molecular Formula	Chemical Class
10.376	Dl-menthol	1.10	$C_{10}H_{20}O$	Cyclohexanols-Menthol
6.953	1,4-cyclohexadiene, 1-methyl-4-(1-methylethyl)-	1.03	$C_{10}H_{16}$	Cyclohexane Monoterpenes/ Gamma-Terpinene
13.071	P-month-8-en-3-ol, acetate	1.03	$C_{12}H_{20}O_2$	Isopulegyl Acetate
9.598	2h-Pyran-3-Ol, 6-Ethenyltetrahydro-2,2,6-Trimethyl-	1.01	$C_{10}H_{18}O_2$	Oxanes/Linalool Oxide Pyranoside

2.2. *Toxicity Studies*

Test oil was safe at 10% *w/w* in the acute cutaneous irritation trial; animals were monitored for three days following the experiment and showed no signs of skin response, inflammation, erythema, irritation, or redness.

2.3. *Percentage of Wound Contraction*

The examination of the excision wound demonstrated a significant and time-dependent decrease in wound area compared to both the reference and control groups. On Day 4, the percentage of wound closure in the MEO group was 45.41 ± 4.70% (* $p < 0.05$), which increased to 68.16 ± 3.44% on Day 8 (*** $p < 0.001$). A marked improvement was observed by Day 12 with 94.86 ± 0.32% closure (*** $p < 0.001$), reaching 99.70 ± 0.13% by Day 16 (**** $p < 0.0001$) and achieving complete closure (100 ± 0.00%) on Day 20 (**** $p < 0.0001$). These values were significantly higher than those observed in the reference and control groups at each corresponding time point, indicating the superior efficacy of MEO in accelerating wound healing (Figures 2 and 3).

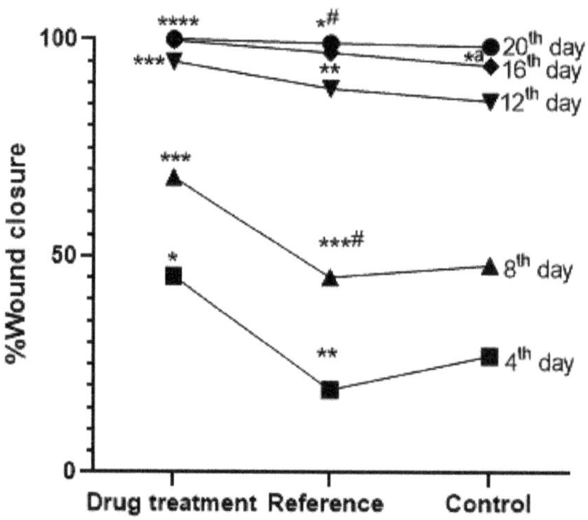

Figure 2. Impact of MEO on wound closure percentage in reference and control groups. $n = 6$; group, **** $p < 0.0001$ MEO vs. control, *** $p < 0.005$ MEO vs. control, ***# $p < 0.005$ MEO vs. reference group, ** $p < 0.05$ MEO vs. reference group, * $p < 0.05$ MEO versus control group, *# $p < 0.05$. MEO vs. reference group, and *a $p < 0.05$ reference vs. control group. Tukey's multiple comparison test was conducted after applying a one-way ANOVA for data analysis. *p*-values below 0.05 are considered significant.

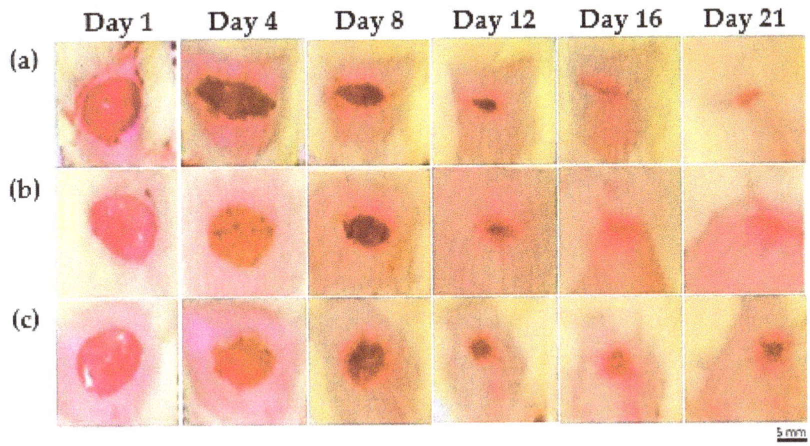

Figure 3. Representative images showing wound healing among the various groups. (**a**) The MEO group, (**b**) reference group, and (**c**) control group showed signs of wound healing throughout time, as seen by typical photos taken between Days 1 and 21. By the conclusion of the observation period, the MEO treatment group had achieved complete epithelialization and shown accelerated wound healing. Scale bar = 5 mm; applies to all panels. Calibration is based on the known initial wound diameter of 20 mm on Day 1.

2.4. Body Weight and Feed Intake

As illustrated in Figures 4 and 5, a clear and consistent increase in body weight and feed intake is observed in the MEO-treated group from the 4th to the 21st day, showing statistically significant differences when compared to the reference and control groups. The body weight gains in the MEO group are marked with increasing significance levels (*** $p < 0.005$ to **** $p < 0.0001$), indicating a robust and progressive improvement over time. In comparison, the reference and control groups exhibited either modest or delayed weight gain, with statistical significance emerging primarily during the later stages (16th and 21st days).

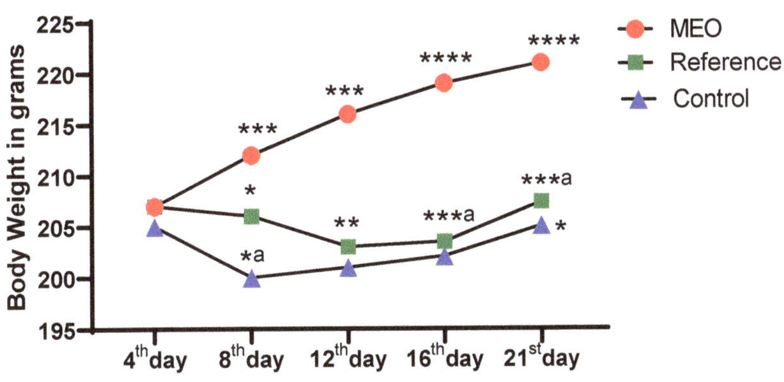

Figure 4. Impact of MEO on body weight compared to the reference and control groups. $n = 6$; mean ± SEM, * $p < 0.05$ MEO vs. reference, *a $p < 0.05$ reference vs. control, ** $p < 0.05$ MEO vs. reference, *** $p < 0.005$ MEO vs. control, and ***a $p < 0.005$ MEO vs. reference group; **** $p < 0.0001$ MEO vs. control group are the corresponding values. Tukey's multiple comparison test was conducted after the data analysis using a one-way ANOVA. p-values below 0.05 are considered statistically significant.

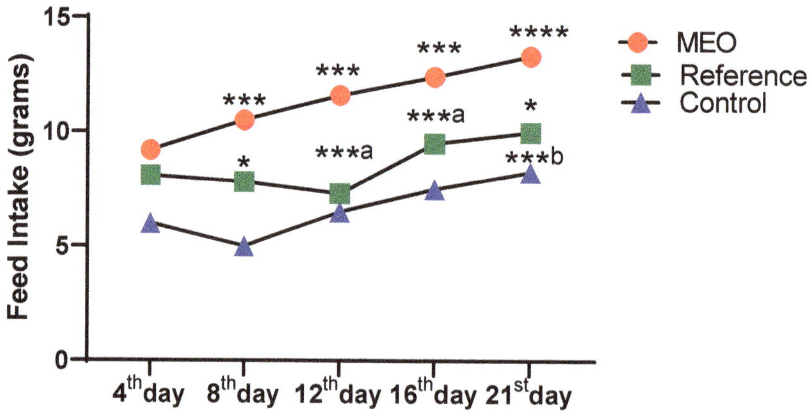

Figure 5. Impact of MEO on body weight compared to the reference and control groups. $n = 6$; mean ± SEM, * $p < 0.05$ MEO vs. reference, *** $p < 0.005$ MEO vs. control, and ***a $p < 0.005$ MEO vs. reference group; ***b $p < 0.001$ reference vs. group and **** $p < 0.0001$ MEO vs. control group are the corresponding values. Tukey's multiple comparison test was conducted subsequent to the data analysis using a one-way ANOVA. p-values below 0.05 are considered statistically significant.

The observed difference in body weight is closely related to feed intake. Each day at 8:00 a.m., feed was weighed and provided to the animals. The next morning, the remaining feed was measured to calculate the daily feed intake. As shown in Figure 5, feed intake also steadily increased in the MEO group, displaying statistically significant differences (*** $p < 0.005$ to **** $p < 0.0001$) across all days when compared to the other groups. In contrast, the reference group showed a moderate increase, and the control group exhibited the least improvement. This pattern highlights a direct correlation between nutritional intake and weight gain, with the MEO group consistently outperforming the others.

The MEO group not only demonstrated enhanced feed consumption and body weight gain but also showed signs of accelerated physiological recovery, suggesting improved metabolic efficiency and superior nutrient assimilation. These findings strongly support the efficacy of MEO in promoting growth and recovery in treated subjects, in contrast to the slower progression observed in the reference and control groups.

2.5. *Effects of MEO on Inflammatory Markers and Wound-Healing Dynamics*

Compared to the reference and control groups, Table 2 shows that on the 21st day, the inflammatory markers IL-1β and TNF-α were markedly higher in injured rats. Treatment with MEO or the standard markedly diminished these heightened inflammatory markers, highlighting their anti-inflammatory effectiveness.

Table 2. Effects of MEO on CD68, IL-1β, and TNF-α against the reference and control groups.

Treatment	IL-1β (pg/mg)	TNF-α (pg/mg)	CD68 (ng/mL)
MEO	658.3 ± 32.70 ***	266.7 ± 33.33 ***	12.67 ± 0.7149 ***
Reference	825 ± 30.96 *	433.3 ± 42.16 *	15.83 ± 0.7032 *
Control	983.3 ± 60.09	650 ± 42.82 **	31.83 ± 1.014 ***

Cytokine levels (IL-1β, TNF-α, and CD68) were measured in serum samples collected on Day 21 post-wounding to assess residual inflammatory activity. Data are presented as mean ± SEM for $n = 6$. ** $p < 0.05$ reference vs. control group, * $p < 0.05$ drug vs. reference, *** $p < 0.005$ drug vs. control, and *** $p < 0.005$ reference vs. control group are the values shown as mean ± SEM for $n = 6$. Tukey's multiple comparison test was performed after a one-way ANOVA was used to analyze the data. p-values of less than 0.05 are regarded as significant.

2.6. *Effect of MEO on CD68 Level in Experimental Rats*

G-protein CD68 functions as a marker for macrophages engaged in tissue repair. The expression level of CD68 in the injured cells of all the test subjects was assessed on Day 21. As seen in Table 2, the untreated control group's CD68 levels were significantly higher than those of the MEO and conventional treatment groups. The MEO group had a much higher reduction in CD68 expression compared to the group undergoing normal pharmaceutical therapy. These data highlight MEO's superior effectiveness in diminishing CD68 levels, demonstrating its strong anti-inflammatory characteristics and essential function in wound healing.

2.7. *Impact on Antioxidant Profile and Oxidative Stress Indicators*

Significant alterations in the levels of oxidative stress markers, ROS and MDA, and antioxidant enzymes, SOD and GSH, were observed in the skin tissues of treated, reference, and control rats, as depicted in Figure 6. By Day 21 post-injury, tissues from the MEO-treated group exhibited a marked increase in SOD activity and GSH levels, indicating enhanced endogenous antioxidant defence. In contrast, the untreated control group showed elevated levels of ROS and MDA, reflecting increased oxidative stress and lipid peroxidation. These findings suggest that the impaired antioxidant defence and accumulation of lipid peroxidation products in the control group contributed to delayed wound healing. Conversely, the MEO-treated group demonstrated a favourable redox status, characterized by reduced oxidative damage and improved antioxidant capacity, which likely facilitated faster and more efficient tissue repair.

2.8. *Results of Histology*

Measurement of Histopathological Changes

A semi-quantitative scoring system was used to evaluate the histopathological changes associated with wound healing. Each tissue sample was assessed for key parameters including collagen deposition, granulation tissue formation, inflammatory cell infiltration, re-epithelialization, and angiogenesis. Scoring was performed on a scale of 0 to 3 (0 = absent, 1 = mild, 2 = moderate, 3 = marked), and the average score for each group was calculated to reflect the overall histological recovery. Higher scores indicated delayed or impaired healing, while lower scores denoted improved tissue regeneration.

Histological evaluations were conducted on tissue sections collected at Day 21 post-wounding using Hematoxylin and Eosin (H&E) staining. All slides were examined in a blinded fashion by an experienced veterinary pathologist who was unaware of the treatment group assignments. This approach ensured the objective assessment of structural integrity and healing dynamics across experimental groups. The final histological scores are presented in Table 3, and representative microscopic images are shown in Figure 7.

Table 3. Effects of MEO on histopathological changes against the reference and control groups.

Changes in Histopathology	Average Score		
	MEO	Reference	Control
Collagen Deposition	1	1	1
Re-epithelialization	3	2	1
Inflammatory Response	0	1	1
Granulation Tissue Formation	2	1	1
Angiogenesis	1	2	3

n = 6; group, measurement of histopathological changes for collagen deposition, re-epithelialization, inflammatory response, granulation tissue formation, and angiogenesis.

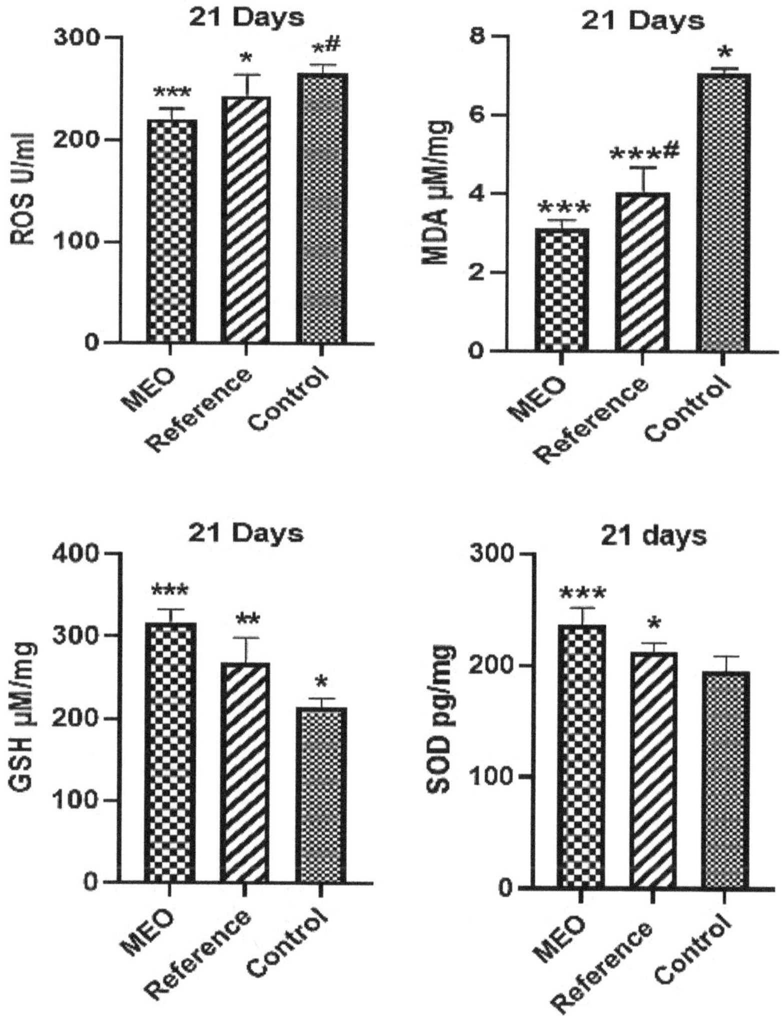

Figure 6. The effects of MEO on ROS, MDA, GSH, and SOD in comparison to the reference and control groups. ** $p < 0.05$ reference compared to control group, *** $p < 0.005$ drug compared to control group, * $p < 0.05$ drug compared to reference group, *# $p < 0.05$ reference compared to control, and ***# $p < 0.005$ reference compared to control group, with $n = 6$ indicating the values, presented as mean ± SEM. Tukey's multiple comparison test was performed following the one-way ANOVA data analysis. p-values of less than 0.05 are considered statistically significant.

2.9. Immunohistochemical Staining

An analysis of the immunohistochemical evaluations of Caspase-3 activation across the groups demonstrates unique patterns linked to wound healing (Figure 8). The MEO-treated cohort's fully healed wound, namely the fibroblasts and immune cells in the granulation tissue, was where caspase 3 was most clearly expressed. The reference group's fully healed wound region shows a modest expression of caspase 3. On the other hand, the control group exhibits very little Caspase-3 expression, which is characterized by a more advanced stage of healing as seen by decreased immune cell activity and fibroblast engagement. The results indicate that MEO treatment influences Caspase-3 expression, possibly promoting wound healing through regulated apoptotic pathways.

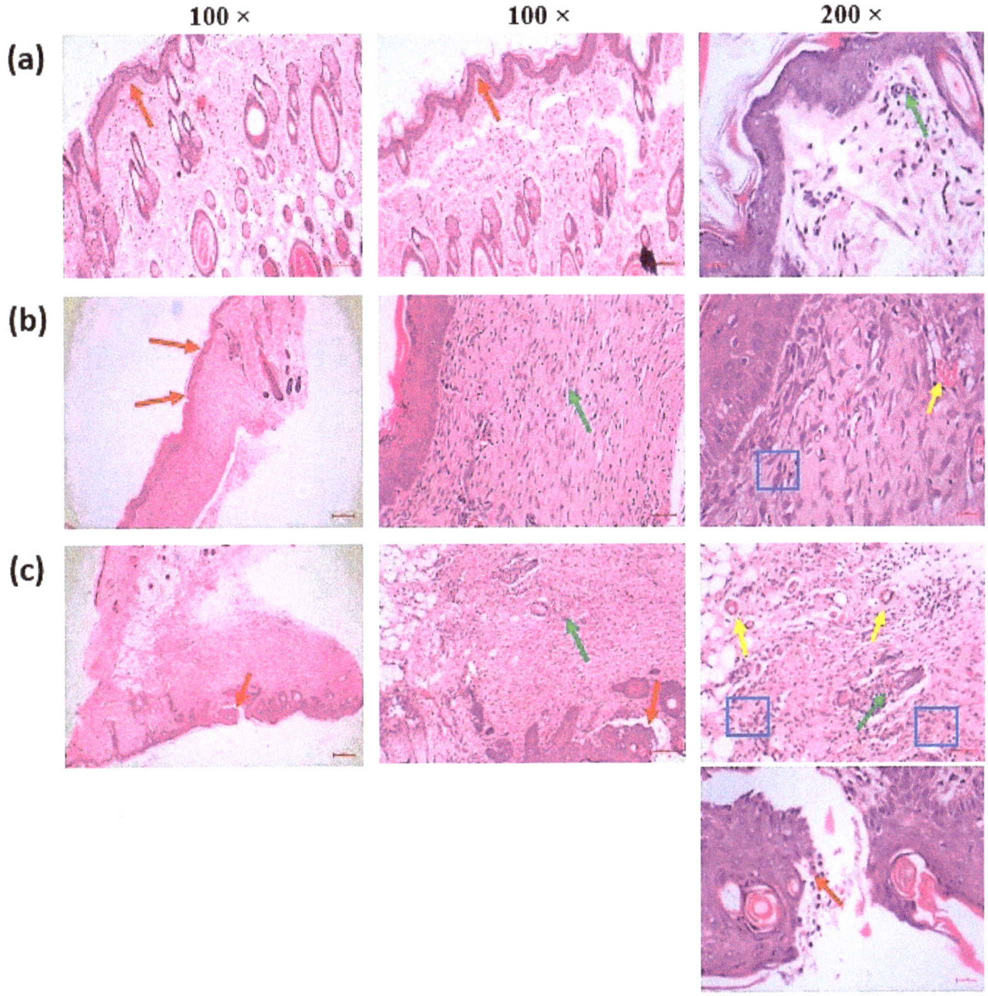

Figure 7. (**a**) MEO treatment—total restoration of the epithelium (red arrow) and dermis, with minimal infiltrating inflammatory cells (green arrow). (**b**) Reference: The impacted areas exhibited complete re-epithelialization alongside epidermal hyperplasia (red arrow) and a moderate inflammatory response, characterized by granulation tissue proliferation in the superficial region adjacent to the injury site (green arrow). Additionally, fewer than five blood vessels per high-power field defined moderate angiogenesis or neovascularization (yellow arrow). The region contiguous to the epidermis was substituted. Fibroblasts (blue square) that make collagen and other extracellular matrix components, a network of tiny blood vessels (yellow arrow—capillaries), and different inflammatory cells (green arrow), primarily plasma cells and lymphocytes, followed by neutrophils, are all part of thick granulation tissue. (**c**) Control: Incomplete wound healing is characterized by inadequate re-epithelialization at the wound site and an overabundance of necrotic debris and inflammatory exudates in the epidermal layers (Red arrow). A considerable inflammatory response with granulation tissue growth was observed in the dermal region around the incision (green arrow), along with pronounced angiogenesis, evidenced by 5 to 10 blood vessels per high-power field (yellow arrow). The area surrounding the epidermal lesion was substituted with granulation tissue, consisting of a network of capillaries (yellow arrow), fibroblasts (blue square) that synthesize collagen and other extracellular matrix components, and various inflammatory cells (green arrow), primarily neutrophils, in addition to plasma cells and lymphocytes.

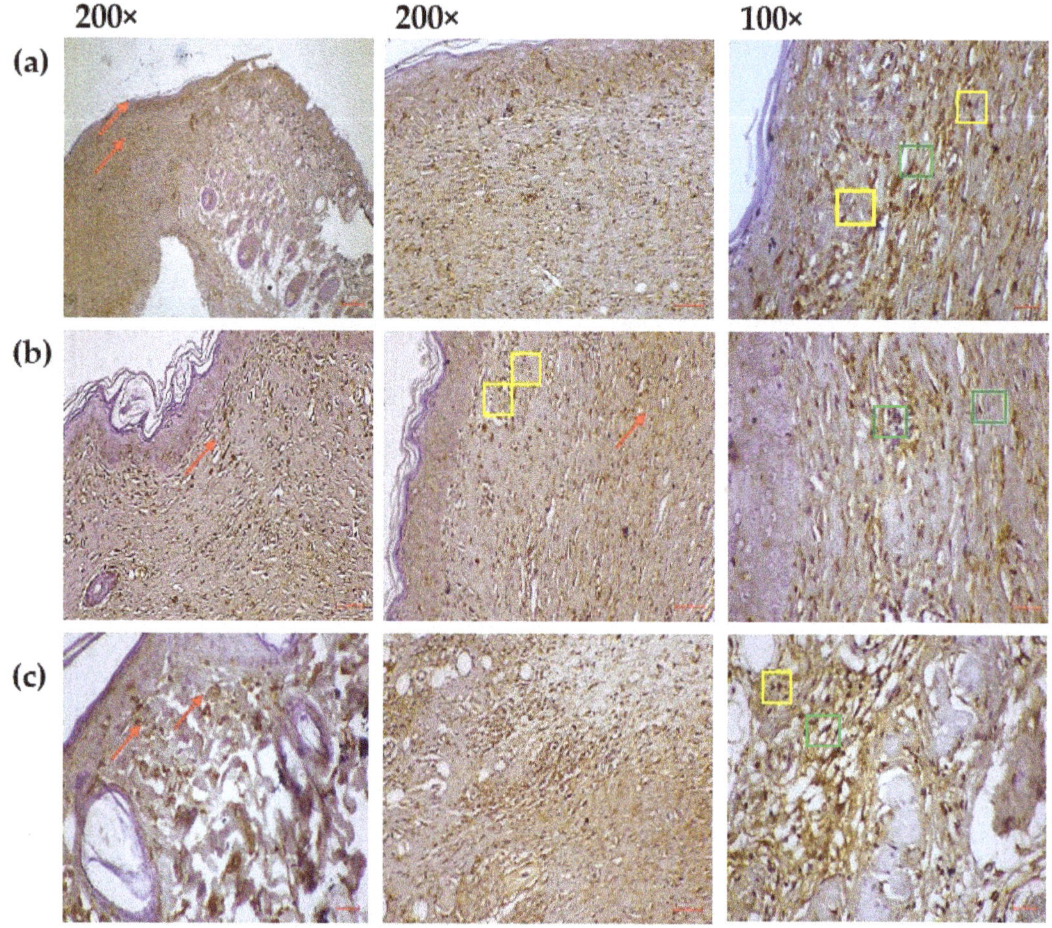

Figure 8. Immunohistochemical assessments of Caspase-3 activation among each of the groups. (**a**) MEO-treated group: Caspase-3 expression appeared at normal levels in the fully re-epithelialized epidermal and dermal regions (indicated by red arrows). Normal nucleo-cytoplasmic staining of caspase-3 was evident in the granulation tissue, particularly within fibroblasts (green square) and among infiltrating immune cells, including neutrophils, plasma cells, and lymphocytes (yellow square), located in both the epidermal and dermal layers. (**b**) Reference group: A moderate level of caspase-3 expression was observed in the healed skin, specifically within the epidermis and dermis (red arrows). Granulation tissue showed moderate nucleo-cytoplasmic caspase-3 localization, primarily in fibroblasts (green square) and immune cells such as neutrophils, plasma cells, and lymphocytes (yellow square), spread across the skin layers. (**c**) Control group: Caspase-3 expression was limited to a mild level in the re-epithelialized epidermis and dermis (red arrows). Weak nucleo-cytoplasmic caspase-3 staining was detected in fibroblasts (green square) and immune cells (yellow square) within the granulation tissue of both skin layers.

3. Discussion

This research is the first evaluation of the wound-healing effectiveness of MEO (*Myristica fragrans*) in a preclinical model. While numerous essential oils, such as those from lavender, tea tree, and eucalyptus, have been extensively studied for their ability to modulate inflammation and stimulate fibroblast activity, MEO appears to exert a broader mechanism of action. Our findings suggest that MEO modulates apoptotic pathways, as indicated by differential Caspase-3 expression in skin tissues, and influences macrophage activity, as supported by changes in serum CD68 levels. These multifaceted effects may collectively enhance wound resolution by attenuating excessive apoptosis and supporting immune cell-driven tissue remodelling. The elevated levels of monoterpene esters and sesquiterpenoids in MEO distinguish it from traditional essential oils, as these bioactive compounds are associated with the inhibition of NF-κB and MAPK, the suppression of COX-2, and the regulation of oxidative stress [19].

In contrast to recognized wound-healing essential oils, such as lavender, tea tree, and clove oil, MEO exhibits a distinctive combination of anti-inflammatory, oxidative stress-regulating, and apoptotic-modulating characteristics. Lavender and tea tree oil primarily function through fibroblast stimulation and microbial inhibition, whereas MEO demonstrates a more extensive, multifaceted impact on wound healing, notably through Caspase-3 inhibition and macrophage polarization [20]. In contrast to eucalyptus and rosemary oil, which primarily mitigate oxidative stress through Nrf2 activation, MEO seems to preserve a delicate equilibrium between oxidative stress reduction and fibroblast viability by inhibiting excessive apoptosis via Caspase-3 inhibition [21].

Additionally, the presence of caryophyllene-type sesquiterpenes and cineole in MEO suggests potential to modulate macrophage activity and favour the shift from pro-inflammatory M1 to reparative M2 phenotypes. This hypothesis is supported by previous preclinical evidence showing that caryophyllene sesquiterpenes, particularly β-caryophyllene, can influence macrophage polarization and dampen inflammatory signalling [22]. While our current study did not directly assess macrophage phenotypes, the observed reduction in pro-inflammatory cytokines (IL-1β and TNF-α) and improved tissue remodelling are consistent with an anti-inflammatory wound environment, which may involve M2 macrophage activity [23]. This immunological transition plays a pivotal role in debris clearance, angiogenesis, and collagen remodelling during the proliferative and remodelling phases of wound healing, thereby enhancing the therapeutic relevance of MEO [24].

Inflammation is a crucial but tightly regulated phase of wound healing. While early inflammatory responses (typically peaking around days 5 to 7) are necessary for microbial clearance and tissue debridement, persistent or unresolved inflammation beyond this window can disrupt tissue regeneration and contribute to chronic wound pathology [25]. In our study, pro-inflammatory cytokines IL-1β and TNF-α were assessed on Day 21 post-wounding to evaluate residual inflammatory activity during the late reparative phase, which is increasingly recognized as a determinant of wound resolution quality. Despite this being a later time point, MEO treatment markedly diminished IL-1β and TNF-α levels, indicating not only a resolution in early inflammation but also a suppression of lingering pro-inflammatory signals that may impair healing. This finding underscores MEO's role in promoting a favourable inflammatory trajectory, not merely during the acute phase but throughout the wound-healing continuum.

Considering that MAPK activation was a critical regulator of IL-1β and TNF-α expression, it is reasonable to propose that MEO mediates its anti-inflammatory effects via the inhibition of these pathways, thereby attenuating cytokine production even at advanced stages of tissue repair [26]. These effects may explain the improved histological outcomes and accelerated epithelialization observed in the MEO group, suggesting an immunomodulatory sustained impact that extends beyond early-phase cytokine suppression.

Moreover, the COX-2 inhibitory potential of MEO is significant, as prostaglandins derived from COX-2 are linked to heightened inflammatory responses in wounds. The presence of linalool, α-terpineol, and γ-terpinene in MEO indicates a pharmacological profile favourable for inflammation reduction and fibroblast viability [27]. Unlike many essential oils traditionally explored for wound healing, MEO exhibits a combination of anti-inflammatory effects, demonstrated by the reduced serum levels of IL-1β and TNF-α and the modulation of macrophage activity, as suggested by decreased CD68 expression [28]. Although the specific transition toward a reparative macrophage phenotype (M2) was not directly assessed, this dual effect suggests a broader immunomodulatory potential that warrants further investigation. Such a combined action is less frequently characterized among other botanical therapies.

Moderate levels of reactive oxygen species (ROS) are essential for cellular signalling and antimicrobial defence; however, excessive oxidative stress disrupts tissue homeostasis, leading to lipid peroxidation, fibroblast apoptosis, and impaired wound healing [29]. MEO demonstrated significant antioxidant activity, as evidenced by increased levels of SOD and GSH, alongside reduced ROS and MDA levels. Excessive ROS production can damage proteins, nucleic acids, and membrane lipids, thereby impairing cell migration and extracellular matrix (ECM) deposition. The observed reduction in ROS in MEO-treated wounds suggests the mitigation of oxidative damage and supports a redox environment favourable for the proliferative phase of wound healing. MDA, a well-established marker of lipid peroxidation and oxidative membrane damage, was also significantly decreased. This reduction indicates the preservation of membrane integrity, a critical requirement for cellular proliferation, migration, and re-epithelialization during wound repair [30].

Glutathione (GSH) is a key intracellular antioxidant involved in redox homeostasis, the detoxification of electrophilic intermediates, and the protection of protein thiol groups. The elevated GSH levels in the MEO-treated group indicate an enhanced cellular capacity to counter oxidative stress, which supports fibroblast viability and effective tissue regeneration [31]. Superoxide dismutase (SOD), although mistakenly referred to as inflammatory by the reviewer, is a primary antioxidant enzyme that catalyzes the dismutation of superoxide radicals into molecular oxygen and hydrogen peroxide. The increased SOD activity observed in the MEO group reflects an upregulation of endogenous antioxidant defences, consistent with a protective cellular response to oxidative challenge [32].

Additionally, the presence of bioactive compounds in MEO—such as caffeic acid derivatives, myristicin, and caryophyllene-type sesquiterpenoids—suggests the potential activation of the Nrf2 signalling pathway, which plays a pivotal role in the transcriptional regulation of antioxidant enzymes and cellular resilience to oxidative damage [33].

The excessive apoptosis of keratinocytes and fibroblasts may hinder wound closure and collagen production. The noted downregulation of Caspase-3 in MEO-treated wounds indicates that MEO protects against apoptosis, thereby promoting cell survival and extracellular matrix deposition. This phenomenon may be ascribed to eugenol, α-terpineol, and derivatives of Shikimic acid, which have been documented to inhibit Caspase-3 activation and enhance fibroblast proliferation [34].

This study emphasizes the modulation of apoptosis as an innovative therapeutic strategy for botanical wound-healing treatments. In contrast to conventional therapies that target solely antioxidant and anti-inflammatory effects, MEO appears to maintain fibroblast integrity by inhibiting excessive apoptotic signalling [35]. No currently available essential oil utilized for wound healing has demonstrated a comparable effect on apoptotic regulation. Nonetheless, further research is required to validate the direct involvement of MEO in apoptotic regulation, utilizing TUNEL staining, Western blot analysis of cleaved Caspase-3, and apoptosis-rescue experiments.

MEO possesses considerable therapeutic potential in wound care and regenerative medicine due to its multi-targeted effects. In contrast to synthetic wound-healing agents that may present risks of cytotoxicity and antibiotic resistance, MEO provides a naturally derived alternative characterized by robust bioactivity and low toxicity. This renders it a promising contender for further advancement in dermatological applications.

Subsequent research should focus on enhancing the therapeutic efficacy and clinical applicability of MEO. A potential approach is the development of MEO-based hydrogels or bioactive dressings, which may offer extended wound protection and the regulated release of bioactive substances. Furthermore, nanocarrier delivery systems, including liposomes and micelles, may be investigated to enhance the bioavailability, stability, and targeted delivery of MEO to wound sites. Moreover, comparative analyses with currently approved wound-healing agents are essential to substantiate the efficacy of MEO and establish it as a credible botanical treatment within contemporary wound management protocols.

4. Materials and Methods

4.1. Animals Used in Experiments

Male adult albino rats weighing 150 and 170 g were removed from the Central Animal House and kept in a controlled environment with a temperature of 25 ± 2 °C and a humidity level of 55%. Rats were systematically observed over 12 h light and dark cycles. Rats were housed in isolation, free from human interaction, and provided with unlimited access to potable water and standard laboratory feed. Every animal experiment must comply with the guidelines set forth by the Experimental Animal Ethics Committee [36]. The Institutional Animal Ethics Committee (IAEC) sanctioned the study procedure (ECM/2021-5306/dated 2 May 2021). The research experiments were conducted according to the guidelines governing the use and care of experimental animals.

4.2. Source of Oil

According to the manufacturer, Allinpro Exporters, India oil was extracted through steam distillation.

4.3. Identification of Compounds in MEO by GC-MS

Essential oil composition was analyzed via gas chromatography–mass spectrometry (GC-MS) utilizing a Shimadzu GCMS-QP2010 Plus system (Shimadzu Corporation, Kyoto, Japan) fitted with an HP-5MS capillary column (30 m, 0.25 mm i.d., 0.25 m film thickness, Agilent Technologies, Santa Clara, CA, USA). The substance was diluted 1:10 (*v*/*v*) in hexane following filtration through a 0.22 µm membrane filter before evaluation. A 1.0 µL aliquot was injected in split mode at a 40:1 split ratio at a temperature of 250 °C. The carrier gas was helium, which flows at a steady 1.0 mL/min. After one minute at 50 °C, the oven temperature was increased by 8 °C per minute until it reached 280 °C, which was maintained for two minutes. Ionization was accomplished using electron impact (EI) at 70 eV while the ion source temperature was maintained at 200 °C. Mass spectra were recorded for a total duration of 31 min within the 40–900 m/z range. The NIST Library, Version 8.0, supplied by the National Institute of Standards and Technology, Gaithersburg, MD, USA, was utilized to compare the mass spectra of chemical compounds for identification purposes.

4.4. Methods of Making Ointment

Ointments were prepared by thoroughly blending 10% *w*/*w* MEO into a soft paraffin base sourced from a certified pharmacy. The mixture was levigated to ensure a smooth ointment texture in the ointment. The standard reference was silver sulfadiazine ointment (1% *w*/*w*), while the negative control was soft paraffin.

4.5. Toxicity Studies

According to OECD guidelines 404 [37], a cohort of ten male Sprague-Dawley rats weighing 250 g and 300 g was utilized to evaluate dermal responses. Rats were divided into two groups, each comprising five individuals. Five rats were used as experimental subjects, while an additional five served as controls. Each rat was individually housed after removing hair from its posterior region using a sterile shaver until a diameter of approximately 20 cm was achieved at the lower mid-position. The rats were permitted to acclimatize in a tranquil environment for 24 h. The test subjects were administered a consistent application of a 10% essential oil solution to the depilated region. One hour was allocated for applying plant extracts to the skin utilizing gauze and non-irritating adhesive tape. After one hour, the substances were eliminated, and distilled water was used to cleanse the skin surface; the level of irritation was then evaluated. Topical evaluations were conducted 24 h post-application and subsequently repeated after 48 and 72 h. Sterile cotton soaked in an adequate amount of sterilized water was used to apply sterile water topically to control rats. The cotton was subsequently encased in gauze and hypoallergenic adhesive tape. The Draize grading system was utilized to assess edema and erythema. Erythema or edema is absent when the score is zero and slightly present when the score is one. A score of two denotes moderate edema, which is characterized by raised skin margins around the affected area. Erythema or moderate-to-severe edema are indicated by a score of 3, while severe erythema or edema are indicated by a score of 4 [38].

4.6. Excision Wound Model

4.6.1. Experimental Design

Three cohorts of mature albino rats ($n = 6$) were utilized in the wound-healing study.
MEO: Test drug treatment of animals (10% w/w MEO).
Reference: Animals receiving a standard dose of 1% silver sulfadiazine.
Control: Control group (treated with soft paraffin).

4.6.2. Wounding Method

A 12 h fast was administered to the adult rats, and then they were given an intraperitoneal anesthetic comprising 50 mg/kg of ketamine and 10 mg/kg of xylazine just before wound preparation. Rats were placed in a prone position on a surgical table. Subsequently, the hair on the back, specifically between the shoulders, was epilated using an electric shaver. The region was subsequently cleaned with 70% ethanol to maintain aseptic conditions and create an excision wound. Within a semi-aseptic environment, a circular incision in the dorsal thoracic region of rats, measuring approximately 2 cm (20 mm), was made. Then, the full thickness of the skin epidermis, dermis, and hypodermis was removed using a knife. The excess blood was mopped up using sterile gauze. The entire incision remained exposed throughout the research, and no treatment was administered to the wounds. To prevent infections, the animals were closely monitored, and any rats showing signs of illness were excluded from the study [39].

4.7. Treatment

Test and standard drugs were applied daily with the help of a sterilized spatula until complete epithelialization. To avoid dosage variations, this was performed with extra caution throughout the day. Before administering the therapies, a tampon saturated with normal saline was used to clean the wound surfaces methodically. The wound area was measured using graph paper at 1, 4, 8, 12, 16, and 21 days post-injury. The epithelialization process is characterized as the flaking of the eschar without any visible wound. The skin surrounding the healed wound and the adjacent tissue was excised on day 21 to perform the histopathological analysis and antioxidant assessment. The tissue was subsequently divided into two equal sections.

4.8. Evaluation Parameters

Percentage wound contraction: Wound contraction was assessed using the Wilson Formula:

$$\% \text{ wound contraction} = (1 - \text{wound area on a particular day/wound area on day 0}) \times 100$$

To document wound progression, the wound margins were initially traced every four days (Days 1, 4, 8, 12, 16, and 21) onto translucent paper using a permanent marker. These tracings were used for planimetric reference. In addition, standardized digital photographs of each wound were captured at the same intervals. The wound area was then calculated using ImageJ software version 1.53k (National Institutes of Health, Bethesda, MD, USA), which provided accurate pixel-based area measurements after appropriate calibration. The combination of manual tracing and digital image analysis allowed for both the visual documentation and precise quantification of wound contraction over time [18].

4.9. Assessment of Biochemistry

4.9.1. Collection of Samples

The EDTA-free tube orbital sinus method was used to extract blood samples from the rats in each group to separate sera for the measurement of CD68, IL-1β, and TNF-α (tumour necrosis factor-alpha) [40]. After collection, the blood was allowed to clot at room temperature and subsequently centrifuged at 3000 rpm for 15 min to obtain serum. The clear supernatant was carefully aspirated and stored at −80 °C until further use. All biochemical measurements were performed using serum samples.

4.9.2. Determination of IL-1β and TNF-α

Following the manufacturer's instructions, a commercial ELISA kit was used to quantify the concentrations of IL-1β and TNF-α in the blood. Cytokine concentrations were measured using a standardized assay and then reported in pg/mL [16]. As the assay kits were optimized for use with serum, normalization to total protein was not required, and concentrations were interpreted directly from standard curves.

4.9.3. Determination of CD68 in the Rat Serum

The collective serum CD68 concentrations in rats were evaluated utilizing a commercial ELISA kit, adhering to the manufacturer's guidelines. The total concentration of macrophage CD68 was quantified using a standard curve and reported in ng/mL [14]. Similarly to cytokines, CD68 quantification was performed directly on serum samples without total protein normalization by kit-specific protocols.

4.9.4. Antioxidant Activity

Skin specimens were homogenized using a glass homogenizer with 1 mL of saline per gram of tissue. After centrifugation of the homogenates in 10,000× *g* for 30 min at 4 °C, the supernatant was stored at −80 °C until analysis. ELISA kits (Andy Hua Tai, Beijing, China) were used to quantify the levels of malondialdehyde (MDA), reactive oxygen species (ROS), superoxide dismutase (SOD), and glutathione (GSH), according to the manufacturer's specifications [15,22].

4.10. Immunohistochemical Staining

The evaluation of cellular mortality in compromised tissue was performed using the immunohistochemical detection of cleaved Caspase-3. Tissue sections were incubated with a primary antibody against Caspase-3 (Anti-Caspase-3 antibody [EPR18297], Abcam, Cambridge, UK) at a dilution of 1:200 overnight at 4 °C. This was followed by incubation with a biotinylated secondary antibody and visualization using the DAB staining. Counter-staining was performed with haematoxylin. Cells exhibiting positive staining appeared brownish-yellow in the cytoplasm, indicating apoptotic activity. For each specimen, the quantity of positive cells was enumerated in three sections and five designated regions of the wound tissues. A quantitative analysis was conducted using Image-Pro Plus 6.0 [41].

5. Conclusions

This study highlights MEO as a multi-targeted wound-healing agent exhibiting anti-inflammatory, antioxidant, and regenerative properties. Compared to previously reported MEO compositions, our oil appears richer in sesquiterpenes and esters, which may enhance cytokine suppression, oxidative stress regulation, and fibroblast survival. While the Caspase-3 pathways are strongly implicated in MEO effects, additional functional studies using pathway inhibitors or gene-silencing approaches are required to establish their definitive role. Future research should also focus on standardizing MEO extraction techniques to optimize its bioactive composition and maximize therapeutic efficacy in wound care and regenerative medicine.

Author Contributions: Y.I.A. conceived and designed research, conducted experiments and wrote the manuscript. K.V. reviewed data and corrected for grammar. All authors have read and agreed to the published version of the manuscript.

Funding: This research was funded by the Deanship of Scientific Research at King Khalid University; Grant number RGP 1/301/45.

Institutional Review Board Statement: The Institutional Animal Ethics Committee (IAEC) at King Khalid University (IAEC) (ECM/2021-5306/Dated 2 May 2021) approved all experimental procedures.

Informed Consent Statement: Not applicable.

Data Availability Statement: Data is contained in the paper.

Acknowledgments: The authors extend their sincere appreciation to the Deanship of Scientific Research at King Khalid University for funding this study through the Small Research Group Project under grant number RGP 1/301/45. We also gratefully acknowledge the technical support and assistance provided by the laboratory staff and research assistants, whose contributions were instrumental in executing various experimental procedures across pharmacological, histological, and biochemical domains.

Conflicts of Interest: The author declares that there are no potential conflicts of interest in this paper.

References

1. Sujatha, P.S.; Pavithran, S.; Sujatha, P.S. Wound Healing Effect of Furfural and Pentadecanal from *Lagerstroemia speciosa* (L.) Pers Acetone Flower extracts against Haemadipsa sylvestris Bite. *J. Adv. Sci. Res.* **2024**, *15*, 12–15.
2. Pereira Beserra, F.; Sergio Gushiken, L.F.; Vieira, A.J.; Augusto Bérgamo, D.; Luísa Bérgamo, P.; Oliveira de Souza, M.; Alberto Hussni, C.; Kiomi Takahira, R.; Henrique Nóbrega, R.; Monteiro Martinez, E.R.; et al. From inflammation to cutaneous repair: Topical application of lupeol improves skin wound healing in rats by modulating the cytokine levels, NF-κB, Ki-67, growth factor expression, and distribution of collagen fibers. *Int. J. Mol. Sci.* **2020**, *21*, 4952. [CrossRef]
3. Ni, X.; Shan, X.; Xu, L.; Yu, W.; Zhang, M.; Lei, C.; Xu, N.; Lin, J.; Wang, B. Adipose-derived stem cells combined with platelet-rich plasma enhance wound healing in a rat model of full-thickness skin defects. *Stem Cell Res. Ther.* **2021**, *12*, 226. [CrossRef] [PubMed]

4. Shenoy, R.R.; Sudheendra, A.T.; Nayak, P.G.; Paul, P.; Kutty, N.G.; Rao, C.M. Normal and delayed wound healing is improved by sesamol, an active constituent of *Sesamum indicum* (L.) in albino rats. *J. Ethnopharmacol.* **2011**, *133*, 608–612. [CrossRef]
5. Kolimi, P.; Narala, S.; Nyavanandi, D.; Youssef, A.A. Innovative treatment strategies to accelerate wound healing: Trajectory and recent advancements. *Cells* **2022**, *11*, 2439. [CrossRef]
6. Pollini, M.; Paladini, F. Antimicrobial silver nanoparticles for wound healing application: Progress and future trends. *Materials* **2019**, *12*, 2540. [CrossRef]
7. Friedman, N.D.; Temkin, E.; Carmeli, Y. The negative impact of antibiotic resistance. *Clin. Microbiol. Infect.* **2016**, *22*, 416–422. [CrossRef]
8. Wagner, W.; Wehrmann, M. Differential cytokine activity and morphology during wound healing in the neonatal and adult rat skin. *J. Cell. Mol. Med.* **2007**, *11*, 1342–1351. [CrossRef]
9. Nieto, G.; Ros, G.; Castillo, J. Antioxidant and antimicrobial properties of rosemary (*Rosmarinus officinalis*, L.): A review. *Medicines* **2018**, *5*, 98. [CrossRef]
10. Falck, C.K. Essential Oils in Veterinary Wound Management: A Review of Current Literature. *AHVMA J.* **2022**, *67*, 11–22.
11. Saini, R.K.; Ranjit, A.; Sharma, K.; Prasad, P.; Shang, X.; Gowda, K.G.M.; Keum, Y.S. Bioactive Compounds of Citrus Fruits: A Review of Composition and Health Benefits of Carotenoids, Flavonoids, Limonoids, and Terpenes. *Antioxidants* **2022**, *11*, 239. [CrossRef] [PubMed]
12. Caballero-Gallardo, K.; Quintero-Rincón, P.; Olivero-Verbel, J. Aromatherapy and Essential Oils: Holistic Strategies in Complementary and Alternative Medicine for Integral Wellbeing. *Plants* **2025**, *14*, 400. [CrossRef]
13. Rosmalia, D.; Marjoni, M.R. Nutmeg (*Myristica fragrans*) Extracts Accelerate Oral Mucosal Wound Healing In Vivo. *J. Angiother.* **2024**, *8*, 1–5.
14. Hoch, C.C.; Petry, J.; Griesbaum, L.; Weiser, T. 1,8-cineole (eucalyptol): A versatile phytochemical with therapeutic applications across multiple diseases. *Biomed. Pharmacother.* **2023**, *170*, 2659. [CrossRef]
15. Anuradha, U.; Bhavana, V.; Chary, P.S.; Kalia, N.P. Exploration of the topical nanoemulgel bearing with ferulic acid and essential oil for diabetic wound healing. *Pathophysiology* **2024**, *31*, 49. [CrossRef]
16. Vitale, S.; Colanero, S.; Placidi, M.; Di Emidio, G.; Tatone, C.; Amicarelli, F.; D'Alessandro, A.M. Phytochemistry and Biological Activity of Medicinal Plants in Wound Healing: An Overview of Current Research. *Molecules* **2022**, *27*, 3566. [CrossRef]
17. Ukaegbu, K.; Allen, E.; Svoboda, K.K.H. Reactive Oxygen Species and Antioxidants in Wound Healing: Mechanisms and Therapeutic Potential. *Int. Wound J.* **2025**, *22*, e70330. [CrossRef]
18. Thangaleela, S.; Sivamaruthi, B.S.; Kesika, P.; Chaiyasut, C. A narrative review on the bioactivity and health benefits of alpha-phellandrene. *Sci. Pharm.* **2022**, *90*, 57. [CrossRef]
19. de Cassia da Silveira e Sá, R.; Andrade, L.N.; de Sousa, D.P. A review on anti-inflammatory activity of monoterpenes. *Molecules* **2013**, *18*, 1227–1254. [CrossRef]
20. Javed, S.; Mangla, B.; Salawi, A.; Sultan, M.H.; Almoshari, Y.; Ahsan, W. Essential Oils as Dermocosmetic Agents, Their Mechanism of Action and Nanolipidic Formulations for Maximized Skincare. *Cosmetics* **2024**, *11*, 210. [CrossRef]
21. Ao, X.; Yan, H.; Huang, M.; Xing, W.; Ao, L.Q.; Wu, X.F.; Pu, C.X.; Zhang, B.Y.; Xu, X.; Liang, H.P.; et al. Lavender essential oil accelerates lipopolysaccharide-induced chronic wound healing by inhibiting caspase-11-mediated macrophage pyroptosis. *Kaohsiung J. Med. Sci.* **2023**, *39*, 511–521. [CrossRef]
22. Gullì, M.; Percaccio, E.; Di Giacomo, S.; Di Sotto, A. Novel Insights into the Immunomodulatory Effects of Caryophyllane Sesquiterpenes: A Systematic Review of Preclinical Studies. *Appl. Sci.* **2022**, *12*, 2292. [CrossRef]
23. Astaneh, M.E.; Fereydouni, N. Nanocurcumin-enhanced zein nanofibers: Advancing macrophage polarization and accelerating wound healing. *Regen. Ther.* **2025**, *28*, 51–62. [CrossRef]
24. Sharifiaghdam, M.; Shaabani, E.; Faridi-Majidi, R.; De Smedt, S.C.; Braeckmans, K.; Fraire, J.C. Macrophages as a therapeutic target to promote diabetic wound healing. *Mol. Ther.* **2022**, *30*, 2891–2908. [CrossRef]
25. Gao, M.; Guo, H.; Dong, X.; Wang, Z.; Yang, Z.; Shang, Q.; Wang, Q. Regulation of inflammation during wound healing: The function of mesenchymal stem cells and strategies for therapeutic enhancement. *Front. Pharmacol.* **2024**, *15*, 1345779. [CrossRef]
26. Liu, T.; Zhang, L.; Joo, D.; Sun, S.C. NF-κB signaling in inflammation. *Signal Transduct. Target. Ther.* **2017**, *2*, 17023. [CrossRef] [PubMed]
27. Ashokkumar, K.; Simal-Gandara, J.; Murugan, M.; Dhanya, M.K.; Pandian, A. Nutmeg (*Myristica fragrans* Houtt.) essential oil: A review on its composition, biological, and pharmacological activities. *Phytother. Res.* **2022**, *36*, 2839–2851. [CrossRef]
28. Trinh, X.T.; Long, N.V.; Van Anh, L.T.; Nga, P.T.; Giang, N.N.; Chien, P.N.; Nam, S.Y.; Heo, C.Y. A Comprehensive Review of Natural Compounds for Wound Healing: Targeting Bioactivity Perspective. *Int. J. Mol. Sci.* **2022**, *23*, 9573. [CrossRef]
29. Venkatesan, K.; Sivadasan, D.; Abderrahmen Al Weslati, M.; Gayasuddin Mouid, M.; Goyal, M.; Bansal, M.; Salama, M.E.M.; Azizullah Ghori, S.; Ahmad, F. Protective Effects of Frankincense Oil on Wound Healing: Downregulating Caspase-3 Expression to Facilitate the Transition from the Inflammatory to Proliferative Phase. *Pharmaceuticals* **2025**, *18*, 407. [CrossRef]

30. Cordiano, R.; Di Gioacchino, M.; Mangifesta, R.; Panzera, C.; Gangemi, S.; Minciullo, P.L. Malondialdehyde as a Potential Oxidative Stress Marker for Allergy-Oriented Diseases: An Update. *Molecules* **2023**, *28*, 5979. [CrossRef]
31. Ribas, V.; García-Ruiz, C.; Fernández-Checa, J.C. Glutathione and mitochondria. *Front. Pharmacol.* **2014**, *5*, 151. [CrossRef]
32. Chidambaram, S.B.; Anand, N.; Varma, S.R.; Ramamurthy, S.; Vichitra, C.; Sharma, A.; Mahalakshmi, A.M.; Essa, M.M. Superoxide dismutase and neurological disorders. *IBRO Neurosci. Rep.* **2024**, *16*, 373. [CrossRef]
33. Zhu, X.; Qiao, T.; Huang, Z.; Jia, G.; Zhao, H.; Chen, X. Caffeic acid improves intestinal barrier function integrity through activation of Nrf2 signaling pathway in weaned piglets and H_2O_2 induced IPEC-J2 cells. *J. Nutr. Biochem.* **2025**, *143*, 109952. [CrossRef]
34. Riwaldt, S.; Corydon, T.J.; Pantalone, D.; Sahana, J.; Wise, P.; Wehland, M.; Krüger, M.; Melnik, D.; Kopp, S.; Infanger, M.; et al. Role of Apoptosis in Wound Healing and Apoptosis Alterations in Microgravity. *Front. Bioeng. Biotechnol.* **2021**, *9*, 679650. [CrossRef]
35. amin Hussen, N.H.; Abdulla, S.K.; Ali, N.M.; Ahmed, V.A.; Hasan, A.H.; Qadir, E.E. Role of antioxidants in skin aging and the molecular mechanism of ROS: A comprehensive review. *Asp. Mol. Med.* **2025**, *5*, 100063. [CrossRef]
36. Khan, F.A.; Khan, N.M.; Ahmad, S.; Nasruddin Aziz, R.; Ullah, I.; Almehmadi, M.; Allahyani, M.; Alsaiari, A.A.; Aljuaid, A. Phytochemical profiling, antioxidant, antimicrobial and cholinesterase inhibitory effects of essential oils isolated from the leaves of Artemisia scoparia and Artemisia absinthium. *Pharmaceuticals* **2022**, *15*, 1221. [CrossRef]
37. Rodrigues, P.M.; Fernandes, A.; Pintado, M.; Tavaria, F.K. A systematic review of natural products for skin applications: Targeting inflammation, wound healing, and photo-aging. *Phytomedicine* **2023**, *112*, 105697.
38. Carson, C.F.; Hammer, K.A.; Riley, T.V. Melaleuca alternifolia (tea tree) oil: A review of antimicrobial and other medicinal properties. *Clin. Microbiol. Rev.* **2006**, *19*, 50–62. [CrossRef]
39. Saddiq, A.; Khayyat, S.A. Chemical and antimicrobial studies of monoterpene: Citral and linalool. *J. King Saud Univ. Sci.* **2010**, *22*, 97–105. [CrossRef]
40. Adhikary, K.; Sarkar, R.; Maity, S.; Sadhukhan, I.; Sarkar, R. Immunomodulation of macrophages in diabetic wound individuals by structurally diverse bioactive phytochemicals. *Pharmaceuticals* **2024**, *17*, 1294. [CrossRef]
41. Dominguez-Verano, P.; Jacobo-Herrera, N.; Sánchez-Cavazos, J.M.; Miranda-Bello, I.; Acosta-Galván, H.A. Chemical composition of Mexicali propolis and its effect on gastric repair in an indomethacin-induced gastric injury murine model. *Antioxidants* **2025**, *14*, 65. [CrossRef] [PubMed]

pharmaceuticals

MDPI

Article

Amaranthus graecizans L. Mitigates Hyperlipidemia-Induced Nonalcoholic Fatty Liver Disease in Experimental Rats: Future Pharmaceuticals

Nadiah S. Alzahrani [1,*], Bayan Aljahdali [2], Aeshah Alhosain [3], Abeer Abdullah Alasmari [4], Touseef Amna [5,*] and Soha Mohamed Yousef [6,7]

1 College of Science, Al-Baha University, Al Baha 65779, Saudi Arabia
2 Department of Home Economics, College of Education, Najran University, Najran 11001, Saudi Arabia; baaljahdali@nu.edu.sa
3 Department of Food Science and Human Nutrition, Qassim University, Buraydah 52571, Saudi Arabia; abhsairn@qu.edu.sa
4 Department of Nutrition and Food Science, King Saud University, Riyadh 11451, Saudi Arabia; 439203421@student.ksu.edu.sa
5 Department of Biology, Faculty of Science, Al-Baha University, Al-Baha 65779, Saudi Arabia
6 Department of Home Economics, Faculty of Specific Education, Fayoum University, Fayoum 63514, Egypt; smy01@fayoum.edu.eg
7 Applied College in Almakhwah, Al-Baha University, Al-Baha 65779, Saudi Arabia
* Correspondence: n.s.alzahrani@bu.edu.sa (N.S.A.); touseefamna@gmail.com (T.A.)

Abstract: Background: Nonalcoholic fatty liver disease (NAFLD) associated with hyperlipidemia is a prevalent metabolic disorder, often triggered by high-fat diets (HFDs) in animal models. *Amaranthus graecizans* L. (AGs), rich in bioactive compounds, offers potential antioxidant and lipid-lowering benefits, making it a candidate for natural liver protection. This study evaluated the protective role of *Amaranthus graecizans* L. against hyperlipidemia-induced NAFLD in rats. **Methods:** Thirty male Wistar rats (150 ± 20 g, 10 weeks old) were split into five groups ($n = 6$ each). A control group received 0.25 mL 0.1% DMSO orally. Four HFD-fed groups included one with only DMSO (0.25 mL) and three supplemented with AG solution (0.25 mL) at 100, 200, or 500 mg/kg body weight. Treatments were given daily via gavage for two months. AGs' nutritional profile, serum lipids, liver function, and liver histology were analyzed. **Results:** AGs contain 21.3% protein, 1.1% fat, 15% fiber, moderate vitamins (ascorbic acid, B-complex), and minerals (high potassium, calcium; low magnesium, phosphorus, sodium). AG-treated rats weighed less than the HFD controls. Unlike the control group (normal lipids, liver function, no steatosis), the HFD rats showed severe hyperlipidemia, liver dysfunction, and steatosis with fat changes. The AG groups exhibited dose-dependent improvements in lipids and liver function; the 200 mg/kg group had reduced fatty changes, and the 500 mg/kg group showed minimal hepatocyte fat. **Conclusions:** *Amaranthus graecizans* L. reduces hyperlipidemia and NAFLD progression in HFD-fed rats, which suggests its potential as a natural liver-protective agent.

Keywords: proximate analysis; lipid profiles; liver function; histological examination

1. Introduction

Nonalcoholic fatty liver disease involves the excessive accumulation of fat in the liver. Important to point out is that, NAFLD is a serious health problem since it may evolve from simple fat accumulation to severely advanced stages. The evolution of NAFLD includes more severe and potentially progressive forms, including the disease that we do and do not consider a form of alcoholic liver disease: nonalcoholic steatohepatitis (NASH). So, when NAFLD becomes more severe, it can lead to fibrosis and cirrhosis, which can be a major problem in public health whenever left untreated [1,2]. The prevalence of NAFLD has significantly increased globally and it affects about 30.05% of the global population [3,4]. NAFLD contributes to advanced liver disease necessitating transplantation and is a key factor in liver-related mortality [2]. It is becoming almost like an epidemic with the rise of type 2 diabetes and obesity [5]. By 2030, NAFLD will probably become the foremost cause of liver transplantation. A more prevalent history of cases also puts the statistics of NAFLD in the Middle East very much on the increase, increasing from 36.53% in 1990 to 42.62% in 2019 [6]. A comprehensive analysis found that NAFLD affects about 16.8% of the population of Saudi Arabia. Obesity rates in the country exceed global norms, likely contributing to the elevated occurrence of NAFLD in this area [7].

Metabolic syndrome (MS) adds to the peril of increased risk of NAFLD. Insulin resistance appears to be the main mechanism behind these above-mentioned processes according to some previous studies [8,9]. The components of metabolic syndrome include systemic hypertension, dyslipidemia, and insulin resistance [9]. Clinical management for metabolic syndrome includes lifestyle modifications such as dietary changes that promote decreased caloric intake; increasing physical activity; and pharmacotherapy aimed at decreasing the risks of dyslipidemia, hyperglycemia, hypertension, and increased LDL-C and decreased HDL-C levels, as well as triglycerides [8,10]. In such cases, functional foods mainly from fruits and vegetables are highly recommended due to their abundance in bioactive compounds, predominantly polyphenols [10,11].

Amaranthus graecizans L. (AGs) is a plant that belongs to the Amaranthaceae family. Originally from the Mediterranean region, this herbaceous plant has now expanded to other parts of the world, including Africa, Asia, and America [12]. AG is consumed as a leafy vegetable in Africa and Asia, whether boiled or stir-fried. Its leaves are high in minerals including iron, calcium, and vitamins, making it an important supplement to local diets, especially in rural regions. The seeds, while less widely utilized, are occasionally collected for their edible grains, which are high in protein and fiber [13]. Recent studies have focused on identifying the therapeutic ingredients of AG [12,13]. Extraction from all parts of AG is expected to possess medicinal properties. Research has been intensified in recent years regarding the nutraceutical and therapeutic possible use of Amaranthus species as functional foods owing to their high antioxidant activity and anti-inflammatory properties [14]. Phytochemical screening of the aerial parts of some AG species has provided evidence of the presence of bioactive components such as steroids, glycosides, alkaloids, phenolic acids, flavonoids, amino acids, betaine, lipids, carotenoids, and catechuic tannins [15].

A review study indicated that these polyphenols could mitigate the effects of obesity and several metabolic problems caused by obesity, such as hypertension, glucose intolerance, and dyslipidemia, while also providing protection against organ damage [14]. The pharmacological effect exhibited by AGs can be attributed to numerous bioactive phytoconstituents as discovered in previous studies [15–17]. A polyphenol-rich diet, Amaranthus being included, seems to provide reasonable protection against several chronic diseases [18]. Dutta and Singh [19] studied the effects of AG leaf extraction on genomic DNA and lipid peroxidation in goat liver, with the findings indicating the significant enhancement in antioxidant levels. The results suggest that elevated antioxidant levels counteract oxidative damage, potentially mitigating degenerative conditions linked to metabolic stress, genotoxicity, and cytotoxicity. However, limited research exists on the protective effects of AGs against hyperlipidemia-induced NAFLD, though plants in the Amaranthaceae family are known for various health and medicinal properties. This highlights the need for in-depth studies to assess AGs' value as a functional food and therapeutic agent. The current investigation examined AGs' ability to safeguard rats from hyperlipidemia-induced NAFLD.

2. Results

2.1. Proximate Composition of *Amaranthus graecizans* L.

Table 1 shows the results of the proximate composition of AG plants. The carbohydrate content of AGs was 31.5%. The AGs have a significant amount of protein (21.3%), while the total fat was 1.1%. The moisture and ash contents in the AGs were 5.15% and 25.6%, respectively. In addition, it was discovered that the AGs contained a high fiber content of (15%).

Table 1. Proximate composition of *Amaranthus graecizans* L. on a dry weight basis (%).

Nutrients	%
Carbohydrates	31.5 ± 0.5
Protein	21.3 ± 0.3
Fat	1.1 ± 0.1
Total fiber	15 ± 0.1
Ash	25.6 ± 0.5
Moisture	5.15 ± 0.5

2.2. Vitamin and Mineral Content of *Amaranthus graecizans* L.

The vitamin and mineral contents of AGs are presented in Table 2. The results outlined that the AGs' powder contained a moderate amount of ascorbic acid and B-complex vitamins (Niacin B3, Thiamine B1, Cobalamin B12, Folic acid B9). In addition, a moderate amount of vitamin A, vitamin E, and vitamin D3 was found in the AGs. The results indicated that AGs' powder contains high amounts of potassium and calcium. However, it contains small amounts of magnesium, phosphorus, and sodium.

Table 2. Vitamin and mineral contents of *Amaranthus graecizans* L. on a dry weight basis.

Vitamins	**μg/mL**
Vitamin C (ascorbic acid)	8.09
Vitamin B1 (Thiamine)	7.16
Vitamin B3(Niacin)	1.39
Vitamin B9 (Folic acid)	6.37
Vitamin B12 (Cobalamin)	1.03
Vitamin A (Retinol)	4.69
Vitamin E (Tocopherol)	69.78
Vitamin D3(Cholecalciferol)	0.085
Minerals	**mg/g**
Magnesium (Mg)	6.55
Potassium (K)	35
Phosphorus (P)	2.5
Sodium (Na)	2.5
Calcium (Ca)	20

2.3. Phenolic Compounds of *Amaranthus graecizans* L.

The result presented in Table 3 shows the phenolic compounds of AGs with their retention times, molecular weights, molecular formulae, and peak area percentages of each compound. The major compound found in AGs was chlorogenic acid (21.20%). The compound with the second largest peak area percentage was gallic acid (16.96%). Some other phenolic compounds were recognized such as rutin (8.71%), rosmarinic acid (6.52%), Vanillin (4.81), Caffeic acid (3.21%), Cinnamic acid (3.01%), p-Coumaric acid (2.69%), Methyl gallate (2.47%), Ferulic acid (2.3%), and Syringic acid (1.22%) as well as catechin and Daidzein (0.59%, 0.54%), respectively (see File S1 in the Supplementary Materials).

Table 3. Phenolic compounds of *Amaranthus graecizans* L. on a dry weight basis.

Compound Name	Formula	* RT (mine)	* MW (g/mol)	Peak Area (%)
Gallic acid	$C_7H_6O_5$	3.557	170.12	16.96
Chlorogenic acid	$C_{16}H_{18}O_9$	4.190	354.31	21.20
Catechin	$C_{15}H_{14}O_6$	4.627	290.26	0.59
Methyl gallate	$C_8H_8O_5$	5.471	184.147	2.47
Caffeic acid	$C_9H_8O_4$	5.850	180.16	3.21
Syringic acid	$C_9H_{10}O_5$	6.342	198.17	1.22
Rutin	$C_{27}H_{30}O_{16}$	6.931	610.517	8.71
p-Coumaric acid	$C_9H_8O_3$	8.522	164.04	2.69
Vanillin	$C_8H_8O_3$	9.070	152.15	4.81
Ferulic acid	$C_{10}H_{10}O_4$	9.642	194.18	2.03
Rosmarinic acid	$C_{18}H_{16}O_8$	11.660	360.318	6.52
Daidzein	$C_{15}H_{10}O_4$	15.658	254.23	0.54
Cinnamic acid	$C_9H_8O_2$	19.162	148.1586	3.01

* RT, retention time; * MW, molecular weight.

2.4. Evaluation of the Body Weight Gain

Rats on an HFD exhibited a notably greater body weight increase than those on a standard diet (SD) (Table 4). In contrast, the HFD-fed rats treated with AGs at doses of 100, 200, and 500 mg/kg showed a substantial decrease in weight gain compared to the untreated HFD group.

Table 4. Effect of AGs on body weight gain in experimental rats.

Group	Body Weight Gain (g)
SD	9.83 ± 02.78
HFD	75.67 ± 11.79 ****
HFD + 100 mg/kg of AGs	49.00 ± 04.04 ++++
HFD + 200 mg/kg of AGs	37.00 ± 09.03 ++++
HFD + 500 mg/kg of AGs	39.00 ± 07.04 ++++

Data are presented as mean ± SD (*n* = 6 rats/group). **** *p*-value < 0.0005; ++++ *p*-value < 0.0001 compared with (HFD) group.

2.5. Effect of AGs on Serum Lipid Profiles

The outcome demonstrated that after 2 months of high-fat diets, the serum levels of lipid profiles were significantly increased in the HFD groups as compared to the controls

(Figure 1A–D). It was found that there was a very significant decrease ($p < 0.0001$) in serum total cholesterol in both the HFD + 200 mg/kg of AG and HFD + 500 mg/kg of AG groups, compared to the HFD group. In addition, all tested doses of AGs (100, 200, 500 mg/kg) decreased the serum TG levels significantly, compared to the HFD groups, with the best result in the HFD + 500 mg/kg of AG group relative to the HFD group concerning the LDL-c levels.

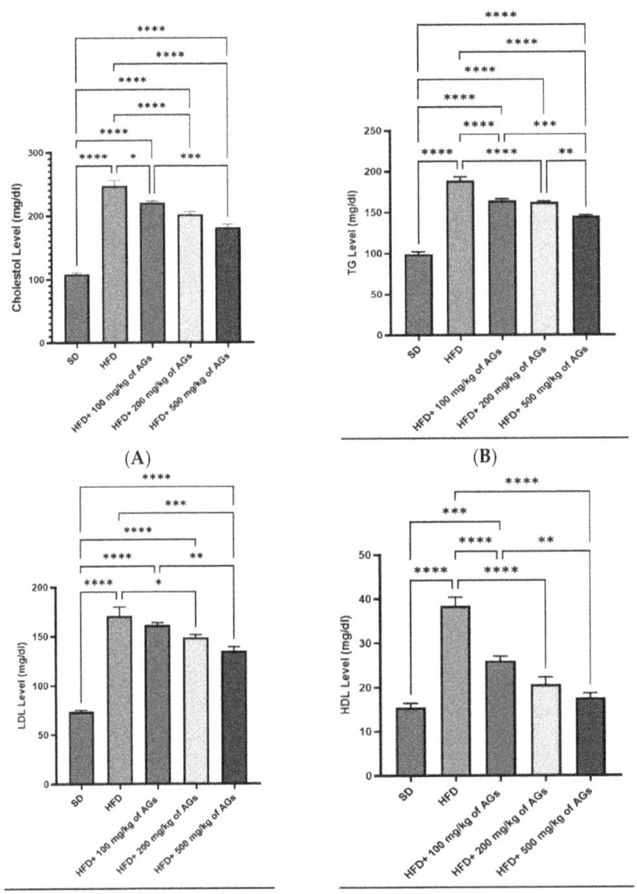

Figure 1. Effect of AG dose-dependent treatment on the following: (**A**) cholesterol levels; (**B**) TG, triglyceride levels; (**C**) LDL-c, low-density lipoprotein cholesterol levels; (**D**) HDL-c, high-density lipoprotein cholesterol levels. The bracket represents statistically significant differences among groups at * p-value < 0.05; ** p-value < 0.005; *** p-value < 0.0005; and **** p-value < 0.0001.

2.6. Effect of AGs on Liver Function

HFD rats that were untreated had elevated serum levels of liver enzymes (ALT, AST, and ALP) compared to the control (Figure 2A–C). Nevertheless, the liver enzymes significantly improved in the HFD-fed animals treated with 100, 200, and 500 mg/kg AGs when compared to HFD alone. Furthermore, the results showed significant increases in the GGT, bilirubin, and total protein levels in the untreated HFD rats as compared to the control rats on standard diet (Figure 2D–F). Yet, there was a significant decrease in these parameters in the HFD rats receiving all tested doses (100, 200, and 500 mg/kg AGs) when compared to HFD alone.

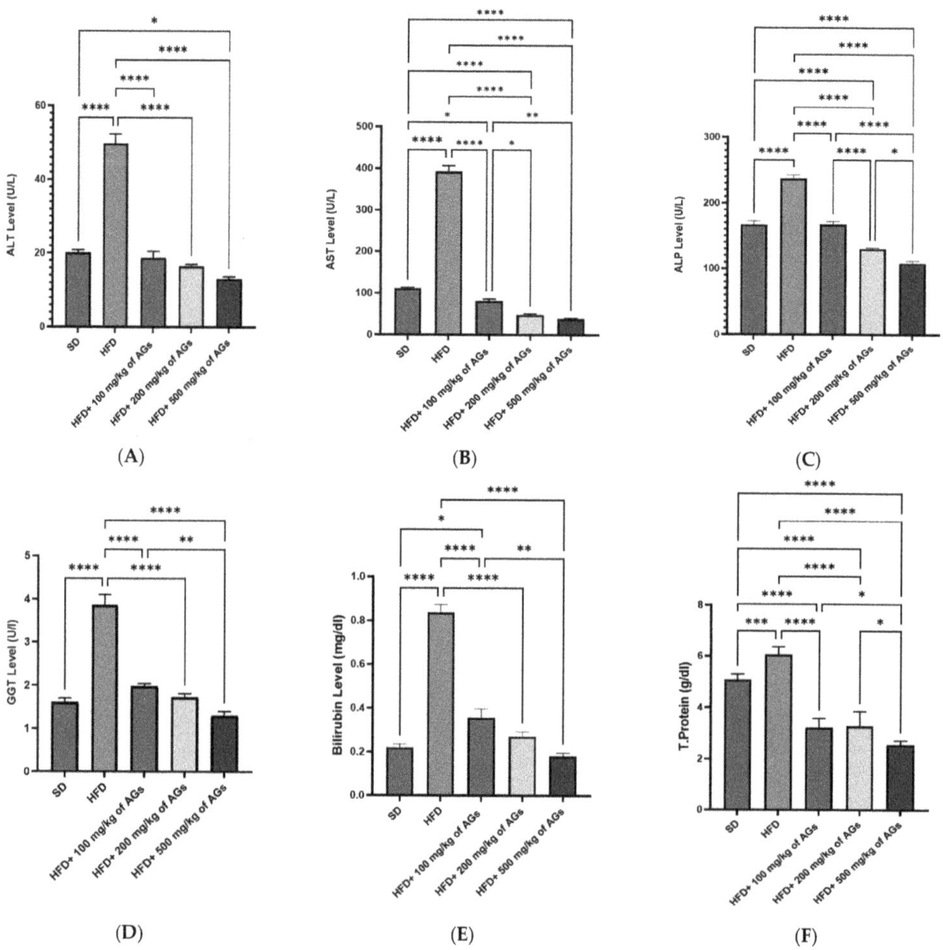

Figure 2. Effect of AG dose-dependent treatment on (**A**) ALT, alanine aminotransferase levels; (**B**) AST, aspartate aminotransferase levels; (**C**) ALP, alkaline phosphatase levels; (**D**) GGT, gamma-glutamyle transferase levels; (**E**) bilirubin levels; (**F**) total protein levels. The bracket represents statistically significant differences among groups at * p-value < 0.05; ** p-value < 0.005; *** p-value < 0.0005; and **** p-value < 0.0001.

2.7. Histological Examination

Histological examinations of the liver tissues are shown in Figures 3 and 4. In the control group (SD), the liver tissue displayed a typical structure, with healthy hepatocytes organized in cords radiating from the central vein and separated by blood sinusoids. In contrast, the HFD group exhibited significant periportal vacuolation, indicative of severe fatty degeneration, along with heightened hepatocyte apoptosis and periportal fibrosis. Moreover, marked degrees of diffuse lobular hepatic fatty changes and changes associated with the presence of large clear vacuoles were shown in the same group. Meanwhile, a decrease in the hepatic vacuolar changes within the cytoplasm of the hepatocytes and a decrease in hepatic apoptotic changes were obvious in the (HFD + 100 mg/kg of AG) group. The same group showed a decrease in the hepatic fatty changes within the cytoplasm of the hepatocytes and also a decrease in the hepatic apoptotic changes. As for the rats of the (HFD + 200 mg/kg of AG) group, liver examination showed focal hepatic fatty changes and with mild periportal fibrosis, a noticeable decrease in the hepatic fatty changes with mild periportal infiltration of inflammatory cells. Regarding the liver examination of the (HFD + 500 mg/kg of AG) group, it showed a marked decrease in hepatic fatty accumulation within the hepatocytes, which are seen with few hepatocytes; while the remaining hepatocytes are within the normal range, a marked decrease in hepatic fatty changes within the hepatocytes is seen. The improvement in liver tissues was noticeable in the AG groups.

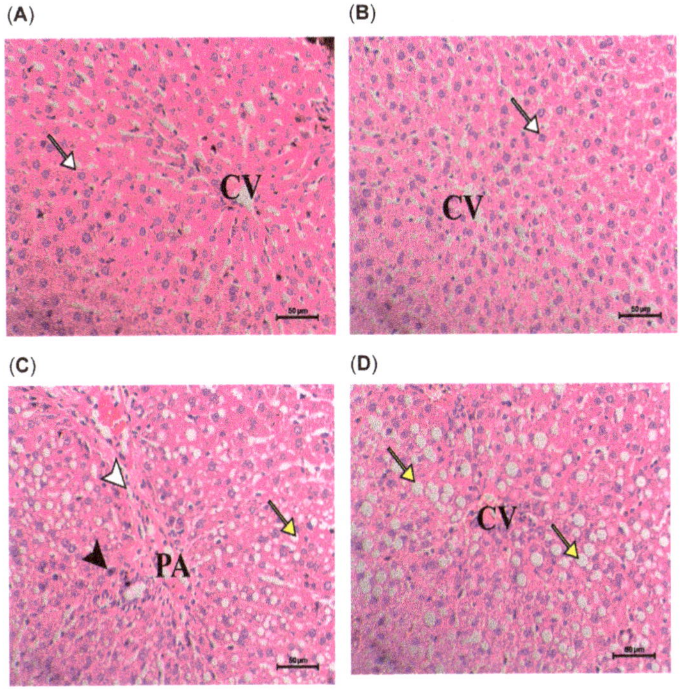

Figure 3. Histological examination of liver for SD and HFD groups of rats. (**A**,**B**) Liver of control animal showing normal hepatic parenchyma consisted of normal hepatocytes (white arrow) arranged in cords around the central vein (CV). (**C**) Liver of HFD animal showing marked degree of periportal hepatic vacuolar changes consistent with severe fatty changes (yellow arrow) associated with increased apoptosis of hepatocytes (black arrowhead) and periportal fibrosis (white arrowhead) (PA portal area). (**D**) Liver of HFD animal showing marked degree of diffuse lobular hepatic fatty changes and changes associated with the presence of large clear vacuoles (yellow arrows).

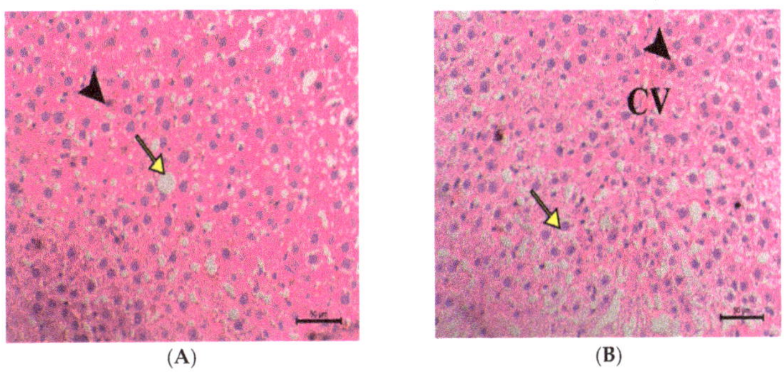

Figure 4. *Cont.*

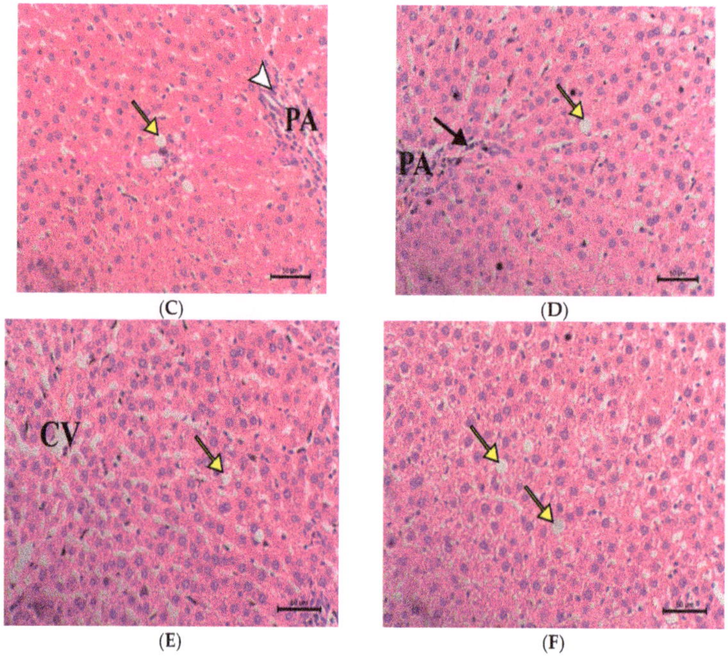

Figure 4. Histological examination of liver for treated groups of rats. (**A**,**B**) Liver of HFD + 100 mg/kg of AGs showing decrease in the hepatic vacuolar changes within the cytoplasm of the hepatocytes (yellow arrow reveals decrease fat vacuoles) and also a decrease in hepatic apoptotic changes (black arrowhead) (CV central vein). (**C**) Liver of HFD + 200 mg/kg of AGs showing focal hepatic fatty changes (yellow arrow) with mild periportal fibrosis (white arrowhead) (PA indicates portal area). (**D**) Liver of HFD + 200 mg /kg of AGs showing noticeable decrease in the hepatic fatty changes (yellow arrow) with mild periportal infiltration of inflammatory cells (black arrow) (PA indicates portal area). (**E**,**F**) Liver of HFD + 500 mg/kg of AGs showing marked decrease in hepatic fatty accumulation within the hepatocytes, which is seen with few hepatocytes (yellow arrow).

3. Discussion

One of the most important organs for metabolic processes such as cholesterol metabolism, gluconeogenesis, and de novo lipogenesis is the liver. The high prevalence of obesity and metabolic syndrome contributes to pathophysiological changes that can cause NAFLD. The recent increases in NAFLD prevalence have become a global health concern [20]. Hyperlipidemia increases in lipogenesis in the liver and steatosis are typical features of HFD-induced NAFLD in experimental rats [21]. It is found that chronic HFD feeding is the most effective means to induce obesity, metabolic abnormalities, and NAFLD in rats [22]. Plants have been widely used to avoid, treat, or even prevent the progression of many ailments such as cancer, cardiovascular, metabolic, and autoimmune diseases owing to their innumerable biological effects such as antioxidant, anti-inflammatory, antimicrobial, and antimutagenic activities [23].

In this study, we propose a dose-dependent treatment strategy for HFD-induced hepatic steatosis in experimental rats by administering different doses of AG plants. In addition, we are establishing that these positive effects are mediated, at least, by hypolipidemic and antioxidant potentials. Obesity was induced by a typical tactic of chronically feeding the experiment rats a high-fat diet [24]. Obesity complications include IR, hypertension, hyperglycemia, and hyperinsulinemia, which may have an adverse effect on general health and accelerate liver damage [25].

The chemical composition of AGs was analyzed to reveal its bioactive compounds. Approximate analyses of AGs were conducted to detect the quantities of carbohydrates, protein, fat, moisture, ash, and total fiber by using different standard methods. The proximate composition of Saudi AGs (Table 2) differs in relativity compared to the African plants, which were found to contain carbohydrate (0%), protein (2.85%), fat (0%), ash (2.20%), and moisture (82%) [26]. The chemical composition of the same plant species at the same stage of growth varies greatly depending on the environment, even if the surrounding is close by. Koutsoukis et al. (2019) explained that could be due to the impact of environmental factors such as climate and ecological concerns [27,28]. In addition, AG plants are composed of many vitamins such as B1, B3, B9, B12, C, A, E, and D3. Also, many crucial minerals were identified in AG plants including Mg, K, P, Na, and Ca (Table 3). They are almost similar to the African AG [26], except for a noticeable difference in the percentage of both vitamin C and E in favor of the Saudi AGs. AGs are nutrient-dense plants that have several advantages for liver health because of their high vitamin, mineral, and antioxidant content. The vitamin A and C content in AGs supports detoxification procedures and shields liver cells from oxidative damage. Additionally, the plant is a robust source of vitamin B, which is vital for metabolism and liver cell regeneration. Furthermore, by boosting enzymatic activity, lowering inflammation, and encouraging detoxification, calcium and magnesium included in AGs are essential for preserving the liver function. This plant is a viable option for promoting liver health and reducing liver-related illnesses because of the combination of these components [14,29,30].

Phenolic compounds, the bioactive compounds in AG's plant, have been identified by HPLC, having 13 polyphenolic compounds, the same number that is also reported by Ishtiaq et al. (2014) and presented in Table 4 [31]. The major compound in the plant is chlorogenic acid (21.20%), which has antioxidants and anti-inflammatory actions [32]. The compound with the next largest peak area percentage was gallic acid (16.96%). Some more phenolic compounds were recognized; these phenolic compounds are in turn protective against several health issues due to their biological activities like antioxidant, antiulcer, anti-inflammatory, hypolipidemic, anti-diabetic, and antitumor [33].

In addition, in this study, the condition known as dyslipidemia was induced by an HFD, characterized by an increase in the circulating levels of LDL-c and TG [34]. On the contrary, the different dosages of AGs inhibited the dose-dependent elevation of lipid levels against anti-hyperlipidemic action. This activity may result from the high acid content of chlorogenic acid and gallic acid, which are both abundantly sourced from this plant, and which lowers the lipid levels via a decreased biosynthesis of LDL-c by the inhibition of 3-hydroxy-3-methylglutaryl-CoA (HMG-CoA), and by decreasing the intestinal absorption of lipids [35,36].

According to further supporting data, chlorogenic acid efficiently lowers fat buildup and enhances lipid metabolism by modifying important enzymes and genes involved in cholesterol homeostasis [37]. Gallic acid's lipid-lowering properties are also attributed to its strong antioxidant and α-glucosidase inhibitory properties. Improved hypolipidemic potential has been associated with increased gallic acid bioactivity via enzymatic transformation [38]. The combined results demonstrate AGs' potential as a natural treatment for dyslipidemia, with the synergistic effects of gallic and chlorogenic acids most likely mediating their benefits.

Additionally, the increase in liver enzyme levels points to the action of an HFD in increasing oxidative stress in rats, something mostly affirmed by many earlier studies [39,40]. But, indeed, oxidative stress was ameliorated in the HFD-fed groups supplemented with different doses of AGs in a dose-dependent manner; AGs' seed thus holds a virtuous promise of possible antioxidant activity. Our results are in the same line with the study performed by Saha et al., which emphasized phenolics' role in hepatoprotection against oxidative damage, thereby helping in the stabilization of cell membrane networks and inhibiting the release and expression of several proinflammatory cytokines such as tumor necrosis factor alpha (TNF-α), transforming growth factor beta (TGF-β), and various interleukins (IL-6, IL-2, and IL-8) [41].

Amaranthus viridis methanol extracts, for example, have demonstrated notable scavenging activities that demonstrate their efficacy as natural antioxidants and possible hepatoprotective agents, highlighting their antioxidant potential [42]. Further highlighting the therapeutic efficacy of Amaranthus species, ethanolic leaf extracts from *Amaranthus gangeticus* showed hepatoprotective benefits through polyphenolic activity [43]. It is well recognized that the phenolic chemicals in AGs, such as gallic acid and chlorogenic acid, are essential for lowering inflammation and oxidative stress. These substances aid in cell membrane stabilization and inhibit the synthesis of interleukins IL-6, IL-2, and IL-8, as well as inflammatory cytokines including TNF-α and TGF-β [41]. Additionally, a study of Amaranthus species highlights the hepatoprotective potential of phenolic components and supports their antioxidant abilities [44]. Further support is provided by research on similar phenolic-rich extracts, such as *Gentiana scabra*, which considerably decreased oxidative stress and liver damage by activating polyphenols like Quercetin and Kaempfero [45]. These results are consistent with the benefits perceived with AGs, pointing to a similar mechanism including anti-inflammatory and free radical scavenging qualities. The combined results show that AGs are viable natural remedies for liver health and oxidative stress management. Its phenolic components are essential for lowering liver enzyme levels and preventing oxidative damage and inflammation.

Several studies have suggested that the serum level of bilirubin is inversely linked with many health conditions such as obesity, metabolic syndrome, T2D, and oxidative stress-mediated diseases due to the increase in the glucuronic UGT1A1 enzyme in the liver among obese subjects that can clear bilirubin from the blood [46,47]. However, a significant increase in bilirubin levels was found among rats fed an HFD, in a similar study performed by Fu et al. (2021), which predicted that subjects would be metabolically healthy [48]. The significant decrease in bilirubin levels was noticed in groups that were fed different doses of AGs, suggesting that it may have bilirubin-lowering ability due to its phenolic compounds and that may occur via the upregulation of hepatic constitutive androstane receptor (CAR) as well as cytochrome P3A1 (CYP3A1) that can facilitate the clearance of bilirubin [49]. AGs' phenolic components may help decrease bilirubin by triggering important liver pathways. By upregulating enzymes such as CYP3A1 and CYP2A5, studies demonstrate how the constitutive androstane receptor (CAR) improves bilirubin elimination [50,51]. Similar effects have been seen by compounds like 6,7-dimethylesculetin, confirming the possible mechanism of AG. Furthermore, bilirubin's connection to enzymatic transcription is highlighted by its control of CYP1A1 through the aryl hydrocarbon receptor (AHR) [52]. These results imply that the phenolic chemicals in AGs may enhance metabolic health, lower oxidative stress, and improve bilirubin metabolism. Alleviated levels of total serum protein were noticed in rats fed an HFD, which are similar to the results of a previous study. Gabuza et al. (2020) suggested an association between the increased serum level of T protein [53] and obesity-related diseases. On the other hand, phenolic compounds such as chlorogenic acid, catechin, and rutin can bind to serum protein such as albumin [54].

The most crucial observation in this study is the ability of our intervention to reverse hepatic steatosis combined with lowering the lipid levels in the HFD-treated rats. However, an HFD causes fats, specifically TG, to be accumulated in the liver due to the excessive influx of free fatty acids from fat tissues, leading to lipotoxicity, mitochondrial impairment, and endoplasmic reticulum stress, which in turn can increase ROS production and inflammation, the two major triggers of NAFLD [41,55]. On the contrary, all polyphenols can attenuate TG accumulation in the hepatocytes by the regulation of lipogenesis, modulation of insulin resistance, controlling of inflammation, and modification of oxidative stress [56], which we found in groups fed AGs, indicating a potent antioxidant and hepatoprotective effect of AG plants due to the presence of many phenolic compounds that have antioxidant properties [57–62]; in addition, both vitamins C and E can function as scavengers of free radicals [63]. Polyphenols, in general, have been revealed to support liver therapy potential by boosting antioxidative defense enzymes via a number of different mechanisms including mediating nuclear factor erythroid 2-related factor 2 (Nrf2) expression and cytochrome P450 2E1 (CYP2E1) expression, alleviating inflammation by downregulating the activity of mitogen-activated protein kinases (MAPK)/nuclear factor kappa B (NF-kB) pathways, and downregulating apoptosis via the manipulation of B-cell lymphoma 2 (Bcl-2)/protein kinase B (AKT)/caspase expression [39]. Otherwise, this could also be due to the high-fiber nature of the AG plant whereby a high-fiber diet can be fermented by the gut microbiota with subsequent augmentation of gut microbiota-derived acetate, which in turn can regulate lipid metabolism during liver diseases [64].

Chronic feeding of a high-fat diet (HFD) to laboratory animals gives rise to hepatic steatosis and dyslipidemia through various pathways. Shortly following HFD feeding, free fatty acids stimulate the synthesis and accumulation of fat droplets within the liver [65]. In the present study, AG treatment lowered hepatic steatosis in the HFD rats compared to the controls, suggesting possible hepatoprotection via improvement in the lipid profile and fatty acid oxidation. AGs led to improved liver histology in the HFD groups. The effect of AGs on liver tissue has not been systematically evaluated previously. However, experimental studies on other Amaranthus species have been studied in animal models and showed significant improvements [66,67].

The potential of numerous plant-based compounds to treat NAFLD has previously been investigated. In both animal models and clinical investigations, green tea (*Camellia sinensis*), which contains the polyphenol epigallocatechin-3-gallate (EGCG), has demonstrated profound liver-protective effects. According to a systematic review report, green tea and its active compounds can enhance antioxidant defense, lower serum triglycerides and LDL cholesterol, and reduce fat accumulation in the liver by activating AMPK and reducing inflammatory markers such as TNF-α and IL-6 [68]. Our research findings are corroborated by an additional study, which determined that the phenolic extract of millet has an anti-hyperlipidemia and anti-steatotic effect on obese rodents [69]. Additionally, in another study conducted on obese rodents, the addition of green tea extract enhanced the body's fat processing, reduced oxidative stress (as evidenced by increased levels of SOD, CAT, and GPx activity), and reduced liver injury, such as the MDA and ALT levels [70]. These findings lend credence to the notion that antioxidants and anti-inflammatory compounds derived from plants can enhance hepatic fat metabolism and mitigate liver damage. These observations are consistent with the results of our investigation, which employed *Amaranthus graecizans*. This clearly implies that the lipid-lowering and liver-protective effects observed may be attributed to the presence of bioactive components such as flavonoids and phenolic compounds.

Conclusively, the inference of this study is that isolated polyphenolic molecules have been reported to normalize the activity of antioxidative enzymes and to ameliorate histopathology by plummeting the inflammatory response by means of tempering oxidative stress, and likewise, by reducing oxidative stress after ischemia–reperfusion liver injury or obstructing hepatotoxicity-derived fibrosis growth in preclinical investigations through downregulating caspase-3, BCL-2, and NF-κB expression whereas it uplifted NRF-2-mediated mitochondrial functions. Likewise, ellagic acid and gallic acids are found in berries and fruits, have been reported to employ shielding effects in liver impairment caused by drug abuse via reducing TNF-mediated inflammation and lipid peroxidation. Alternatively, various plant-derived bioactive compounds may directly avert NAFLD and hepatic steatosis by lessening de novo lipogenesis via the direct downregulation of sterol regulatory element-binding protein 1c (SREBP-1c), increasing FA oxidation through upregulating PPAR receptor and improving insulin sensitivity, and decreasing intestinal lipid absorption.

Nevertheless, some limitations remain in this investigation. Herein, we used AG plants grown in the Al-Baha region; it would be very interesting to examine AG plants from other parts of Saudi Arabia. Furthermore, more well-designed research to investigate the molecular processes underlying these effects is strongly encouraged, such as targeting adipose and hepatic lipid regulators such as AMPK, SREBPs, and PPARs. Furthermore, our work emphasizes the importance of AG plant components as antioxidants, although we were unable to pursue this further. Consequently, it will be a fantastic topic for future research considering diverse parameters.

4. Materials and Methods

4.1. Chemical Reagents

Reagents used included ethanol (95%), petroleum ether, trifluoroacetic acid (0.05%), sodium carbonate, glucose, sulfuric acid (98%), sodium hydroxide, boric acid, hydrochloric acid (37%), and Tashiro's indicator (pH 4.4–5.8), all obtained from Sigma-Aldrich (St. Louis, MO, USA).

4.2. Preparation of AG Powder

Amaranthus graecizans L. (AGs) was obtained from a local market in Al-Baha, Saudi Arabia. The plant was air-dried following Alibas [71], then ground into a fine powder using a 750-Watt Master Class Sanyo Mixer Grinder, Tokyo, Japan. The powder was stored in a clean, dry environment throughout the study.

4.3. Experimental Animals

Thirty male Wistar rats (150 ± 20 g, 10 weeks old) were housed under controlled conditions (22 ± 2 °C, 50% humidity, 12/12 h light/dark cycle) for a one-week acclimatization period with free access to food and water.

4.4. Diet Preparation

Control (SD) and high-fat diets (HFDs) were procured from Research Diets, New Brunswick, NJ, USA (Cat. No. D12450H and D12451, respectively). Table 5 details their nutritional composition.

Table 5. Energy in the diet of control and high-fat diet groups.

	SD (D12450H)		HFD (D12451)	
	gm%	**Kcal%**	**gm%**	**Kcal%**
Carbohydrate	67.3	70%	41	35%
Proteins	19.2	20%	24	20%
Fat	4.3	10%	24	45%
Others	9.7	-	11	-
Total (Kcal/gm)	100 (3.85 Kcal/g)		100 (4.73 Kcal/g)	

4.5. Experimental Design

Rats were divided into five groups (n = 6 each): (1) SD + 0.25 mL 0.1% DMSO (control); (2) HFD + 0.25 mL 0.1% DMSO; (3–5) HFD + AG solution (0.25 mL) at 100, 200, or 500 mg/kg body weight, respectively, as per Zeashan et al. [72]. Treatments were administered daily via gavage for two months. Body weights were recorded weekly. After overnight fasting, rats were anesthetized (90 mg/kg ketamine, 10 mg/kg xylazine) [73], and 1 mL blood was collected via cardiac puncture, centrifuged (3000 rpm, 10 min), and serum stored at −20 °C. Livers were harvested post-euthanasia and preserved in 10% formalin.

4.6. Proximate Analysis

4.6.1. Carbohydrates

Carbohydrate content was measured using the Hedge and Hofreiter [74] method. A 100 mg sample in a boiling tube was mixed with 5 mL of 2.5 N HCl and hydrolyzed in a water bath for 3 h. After cooling at room temperature, sodium carbonate was added until bubbling stopped. The solution was diluted to 100 mL with distilled water and centrifuged. Glucose standards of varying concentrations were prepared alongside. Aliquots (0.5 mL) of both sample and standards were adjusted to 1 mL with distilled water, mixed with 4 mL anthrone reagent, and heated in a boiling water bath for 8 min, shifted from green to dark green to indicate glucose. After rapid cooling, absorbance was read at 630 nm using a spectrophotometer. Carbohydrate content was determined from the glucose standard curve as follows:

Amount of carbohydrates present in 100 mg of the sample = (mg of glucose/volume of the test sample) × 100.

4.6.2. Crude Protein

Crude protein was assessed using the Kjeldahl method [75], converting total nitrogen (N) to protein with a factor. For digestion, 5 g of the sample was placed in a flask with 20 mL concentrated sulfuric acid and a Kjeldahl catalyst (0.3% $CuSO_4 \cdot 5H_2O$ catalyst in 1000 mL solution). The mixture was heated at 350–380 °C for 3 h until partially whitened, then cooled and mixed with sodium hydroxide, turning blue to signal digestion completion. After adding 100 mL water, the solution was distilled with 50 mL 50% sodium hydroxide. Ammonia released was captured in 50 mL 4% boric acid with 6–7 drops of Tashiro's indicator, shifting from reddish-violet to green (pH 4.4–5.8) as ammonium borate formed. This was titrated with 0.25 M HCl until a faint violet hue appeared. Nitrogen was calculated as follows:

$$\%\ \text{Nitrogen (N)} = [(\text{mL standard acid} - \text{mL blank}) \times \text{N of acid} \times 1.4007/\text{weight of sample (g)}] \times 100$$

$$\%\ \text{protein} = \text{N}\% \times \text{F (where F is the conversion factor equal to 6.25)}$$

4.6.3. Total Fat Content

Total fat content was measured using the hydrolysis method as per the AOAC Official Method 966.01 [76]. A 50 mL screw-top test tube with 1 g of AG powder was mixed with 1 mL ethanol, followed by 5 mL HCl. The mixture was heated to 75.5 °C for 40 min, shaken occasionally, then cooled to room temperature. Next, 5 mL ethanol, 12 mL anhydrous ether, and 12 mL petroleum ether were added sequentially, with shaking after each addition. After settling, the top ether layer was separated, transferred to a 150 mL beaker via a Pasteur pipette and filter paper, and repeated thrice with 8 mL ether each time. The extract was evaporated on a low-heat hot plate for 1 h, then heated at 135 °C for 10 min, cooled in a desiccator, and weighed. Fat percentage was calculated as follows:

$$\% \text{ Fat} = [(\text{Weight of beaker and fat} - \text{tared beaker weight})/\text{Sample weight})] \times 100$$

4.6.4. Moisture

Moisture content of AGs was assessed using ICC Standard No. 110/1 (1976) [77]. A pre-weighed, dry crucible with 2 g of sample was heated to 130–133 °C, cooled in a desiccator, and reweighed. Heating continued until a constant weight was achieved. Moisture percentage was calculated as follows:

$$MC\% = (w2 - w1) - (w1 - w3)\,(w2 - w1) \times 100\%$$

w1 = weight of empty crucible. w2 = weight of crucible with sample. w3 = weight of crucible with dry sample.

4.6.5. Ash

Ash content was determined following ICC Standard No. 104/1 (1990) [78]. A pre-weighed dry porcelain crucible with 2 g of sample was incinerated in a muffle furnace at 900 °C, for approximately 3 h until light gray ash formed. After cooling in a desiccator, the crucible was reweighed. Ash percentage was calculated using the formula:

$$AC\% = [(w2 - w1)/w3] \times 100\%$$

AC = ash content. w1 = weight of empty crucible. w2 = weight of crucible after incineration. w3 = weight of the fresh sample

4.7. Micronutrient Analysis

4.7.1. Vitamins

HPLC was conducted on an (Agilent 1260 system, Santa Clara, CA, USA) with an Eclipse C8 column (4.6 mm × 150 mm, 5 µm). The mobile phase, 0.01% TFA: methanol (70:30), flowed isocratically at 1 mL/min. A multi-wavelength detector monitored 248 nm. Samples (10 µL) were injected, and the column was kept at 40 °C.

4.7.2. Minerals

Metal ion levels were measured using an Agilent 5100 SVDV ICP-OES (Serial No. MY15180008, Santa Clara, CA, USA). Dried samples (1 g) were digested in 250 mL Erlenmeyer flasks with 50 mL 20% HNO_3, stirred, and heated at 70–85 °C for 48 h, with extra HNO_3 added to maintain volume. Post-digestion, extracts were filtered (Nalgene, Thermo Scientific, Rochester, NY, USA), cooled, diluted to 100 mL with deionized water (Milli-Q, Ion Exchange Arabia, Jeddah, Saudi Arabia) and analyzed by ICP-OES. Glassware was rinsed thrice with 20% HNO_3 and deionized water. Analysis used a PFA-ST/Peltier-cooled spray chamber at 1500 W RF power, with gas flow of 15 L/min (plasma), 1 L/min (nebulizer), and 0.83–0.88 L/min (auxiliary). The chamber was kept at 2 °C, pump speed at 0.5 mL/min, using nickel cones and dual lens/outlines detection. Scanning was in peak hopping mode (1 sweep/reading, 10 points/peak, 1 reading/replicate), performed in triplicate.

4.8. Phenolic Compounds

The phenolic compounds were analyzed using an Agilent 1260 series HPLC system (Santa Clara, CA, USA). Separation was achieved with a Zorbax Eclipse Plus C8 column (4.6 mm × 250 mm, 5 µm particle size). The mobile phase comprised water (A) and acetonitrile (B), both containing 0.05% trifluoroacetic acid, delivered at a flow rate of 0.9 mL/min. A linear gradient was applied as follows: 82% A from 0 to 18 min, maintained at 82% A from 18 to 24 min, reduced to 60% A from 11 to 18 min, then returned to 82% A at 0 min. Detection occurred at 280 nm using a multi-wavelength detector. Each sample was injected with 5 µL volume, and the column was kept at 40 °C.

4.9. Biochemical Analysis

Serum cholesterol levels were evaluated with a kit designed for rats (Cat. No. MBS168179, MyBioSource, San Diego, CA, USA). Serum triglyceride (TG) amounts were determined using a specialized rat assay (Cat. No. 10010303, Cayman Chemical, Ann Arbor, MI, USA). Levels of high-density lipoprotein cholesterol (HDL-c) and low-density lipoprotein cholesterol (LDL-c) were measured with colorimetric kits (Cat. No. K613-100, BioVision, Milpitas, CA, USA). Liver enzymes' alanine aminotransferase (ALT) and aspartate aminotransferase (AST) were quantified with ELISA assays (Cat. No. MBS8801684 and MBS8804612, MyBioSource, San Diego, CA, USA). Activities of alkaline phosphatase (ALP) and gamma-glutamyl transferase (GGT) were assessed using Abcam kits (Cat. No. ab8336 and ab241029, Shanghai, China). Total bilirubin and protein concentrations were determined with kits (Cat. No. MBS730053 and MBS3808613, MyBioSource, San Diego, CA, USA). All steps adhered to supplier protocols, using samples from six rats per group.

4.10. Histopathology

Liver sections (4 µm) were fixed in 10% formalin, dehydrated, paraffin-embedded, stained with hematoxylin–eosin, and examined under a light microscope (Olympus, Tokyo, Japan) by an independent researcher.

4.11. Ethical Approval

The study was approved by Al-Baha University's Research Ethics Committee (Ref. No. 46110115).

4.12. Statistical Analysis

Data were analyzed using GraphPad Prism 8 software with one-way ANOVA and Tukey's post hoc test. Statistical significance was set at $p < 0.05$.

5. Conclusions

This study indicates that HFD triggers hyperlipidemia, liver damage, and fat accumulation in the liver. Administering AGs at different doses markedly reduced the serum levels of total cholesterol, TG, and LDL-C, while enhancing liver function and improving liver tissue structure. These results provide scientific support for AGs as an antioxidant and lipid-lowering agent in HFD-fed rats, mainly attributable to their rich polyphenolic compounds. Future research should prioritize human clinical trials to validate the safety and effectiveness of AGs for managing NAFLD. Additional studies exploring its mechanisms and optimal doses will strengthen its therapeutic potential. Moreover, AGs could gain traction as a natural remedy through the development of functional foods and the promotion of sustainable farming practices.

Supplementary Materials: The following supporting information can be downloaded at: https://www.mdpi.com/article/10.3390/ph18081196/s1, File S1: HPLC profile of AGs plant.

Author Contributions: Conceptualization, N.S.A.; methodology, N.S.A.; software, B.A.; validation, A.A., A.A.A. and N.S.A.; formal analysis, B.A.; investigation, A.A. and T.A.; resources, A.A.A.; data curation, A.A.; writing—original draft preparation, A.A.A.; writing—review and editing, T.A. and

S.M.Y., visualization, B.A.; supervision, S.M.Y.; project administration, N.S.A.; funding acquisition, A.A. All authors have read and agreed to the published version of the manuscript.

Funding: This research received no specific grant from any funding agency.

Institutional Review Board Statement: This study was approved by the Al-Baha university research ethics committee (Ref.No.46110115, approval date 19 December 2024).

Informed Consent Statement: Not applicable.

Data Availability Statement: The datasets used and analyzed during the current study are available from the corresponding author on reasonable request.

Conflicts of Interest: The authors declare no conflicts of interest.

References

1. Machado, M.V.; Diehl, A.M. Pathogenesis of nonalcoholic steatohepatitis. *Gastroenterology* **2016**, *150*, 1769–1777. [CrossRef]
2. Powell, E.E.; Wong, V.W.-S.; Rinella, M. Non-alcoholic fatty liver disease. *Lancet* **2021**, *397*, 2212–2224. [CrossRef]
3. Younossi, Z.M.; Golabi, P.; Paik, J.M.; Henry, A.; Van Dongen, C.; Henry, L. The global epidemiology of nonalcoholic fatty liver disease (NAFLD) and nonalcoholic steatohepatitis (NASH): A systematic review. *Hepatology* **2023**, *77*, 1335–1347. [CrossRef]
4. Younossi, Z.M.; Kalligeros, M.; Henry, L. Epidemiology of metabolic dysfunction associated steatotic liver disease. *Clin. Mol. Hepatol.* **2024**, *31*, S32–S50. [CrossRef] [PubMed]
5. Ahmed, A.; Wong, R.J.; Harrison, S.A. Nonalcoholic fatty liver disease review: Diagnosis, treatment, and outcomes. *Clin. Gastroenterol. Hepatol.* **2015**, *13*, 2062–2070. [CrossRef] [PubMed]
6. Miao, L.; Targher, G.; Byrne, C.D.; Cao, Y.Y.; Zheng, M.H. Current status and future trends of the global burden of MASLD. *Trends Endocrinol. Metab.* **2024**, *35*, 697–707. [CrossRef] [PubMed]
7. Salem, V.; AlHusseini, N.; Abdul Razack, H.I.; Naoum, A.; Sims, O.T.; Alqahtani, S.A. Prevalence, risk factors, and interventions for obesity in Saudi Arabia: A systematic review. *Obes. Rev.* **2022**, *23*, e13448. [CrossRef]
8. Grundy, S.M. Metabolic syndrome update. *Trends Cardiovasc. Med.* **2016**, *26*, 364–373. [CrossRef]
9. Prasad, H.; Ryan, D.A.; Celzo, M.F.; Stapleton, D. Metabolic syndrome: Definition and therapeutic implications. *Postgrad. Med.* **2012**, *124*, 21–30. [CrossRef]
10. Mohamed, S. Functional foods against metabolic syndrome (obesity, diabetes, hypertension and dyslipidemia) and cardiovascular disease. *Trends Food Sci. Technol.* **2014**, *35*, 114–128. [CrossRef]
11. Chiva-Blanch, G.; Badimon, L. Effects of polyphenol intake on metabolic syndrome: Current evidences from human trials. *Oxidative Med. Cell. Longev.* **2017**, *2017*, 5812401. [CrossRef] [PubMed]
12. Sarker, U.; Lin, Y.P.; Oba, S.; Yoshioka, Y.; Hoshikawa, K. Prospects and potentials of underutilized leafy amaranths as vegetable use for health-promotion. *Plant Physiol. Biochem.* **2022**, *182*, 104–123. [CrossRef] [PubMed]
13. Peña, N.; Minguez, S.; Escobar, J.D. Current production scenario and functional potential of the whole amaranth plant: A review. In *Agricultural Sciences*; Waisundara, V.Y., Ed.; IntechOpen: London, UK, 2024; Volume 5, ISBN 978-1-83768-606-3.
14. Jimoh, M.O.; Okaiyeto, K.; Oguntibeju, O.O.; Laubscher, C.P. A systematic review on Amaranthus-related research. *Horticulturae* **2022**, *8*, 239. [CrossRef]
15. Peter, K.; Gandhi, P. Rediscovering the therapeutic potential of Amaranthus species: A review. *Egypt. J. Basic Appl. Sci.* **2017**, *4*, 196–205. [CrossRef]
16. Sharma, N.; Gupta, P.C.; Rao, C.V. Nutrient content, mineral content and antioxidant activity of *Amaranthus viridis* and *Moringa oleifera* leaves. *Res. J. Med. Plant* **2012**, *6*, 253–259. [CrossRef]
17. Bagepalli, S.A.K.; Kuruba, L.; Jayaveera, K. Comparative antipyretic activity of methanolic extracts of some species of *Amaranthus*. *Asian Pac. J. Trop. Biomed.* **2011**, *1*, S47–S50. [CrossRef]
18. Venskutonis, P.R.; Kraujalis, P. Nutritional components of amaranth seeds and vegetables: A review on composition, properties, and uses. *Compr. Rev. Food Sci. Food Saf.* **2013**, *12*, 381–412. [CrossRef]
19. Dutta, A.; Singh, M. Comparative analysis of aqueous extracts of amaranth and coriander in scavenging free radical activity and protection of DNA against oxidative damage. *Chiang Mai J. Sci.* **2011**, *38*, 560–571.
20. Semmler, G.; Datz, C.; Trauner, M. Eating, diet, and nutrition for the treatment of non-alcoholic fatty liver disease. *Clin. Mol. Hepatol.* **2023**, *29*, S244–S260. [CrossRef]
21. Carmiel-Haggai, M.; Cederbaum, A.I.; Nieto, N. A high-fat diet leads to the progression of non-alcoholic fatty liver disease in obese rats. *FASEB J.* **2005**, *19*, 136–138. [CrossRef]

22. de Moura e Dias, M.; dos Reis, S.A.; da Conceição, L.L.; Sediyama, C.M.N.d.O.; Pereira, S.S.; de Oliveira, L.L.; Gouveia Peluzio, M.d.C.; Martinez, J.A.; Milagro, F.I. Diet-induced obesity in animal models: Points to consider and influence on metabolic markers. *Diabetol. Metab. Syndr.* **2021**, *13*, 32. [CrossRef]
23. Dincheva, I.; Badjakov, I.; Galunska, B. New insights into the research of bioactive compounds from plant origins with nutraceutical and pharmaceutical potential. *Plants* **2023**, *12*, 258. [CrossRef] [PubMed]
24. Marques, C.; Meireles, M.; Norberto, S.; Leite, J.; Freitas, J.; Pestana, D.; Faria, A.; Calhau, C. High-fat diet-induced obesity rat model: A comparison between Wistar and Sprague-Dawley rat. *Adipocyte* **2015**, *5*, 11–21. [CrossRef] [PubMed]
25. Godoy-Matos, A.F.; Silva Júnior, W.S.; Valerio, C.M. NAFLD as a continuum: From obesity to metabolic syndrome and diabetes. *Diabetol. Metab. Syndr.* **2020**, *12*, 60. [CrossRef] [PubMed]
26. Emmanuel, O.C.; Babalola, O.O. Amaranth production and consumption in South Africa: The challenges of sustainability for food and nutrition security. *Int. J. Agric. Sustain.* **2022**, *20*, 449–460. [CrossRef]
27. Koutsoukis, C.; Roukos, C.; Demertzis, P.G.; Kandrelis, S.; Akrida-Demertzi, K. The variation of the chemical composition of the main plant species in a subalpine grassland in northwestern Greece. *Legume Sci.* **2019**, *1*, e23. [CrossRef]
28. Pant, P.; Pandey, S.; Dall'Acqua, S. The influence of environmental conditions on secondary metabolites in medicinal plants: A literature review. *Chem. Biodivers.* **2021**, *18*, e2100345. [CrossRef]
29. Maurya, N.K.; Arya, P. Amaranthus grain nutritional benefits: A review. *J. Pharmacogn. Phytochem.* **2018**, *7*, 2258–2262.
30. Schmidt, D.; Verruma-Bernardi, M.R.; Forti, V.A.; Borges, M.T.M.R. Quinoa and amaranth as functional foods: A review. *Food Rev. Int.* **2023**, *39*, 2277–2296. [CrossRef]
31. Ishtiaq, S.; Ahmad, M.; Hanif, U.; Akbar, S.; Mehjabeen Kamran, S.H. Phytochemical and in vitro antioxidant evaluation of different fractions of *Amaranthus graecizans* subsp. silvestris (Vill.) Brenan. *Asian Pac. J. Trop. Med.* **2014**, *7*, S342–S347. [CrossRef]
32. Wang, L.; Pan, X.; Jiang, L.; Chu, Y.; Gao, S.; Jiang, X.; Zhang, Y.; Chen, Y.; Luo, S.; Peng, C. The biological activity mechanism of chlorogenic acid and its applications in food industry: A review. *Front. Nutr.* **2022**, *9*, 943911. [CrossRef]
33. Shehab, N.G.; Abu-Gharbieh, E.; Bayoumi, F.A. Impact of phenolic composition on hepatoprotective and antioxidant effects of four desert medicinal plants. *BMC Complement. Altern. Med.* **2015**, *15*, 401. [CrossRef]
34. Németh, K.; Tóth, B.; Sarnyai, F.; Koncz, A.; Lenzinger, D.; Kereszturi, É.; Visnovitz, T.; Kestecher, B.M.; Osteikoetxea, X.; Csala, M.; et al. High fat diet and PCSK9 knockout modulates lipid profile of the liver and changes the expression of lipid homeostasis related genes. *Nutr. Metab.* **2023**, *20*, 19. [CrossRef]
35. Meng, S.; Cao, J.; Feng, Q.; Peng, J.; Hu, Y. Roles of chlorogenic acid on regulating glucose and lipids metabolism: A review. *Evid. Based Complement. Altern. Med.* **2013**, *2013*, 801457. [CrossRef] [PubMed]
36. Zhang, Z.; Yang, R.; Zi, Z.; Liu, B. A new clinical age of aging research. *Trends Endocrinol. Metab.* **2024**, *36*, 440–458. [CrossRef] [PubMed]
37. Freitas, R.A.M.S. Avaliação de Biodisponibilidade e Mecanismos de Ação Hipocolesterolemizante de Peptídeos do Amaranto (*Amaranthus cruentus* L. BRS-Alegria). Ph.D. Thesis, Universidade de São Paulo, São Paulo, Brazil, 2018.
38. Jeong, Y.H.; Kim, T.H. Evaluation of radical scavenging and α-glucosidase inhibitory effects of gallic acid reactants using polyphenol oxidase. *J. Korean Soc. Food Sci. Nutr.* **2016**, *45*, 1385–1390. [CrossRef]
39. Li, S.; Tan, H.Y.; Wang, N.; Cheung, F.; Hong, M.; Feng, Y. The potential and action mechanism of polyphenols in the treatment of liver diseases. *Oxidative Med. Cell. Longev.* **2018**, *2018*, 8394818. [CrossRef]
40. Wang, J.; Jiang, Y.; Jin, L.; Qian, C.; Zuo, W.; Lin, J.; Xie, L.; Jin, B.; Zhao, Y.; Huang, L.; et al. Alantolactone attenuates high-fat diet-induced inflammation and oxidative stress in non-alcoholic fatty liver disease. *Nutr. Diabetes* **2024**, *14*, 41. [CrossRef]
41. Saha, P.; Talukdar, A.D.; Nath, R.; Sarker, S.D.; Nahar, L.; Sahu, J.; Choudhury, M.D. Role of natural phenolics in hepatoprotection: A mechanistic review and analysis of regulatory network of associated genes. *Front. Pharmacol.* **2019**, *10*, 509. [CrossRef]
42. Jadhav, V.; Biradar, S. Evaluation of antioxidant activity of *Amaranthus viridis* L. methanolic extract. *Int. J. Pharm. Bio Sci.* **2016**, *6*, 150–153. [CrossRef]
43. Sarker, U.; Ercisli, S. Salt eustress induction in red amaranth (*Amaranthus gangeticus*) augments nutritional, phenolic acids and antiradical potential of leaves. *Antioxidants* **2022**, *11*, 2434. [CrossRef]
44. Adegbola, P.I.; Adetutu, A.; Olaniyi, T.D. Antioxidant activity of *Amaranthus* species from the Amaranthaceae family—A review. *S. Afr. J. Bot.* **2020**, *133*, 111–117. [CrossRef]
45. Ko, H.J.; Chen, J.H.; Ng, L.T. Hepatoprotection of *Gentiana scabra* extract and polyphenols in liver of carbon tetrachloride-intoxicated mice. *J. Environ. Pathol. Toxicol. Oncol.* **2011**, *30*, 179–187. [CrossRef]
46. Žiberna, L.; Jenko-Pražnikar, Z.; Petelin, A. Serum bilirubin levels in overweight and obese individuals: The importance of anti-inflammatory and antioxidant responses. *Antioxidants* **2021**, *10*, 1352. [CrossRef]
47. Kipp, Z.A.; Xu, M.; Bates, E.A.; Lee, W.H.; Kern, P.A.; Hinds, T.D. Bilirubin levels are negatively correlated with adiposity in obese men and women, and its catabolized product, urobilin, is positively associated with insulin resistance. *Antioxidants* **2023**, *12*, 170. [CrossRef] [PubMed]

48. Fu, K.; Wang, C.; Ma, C.; Zhou, H.; Li, Y. The potential application of Chinese medicine in liver diseases: A new opportunity. *Front. Pharmacol.* **2021**, *12*, 771459. [CrossRef] [PubMed]
49. Maity, S.; Nag, N.; Chatterjee, S.; Adhikari, S.; Mazumder, S. Bilirubin clearance and antioxidant activities of ethanol extract of Phyllanthus amarus root in phenylhydrazine-induced neonatal jaundice in mice. *J. Physiol. Biochem.* **2013**, *69*, 467–476. [CrossRef] [PubMed]
50. Huang, W.; Zhang, J.; Chua, S.S.; Qatanani, M.; Han, Y.; Granata, R.; Moore, D.D. Induction of bilirubin clearance by the constitutive androstane receptor (CAR). *Proc. Natl. Acad. Sci. USA* **2003**, *100*, 4156–4161. [CrossRef]
51. Kim, S.D.; Morgan, L.; Hargreaves, E.; Zhang, X.; Jiang, Z.; Antenos, M.; Li, B.; Kirby, G.M. Regulation of cytochrome P450 2a5 by *Artemisia capillaris* and 6,7-dimethylesculetin in mouse hepatocytes. *Front. Pharmacol.* **2021**, *12*, 730416. [CrossRef]
52. Sinal, C.J.; Bend, J.R. Aryl hydrocarbon receptor-dependent induction of Cyp1a1 by bilirubin in mouse hepatoma Hepa 1c1c7 cells. *Mol. Pharmacol.* **1997**, *52*, 590–599. [CrossRef]
53. Gabuza, K.B.; Sibuyi, N.R.S.; Mobo, M.P.; Madiehe, A.M. Differentially expressed serum proteins from obese Wistar rats as a risk factor for obesity-induced diseases. *Sci. Rep.* **2020**, *10*, 12415. [CrossRef]
54. Diniz, A.; Escuder-Gilabert, L.; Lopes, N.P.; Villanueva-Camañas, R.M.; Sagrado, S.; Medina-Hernández, M.J. Characterization of interactions between polyphenolic compounds and human serum proteins by capillary electrophoresis. *Anal. Bioanal. Chem.* **2008**, *391*, 625–632. [CrossRef]
55. Westerbacka, J.; Lammi, K.; Häkkinen, A.M.; Rissanen, A.; Salminen, I.; Aro, A.; Yki-Järvinen, H. Dietary fat content modifies liver fat in overweight nondiabetic subjects. *J. Clin. Endocrinol. Metab.* **2005**, *90*, 2804–2809. [CrossRef]
56. Abenavoli, L.; Larussa, T.; Corea, A.; Procopio, A.C.; Boccuto, L.; Dallio, M.; Federico, A.; Luzza, F. Dietary polyphenols and non-alcoholic fatty liver disease. *Nutrients* **2021**, *13*, 494. [CrossRef] [PubMed]
57. Liang, N.; Kitts, D. Role of chlorogenic acids in controlling oxidative and inflammatory stress conditions. *Nutrients* **2015**, *8*, 16. [CrossRef] [PubMed]
58. Badhani, B.; Sharma, N.; Kakkar, R. Gallic acid: A versatile antioxidant with promising therapeutic and industrial applications. *RSC Adv.* **2015**, *5*, 27540–27557. [CrossRef]
59. Pravin, B.; Nanaware, V.; Ashwini, B.; Wondmie, G.F.; Jardan, Y.A.B.; Bourhia, M. Assessing the antioxidant properties of naringin and rutin and investigating their oxidative DNA damage effects in breast cancer. *Sci. Rep.* **2024**, *14*, 15314. [CrossRef] [PubMed]
60. Aldoghachi, F.E.H.; Noor Al-Mousawi, U.M.; Shari, F.H. Antioxidant activity of rosmarinic acid extracted and purified from *Mentha piperita*. *Arch. Razi Inst.* **2021**, *76*, 1279–1287. [CrossRef]
61. Kumar, U.; Kumar, I.; Singh, P.K.; Yadav, J.S.; Dwivedi, A.; Singh, P.; Mishra, S.; Sharma, R.K. Total phenolic content and antioxidant activities in methanol extracts of medicinal herbs from Indo-Gangetic plains of India. *J. Appl. Biol. Biotechnol.* **2024**, *12*, 89–99. [CrossRef]
62. Olubukola Sinbad, O.; Folorunsho, A.A.; Olabisi, O.L.; Abimbola Ayoola, O.; Johnson Temitope, E. Vitamins as antioxidants. *J. Food Sci. Nutr. Res.* **2019**, *2*, 214–235. [CrossRef]
63. Kruk, J.; Aboul-Enein, B.H.; Duchnik, E.; Marchlewicz, M. Antioxidative properties of phenolic compounds and their effect on oxidative stress induced by severe physical exercise. *J. Physiol. Sci.* **2022**, *72*, 19. [CrossRef] [PubMed]
64. Maciejewska-Markiewicz, D.; Stachowska, E.; Hawryłkowicz, V.; Stachowska, L.; Prowans, P. The role of resolvins, protectins and marensins in non-alcoholic fatty liver disease (NAFLD). *Biomolecules* **2021**, *11*, 937. [CrossRef] [PubMed]
65. Xu, Z.J.; Fan, J.G.; Ding, X.D.; Qiao, L.; Wang, G.L. Characterization of high-fat, diet-induced, non-alcoholic steatohepatitis with fibrosis in rats. *Dig. Dis. Sci.* **2010**, *55*, 931–940. [CrossRef]
66. Al-Dosari, M.S. The effectiveness of ethanolic extract of *Amaranthus tricolor* L.: A natural hepatoprotective agent. *Am. J. Chin. Med.* **2010**, *38*, 1051–1064. [CrossRef] [PubMed]
67. Ashok Kumar, B.S.; Lakshman, K.; Jayaveera, K.N.; Sheshadri Shekar, D.; Nandeesh, R.; Velmurugan, C. Chemoprotective and antioxidant activities of methanolic extract of *Amaranthus spinosus* leaves on paracetamol induced liver damage in rats. *Acta Medica Salin.* **2010**, *39*, 68–74. [CrossRef]
68. Mahmoodi, M.; Hosseini, R.; Kazemi, A.; Ofori-Asenso, R.; Mazidi, M.; Mazloomi, S.M. Effects of green tea or green tea catechin on liver enzymes in healthy individuals and people with nonalcoholic fatty liver disease: A systematic review and meta-analysis of randomized clinical trials. *Phytother. Res.* **2020**, *34*, 1587–1598. [CrossRef]
69. Alzahrani, N.S.; Alshammari, G.M.; El-Ansary, A.; Yagoub, A.E.A.; Amina, M.; Saleh, A.; Yahya, M.A. Anti-Hyperlipidemia, Hypoglycemic, and Hepatoprotective Impacts of Pearl Millet (*Pennisetum glaucum* L.) Grains and Their Ethanol Extract on Rats Fed a High-Fat Diet. *Nutrients* **2022**, *14*, 1791. [CrossRef]
70. Bose, M.; Lambert, J.D.; Ju, J.; Reuhl, K.R.; Shapses, S.A.; Yang, C.S. The major green tea polyphenol, (-)-epigallocatechin-3-gallate, inhibits obesity, metabolic syndrome, and fatty liver disease in high-fat–fed mice. *J. Nutr.* **2008**, *138*, 1677–1683. [CrossRef]
71. Alibas, I. Microwave, vacuum, and air-drying characteristics of collard leaves. *Dry. Technol.* **2009**, *27*, 1266–1273. [CrossRef]
72. Zeashan, H.; Amresh, G.; Singh, S.; Rao, C.V. Hepatoprotective activity of *Amaranthus spinosus* in experimental animals. *Food Chem. Toxicol.* **2008**, *46*, 3417–3421. [CrossRef]

73. Kim, H.C.; Song, J.M.; Kim, C.J.; Yoon, S.Y.; Kim, I.R.; Park, B.S.; Shin, S.H. Combined effect of bisphosphonate and recombinant human bone morphogenetic protein 2 on bone healing of rat calvarial defects. *Maxillofac. Plast. Reconstr. Surg.* **2015**, *37*, 16. [CrossRef]
74. Hedge, J.; Hofreiter, B.; Whistler, R. *Carbohydrate Chemistry*; Academic Press: New York, NY, USA, 1962; pp. 371–380.
75. Kjeldahl, J. New method for the determination of nitrogen. *Sci. Am.* **1883**, *16*, 6470. [CrossRef]
76. Agroindustriais, P. Official methods of analysis of the Association of Official Analytical Chemists. In *Caracterização Propagação e Melhor Genético Pitaya Comer e Nativa Cerrado*; AOAC: Rockville, MD, USA, 2013; Volume 26, p. 62.
77. *ICC-Standard No. 110/1*; Determination of the Moisture Content of Cereals and Cereal Products (Practical Method). International Association for Cereal Chemistry (ICC): Vienna, Austria, 1976.
78. *ICC 104/1*; Determination of Ash in Cereals and Cereal Products. International Association for Cereal Chemistry (ICC): Vienna, Austria, 1990.

pharmaceuticals MDPI

Case Report

Harnessing the Interactions of Wound Exudate Cells with Dressings Biomaterials for the Control and Prognosis of Healing Pathways

Shirin Saberianpour [1,2], Gianluca Melotto [1,3], Lucy Redhead [1,3], Nadia Terrazzini [1,2], Jaqueline Rachel Forss [1,3] and Matteo Santin [1,2,*]

1 Centre for Regenerative Medicine and Devices, University of Brighton, Huxley Building Lewes Road, Brighton BN2 4GJ, UK; s.saberianpour@brighton.ac.uk (S.S.); g.melotto@brighton.ac.uk (G.M.); l.redhead@brighton.ac.uk (L.R.); n.terrazzini@brighton.ac.uk (N.T.); j.forss@brighton.ac.uk (J.R.F.)
2 School of Applied Sciences, University of Brighton, Huxley Building Lewes Road, Brighton BN2 4GJ, UK
3 School of Health and Sport Sciences, University of Brighton, Falmer Campus, Village Way, Brighton BN1 9PH, UK
* Correspondence: m.santin@brighton.ac.uk

Abstract: The global socioeconomic challenge generated by wounds requires an understanding of healing and non-healing pathways in patients. Also, the interactions occurring between the wound dressing biomaterials with cells relevant to the healing process have not been sufficiently investigated, thus neglecting the role that wound dressing composition can play in healing. Through the study of six cases of acute surgical wounds, the present work analyses the early (24 h post-surgery) interactions of biochemical and cellular components with (i) Atrauman, a device made of knitted woven synthetic polymeric fibre when used as a primary dressing, and (ii) Melolin, a hydrocolloid engineered as two layers of synthetic and cellulose non-woven fibres when used as a secondary dressing. A pathway towards healing could be observed in those cases where endoglin-expressing cells and M2 macrophages were retained by Atrauman fibres at the interface with the wound bed. On the contrary, cases where the secondary dressing Melolin absorbed these cell phenotypes in its mesh resulted in a slower or deteriorating healing process. The data obtained indicate that a subtraction of progenitor cells by Melolin may impair the healing process and that the analysis of the retrieved wound dressings for biomarkers expressed by cells relevant to wound healing may become an additional tool to determine the patient's prognosis.

Keywords: wound dressings; inflammatory cells; progenitor cells; biocompatibility; prognosis

1. Introduction

Wound healing is a unanimously recognised clinical and socioeconomic problem on a global scale [1]. Wounds are broadly categorised as acute or chronic, the former mostly resulting in healing, while the latter fails to repair for weeks, months or years, leading to a deterioration of patient quality of life and, in a significant number of cases, to amputations and death [2]. It is known that the healing process of both acute and chronic wounds can be affected by a range of patient comorbidities and by infections.

In response to this growing clinical need, a range of wound dressings have been made available that differ from each other in their chemical composition, engineering and presence of therapeutic compounds, such as, for example, antibacterial agents [3]. The main approaches to the development of these devices are (i) engineering solutions to protect the wound from traumas (e.g., dressing made of knitted polymeric fibres) and bacterial colonisation (i.e., an oxygen-permeable polymeric film barrier) or (ii) engineering one or more absorbent layers to absorb the exudate while keeping the wound moist by the same oxygen-permeable polymeric film preventing bacterial invasion of the wound [4]. In fact, wound moisture is widely considered a prerequisite to maintaining the appropriate environment for the wound-healing process. These dressings can be used as such or in combination. In the latter case, they are referred to as primary and secondary dressings, whereby the primary dressing is often a mechanically resilient, knitted dressing, and the secondary is a hydrogel or hydrocolloid able to absorb excesses of wound exudate [5]. Typical wound dressings used as primary and secondary devices are Atrauman and Melolin [6,7]. Atrauman is a non-medicated tulle dressing consisting of water-repellent polyester fibres impregnated with fatty acids and recommended for use in combination with a secondary dressing [6]. While the engineered polyethylene fibres provide protection to fragile wounds, the triglycerides impregnation ensures low adhesion, thus reducing their disruption [6]. Melolin is a multi-layered device recommended for moderate wound exudates, where a film of polyethylene terephthalate protects a two-layer absorbent component, including a mixture of cotton and polyacrylonitrile fibres combined with a layer of non-woven cellulose fabric [7]. These two types of dressings are among the most used devices alongside dressings made of either synthetic (e.g., polyacrylic acids, polymethyl methacrylates) or natural polymers (e.g., alginate, carboxymethylcellulose) [5].

Currently, clinicians choose the dressings and consider their combination according to accepted wound classifications and, in particular, to the type of wound exudate, i.e., limited, moderate or large exudate volumes [8–10]. In this framework, the lack of consistent clinical outcomes deriving from the use of these devices has prompted studies aiming at the assessment of wound dressing efficacy, these being mainly based on clinical parameters [11–13].

An analysis of the many case studies and randomised clinical trials published over a few decades clearly shows that few of these investigations have focussed on the potential effects that wound dressings, as any other medical implants in contact with body fluids, may have on the healing process [14,15]. Indeed, unlike other clinical areas where the biocompatibility of implants has been studied at the level of interactions between biochemical and cellular components of the body fluid with the surface of the implant, the technological development and clinical use of wound dressings appear to have neglected the process known as the 'foreign body response to implants' [16]. Such a concept is based on data showing that, upon contact with the body fluid, the physicochemical properties of any implanted biomaterial (e.g., hydrophilicity/hydrophobicity, electric charges) can lead to the adsorption of proteins and consequent change of their conformation that makes them recognised by the inflammatory cells as antigens and to the consequent protracted activation of inflammatory cells leading to a chronic inflammatory status and to either the lack of healing or the formation of scar tissue.

It is argued that the study of the interactions of these biochemical and cellular components with the wound dressing biomaterials is not only important to ascertain their biocompatibility and prompt the development of new devices, but also has a potential value in identifying new biological markers of healing or not healing that can assist clinicians in their assessment of wounds and in their consequent choice of the best treatment, in a way that is more accurate than the current clinical parameters [17].

A biological marker, also referred to as a biomarker, serves as an indicator of the condition of a biological system [18]. Historically, parameters such as the erythrocyte sedimentation rate (ESR), C-reactive protein and albumin levels have been employed to evaluate the possibility of recovery and the presence of infections. Studies have identified various cellular processes and signalling molecules linked to wound healing, and it has been suggested that the clinical assessment of these agents in wounds may enable the wound prognosis thus hinting at their potential utilisation as biomarkers [19–24]. TNF-α, interleukins (e.g., IL-1, IL-6) and growth factors (e.g., platelet-derived growth factor, PDGF-BB) are secreted by cells such as macrophages, neutrophils, fibroblasts and platelets [25–27]. Research has demonstrated that elevated levels of several types of cytokines, exceeding the normal range, are frequently detected in non-healing wounds [28]. Additionally, evidence suggests that the administration of growth factors such as PDGF may expedite the healing process for persistent, non-healing wounds [27]. Nevertheless, the identification of a biomarker or a panel of biomarkers that is, at the same time, reliable and suited to clinical use remains an unmet challenge. For example, IL-6 lacks a reliable, predictive value for both favourable and unfavourable outcomes [26]. Consequently, these factors are seldom utilised in the assessment of wounds. More recent advances in genomics, proteomics, and molecular pathology have unveiled numerous potential biomarkers of clinical importance (e.g., microRNAs, long non-coding RNAs, and circular RNAs), but the technically complex, time-consuming and relatively expensive character of these techniques make them not implementable in clinical settings [29]. Likewise, the adhesion and activation of inflammatory cells such as neutrophils and macrophages are known to be affected upon adhesion with medical implants [16]. Despite that studies of neutrophils and macrophage interactions with wound dressings have been widely advocated [30,31], the systematic study of their interactions with wound dressings with different physicochemical properties, their phenotypical changes and potential harnessing as biomarkers of wound healing have not been sufficiently explored.

The aim of this study is to demonstrate, through six cases of toenail-surgery acute wounds in subjects with no ascertained relevant comorbidities, that the contact of the wound exudate with the biomaterials of primary and secondary dressings with different physicochemical properties leads to their interactions with biomolecules and cells inducing changes that can either favour or impair the healing process. The study of these interactions and the changes they induce in biomolecules and cells in relation to the final clinical outcome also paves the way towards the identification of specific biomarkers of healing or non-healing thus making the retrieved wound dressings a potentially accurate and clinically suitable prognostic tool helping clinicians to implement appropriate treatments by anticipating the pathway entered by the healing process.

2. Results

The clinical assessment and biochemical and cellular analyses of each patient were examined individually and linked to the final clinical outcomes. Participants' demographic data and initial clinical assessment are reported in Table 1.

Table 1. Participants' demographic data and initial clinical assessment.

Patients	Age	Gender	Body Mass Index	Smoking	Diabetic	Martinez-Nova's Classification Visit 1
Case 1	20	Female	31.9	No	No	IIB
Case 2	19	Male	24.5	No	No	IIB
Case 3	49	Female	28.4	No	No	IIA
Case 4	62	Male	28.1	No	No	III
Case 5	36	Female	24.2	No	No	Unstageable
Case 6	17	Female	18.8	No	No	IIB

All patients showed monofilament scores of 10 in both LF and RF, ruling out any significant sensory loss. The Doppler analysis revealed a biphasic RF DP, a triphasic RF PT, a biphasic LF DP, and a biphasic LF PT, denoting an absence of peripherical arterial disease.

With the exception of Case 5, where a total nail avulsion was performed, all other patients underwent partial avulsion. Pre- and post-surgery wound areas were measured at each visit (Table 2), and healing progression evaluated as a percentage of the wound reduction or increase after the surgical procedure (Figure 1).

Table 2. Participants' wound area size as measured at each visit.

Participant n.	Visit 1 Wound Area	Visit 2 Wound Area *	Visit 3 Wound Area
Case 1	23.4 mm^2	27.4 mm^2	22.7 mm^2 (−17.6%)
Case 2	59.0 mm^2	78.5 mm^2	45.2 mm^2 (−42.4%)
Case 3	6.9 mm^2	29.6 mm^2	10.7 mm^2 (−63.9%)
Case 4	75 mm^2	160 mm^2	136 mm^2 (−15%)
Case 5	39.8 mm^2	50.7 mm^2	70.4 mm^2 (+38.9%)
Case 6	47.7 mm^2	48.1 mm^2	45.5 mm^2 (−5.4)

* Visit 2 wound areas refers to measurement post-surgery.

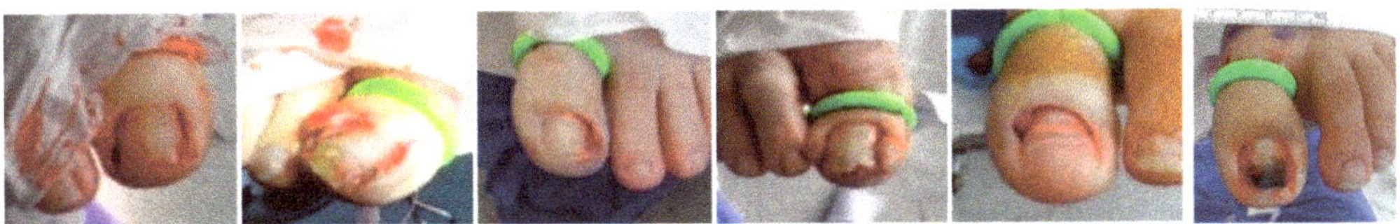

Figure 1. Participants' wounds immediately after surgical procedures at Visit 2.

2.1. Case 1

A 20-year-old female with a BMI of 31.9, no history of diabetes or smoking and an IGTN of the fibular sulcus of the right hallux stage IIB (Table 1). At Visit 1, the patient's wound was treated with Melolin as wound dressing, and she was recommended to regularly change the same dressing.

The patient returned five weeks later for surgery. At this stage, the wound did not show any sign of infection or of any other abnormal features, and a moderate exudate volume was observed. After surgery was performed (Figure 1, Case 1), primary and secondary dressings were applied. After one day, the patient returned for the final removal of the dressing prior to discharge with a wound area reduction of 17.6% (Table 2, Case 1).

The overall protein concentration in the wound exudate was maintained constant across the three visits (ca. 15 mg/mL), but a gradual and sharp increase in the concentration of proteins absorbed by Melolin was observed with values ranging from 3.89 mg/mL in Visit 2 retrieved dressing to 78.80 mg/mL at Visit 3 retrieved dressing (Figure 2). The Atrauman applied at Visit 2 showed to have absorbed proteins at a concentration of 11.96 mg/mL (Figure 2). The analysis of the protein species, focussing on two cytokines relevant to acute inflammation (TNFα and IL-6), showed different concentration profiles (Figure 3A,B, Patient 1). In particular, the pro-inflammatory cytokine TNFα that was found at a concentration of 180.76 ± 18.02 pg/mL at Visit 1 reached a peak of 320.9 ± 44.59 pg/mL at Visit 2 and underwent a significant reduction of its concentration at Visit 3 46.51 ± 11.69 pg/mL (Figure 3A). Relatively lower concentrations of this pro-inflammatory factor were found in the Melolin absorbent layer at Visit 2 (66.46 ± 5.25 pg/mL) and Visit 3 (53.68 ± 5.08 pg/mL). Similar concentration levels were eluted from the primary dressing Atrauman at Visit 3 (58.20 ± 7.93 pg/mL).

IL-6 profiles differed from those of the TNFα in both the exudate and dressings (Figure 3B, Patient 1). In particular, the concentration levels of this cytokine remained constant in the exudate and both the dressings across the visits with values at around 200 pg/mL, but for the concentration level found in Atrauman and Melolin at Visit 3, the concentration levels were 280.38 ± 21.84 pg/mL and 325.21 ± 17.96 pg/mL, respectively.

PDGF-BB levels in the exudates collected at Visit 2 and Visit 3 showed relatively low concentrations ranging from 64 to 71 pg/mL (Figure 3C, Patient 1). This factor seemed to be captured at similar concentration levels by both Atrauman (Visit 3: 51.95 ± 23.61 pg/mL) and Melolin (Visit 2: 77.72 ± 39.99 pg/mL, Visit 3: 80.06 ± 32.67 pg/mL).

This patient showed a very low cell count in the exudate of the first visit (12,353/100 µL) that gradually increased during the healing process to reach 1,494,000 cells/100 µL (Table 3). The immunostaining of the exudate at Visit 3 showed a uniform presence of all the cell phenotypes investigated (Figure 4, Case 1), while the analysis of the same phenotypes in contact with the primary and secondary dressing showed higher cell densities with cells forming aggregates, particularly in the case of their adhesion on the Atrauman fibres (Figure 5, Case 1).

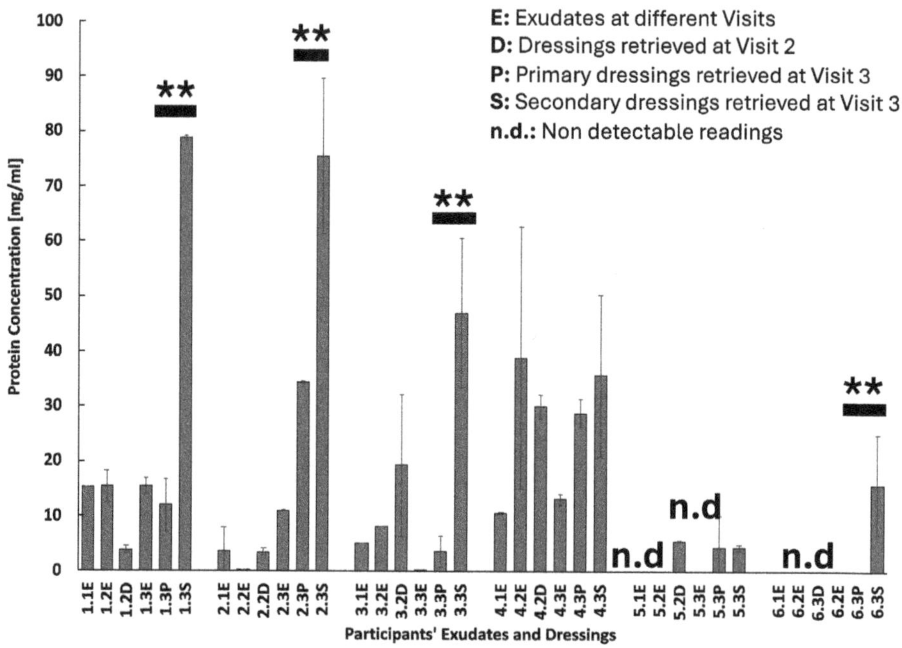

Figure 2. Protein concentration levels in exudates (E) and primary or secondary dressings (D, P, S) at different visits. Numbers indicate participant's case study number and Visit number (e.g., 1.1E: Participant 1, Visit 1, Exudate). Statistical analysis was performed only on primary and secondary dressings protein levels at Visit 3. ** indicates statistically significant differences at $p \leq 0.01$. Tests were performed by a Bradford assay and optical density values were converted into mg/mL through a standard curve obtained by measuring different concentrations of bovine serum albumin (BSA).

Table 3. Participants' cell numbers in exudates at different visits.

	Exudate Cell Number (in 100 µL)		
	Visit 1	**Visit 2**	**Visit 3** *
Case 1	12,352	58,800	1,494,000 (2540%)
Case 2	21,851	766,451	540,800 (70%)
Case 3	5468	12,404	5125 (41.3%)
Case 4	210,370	374,375	137,666 (36.8%)
Case 5	666,000	232,142	403,571 (173.8%)
Case 6	20,833	6,666	150,000 (2250%)

* Percentages refer to cell number changes from Visit 2 to Visit 3.

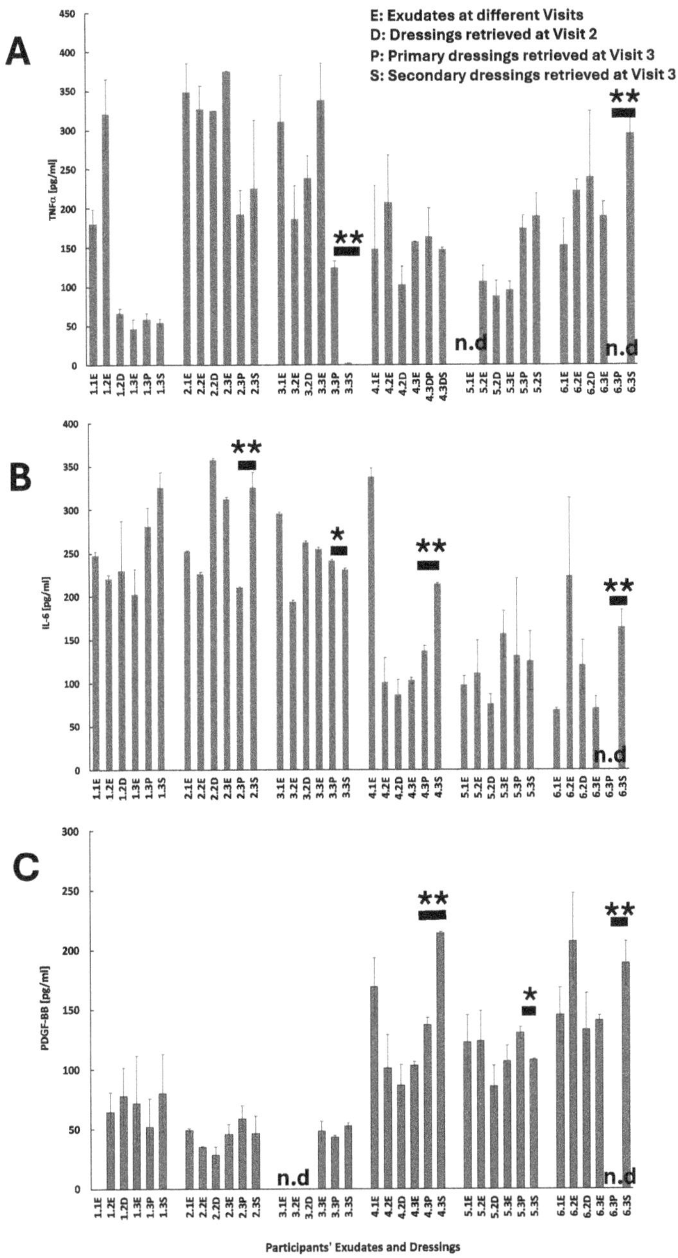

Figure 3. Participants' levels of cytokines in exudates and retrieved dressings. (**A**) TNFα, (**B**) IL-6, (**C**) PDGF-BB. Statistical analysis was performed only on primary and secondary dressings cytokine and growth factor levels at Visit 3. * indicates statistically significant differences at $p \leq 0.05$. ** indicates statistically significant differences at $p \leq 0.01$. n.d. indicates not detectable values.

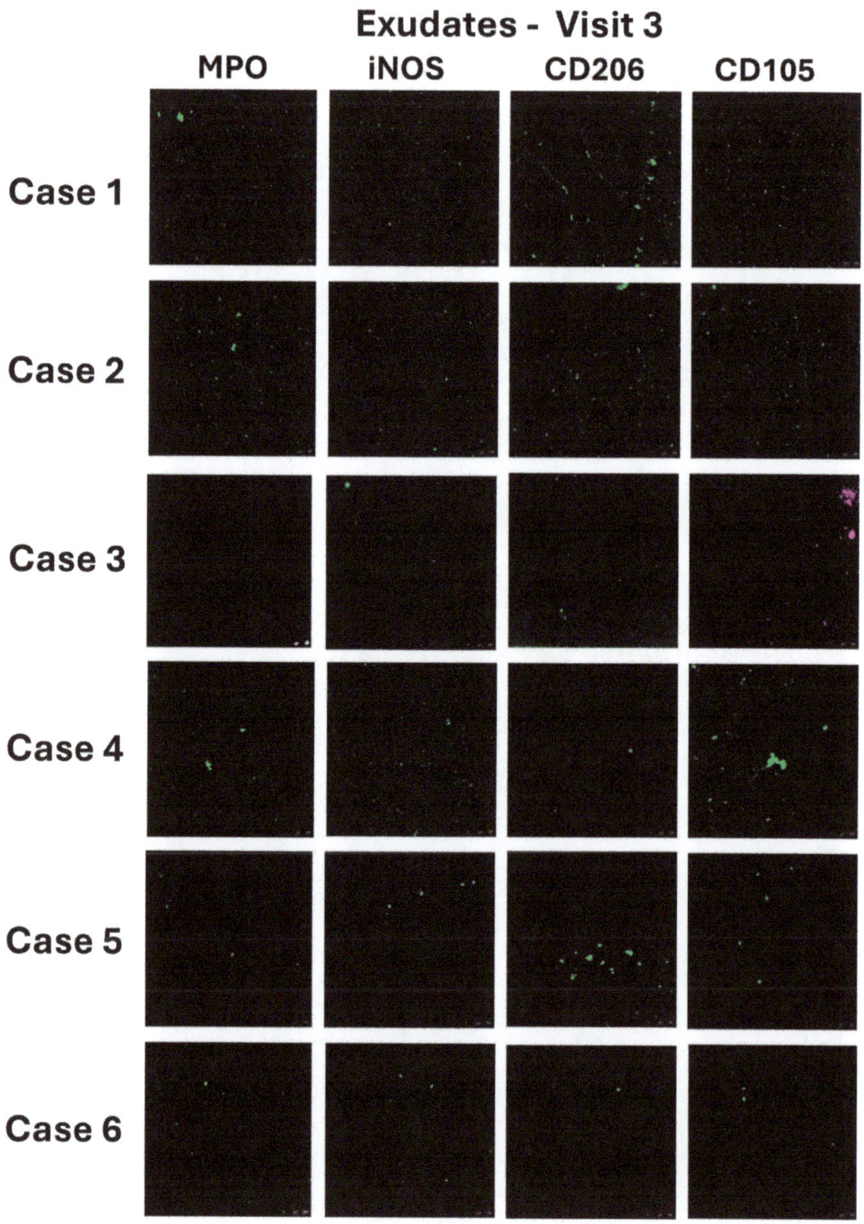

Figure 4. Immunostaining of patients' exudates at Visit 3 (24 sh post-surgery). MPO: Neutrophil and platelet marker (myeloperoxidase), iNOS (nitric oxide synthase): M1 pro-inflammatory macrophages, CD206: M2 macrophage regenerative phenotype, CD105: progenitor cells. Scale bars = 100 μm. Wound exudates were diluted in PBS, applied to glass slides by smearing, fixed with paraformaldehyde, incubated with 3% *w*/*v* BSA blocking solution and finally stained with primary and fluorophore-tagged secondary antibodies.

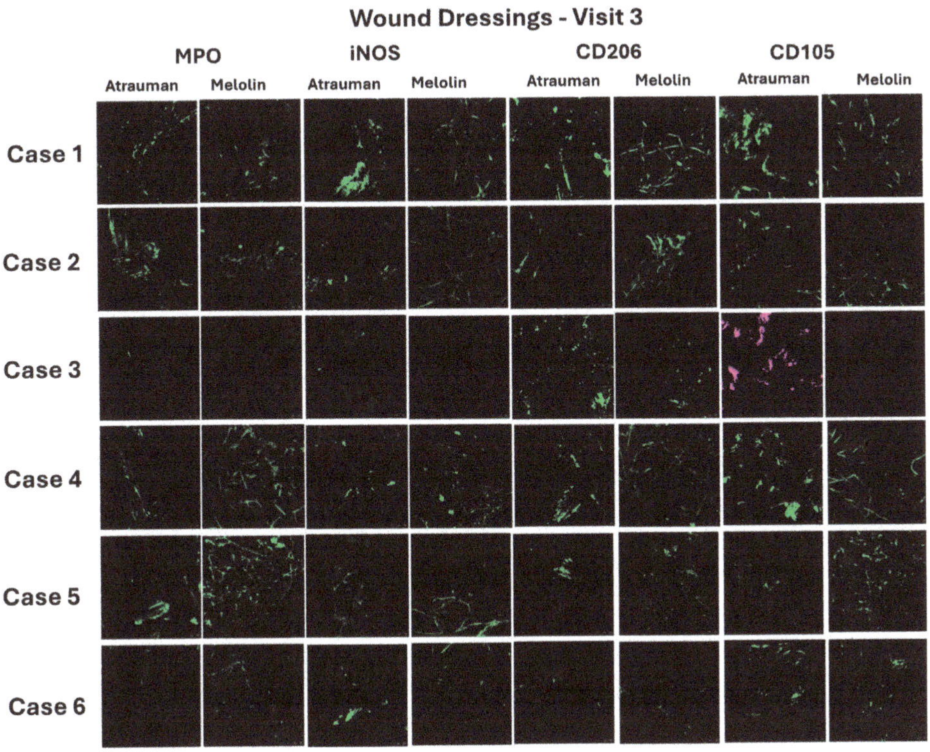

Figure 5. Immunostaining of patients' primary and secondary wound dressings removed at visit 3 (24 h post-surgery). MPO: Neutrophil and platelet marker (myeloperoxidase), iNOS (nitric oxide synthase): M1 pro-inflammatory macrophages, CD206: M2 macrophage regenerative phenotype, CD105: progenitor cells. Case 3's CD105^{+} cells were stained in purple to highlight the differences with all the other cases. Scale bars = 100 μm. Withdrawn dressings were copiously washed with PBS, fixed with paraformaldehyde, incubated with 3% *w*/*v* BSA blocking solution and finally stained with primary and fluorophore-tagged secondary antibodies.

2.2. *Case 2*

A 19-year-old male with a BMI of 24.5, a previous smoker with no history of diabetes and with an IGTN of the fibular sulcus of the right hallux stage IIB (Table 1) visited and treated with Melolin returned for surgery after 10 days. The wound after surgery (Figure 1, Case 2) was dressed with Atrauman as a primary wound dressing and Melolin as a secondary wound dressing. After one day, the patient returned to clinics for final treatment and discharge, showing a wound area reduction of 42.4% (Table 2).

This patient also showed a relatively low concentration of proteins in the exudate during the first two visits and an increase at levels similar to those of Case 1 at Visit 3 (11 mg/mL) (Figure 2). The values of protein concentrations absorbed by Melolin at Visits 2 and 3 were also consistent with the values of Case 1, but higher concentrations were measured in Atrauman (34.33 mg/mL) (Figure 2). This patient showed constantly higher levels of TNFα in the exudates of the three visits (>300 pg/mL, Figure 3A, Patient 2), with dressings absorbing levels of this pro-inflammatory cytokine relatively higher than in Case 1 (Figure 3A, Cases 1 and 2). In the case of IL-6, the concentrations were at levels similar to Case 1, but for the last visit, the Case 2 patient showed an increase in this cytokine (Figure 3B, Case 2). Melolin showed higher concentrations of IL-6 than Atrauman at Visit 3, the latter absorbing lower levels than those observed on the same biomaterial in Patient 1 (Figure 3B, 2.3P and 2.3S).

This patient showed concentration levels of PDGF-BB in all exudates and dressings similar to Case 1 (Figure 3C, Cases 1 and 2).

The number of cells in the exudate of this patient over the three visits sharply increased between Visits 1 and 2 to then undergo a relative decrease at Visit 3 (Table 3, Visit 1: 21,851 cells/100 μL; Visit 2: 766,451 cells/100 μL; Visit 3: 540,800 cells/100 μL). The immunohistochemistry of the exudates and retrieved dressings at Visit 3 were similar to that of Case 1, showing all phenotypes consistently observed (Figures 4 and 5, Case 2).

2.3. Case 3

A 49-year-old female with a BMI of 28.4, a previous smoker with no history of diabetes and an IGTN of the fibular sulcus of left hallux stage IIA (Table 1) was treated with Melolin and returned for surgery after 3 days (Figure 1, Case 3). After one day, the patient returned to clinics for final medication and discharge, showing a reduction of the wound area of 63.9% (Table 2).

This patient showed low protein concentrations in the exudates collected during the three visits with a peak observed at Visit 2 (Visit 1: 5 mg/mL, Visit 2: 8 mg/mL, Visit 3: 0.05 mg/mL), concentration levels were absorbed by Melolin as per Case 1 and 2 (Visit 1: 19 mg/mL, Visit 2: 47 mg/mL), but lower protein concentrations were found in both Atrauman (3.64 mg/mL) and Melolin (ca. 48 mg/mL) at Visit 3 (Figure 2, Case 3).

In this patient, the relatively high levels of TNFα and IL-6 observed in the exudate at Visit 1 dropped significantly at Visit 2, where Melolin appeared to have absorbed concentrations of these two pro-inflammatory cytokines but returned to high values after surgery as their levels were higher at Visit 3 in the exudate and in the two dressings (Figure 3A,B, Case 3).

Noticeably, this patient showed non-detectable levels of PDGF-BB in the exudates of Visits 1 and 2, while the levels of this growth factor were similar to those of the other previous patients at Visit 3 (Figure 3C, Case 3).

Case 3 also showed very low levels of cell numbers in the exudate with a peak detected at Visit 2 (Table 3, Visit 1: 5468 cells/100 μL; Visit 2: 12,404 /100 μL; Visit 3: 5125/100 μL). Consistently, the characterisation of the cell subpopulations in the exudate of this patient at Visit 3 showed scarce traces of all the cell phenotypes with the exception of the $CD105^+$ progenitor cells that appeared as both single cells and aggregates (Figure 4, Case 3). High levels of adhesion of this type of cells and of the $CD206^+$ M2 macrophages were observed in the Atrauman retrieved at Visit 3, but no cell adhesion was detected in Melolin (Figure 5, Case 3).

2.4. Case 4

A 62-year-old male with a BMI of 28.1, no history of diabetes or smoking and an IGTN of both fibular and tibial sulcus of the right hallux stage III (Table 1) was treated with Melolin and returned for surgery after five weeks. After surgery (Figure 1, Case 4), Atrauman and Melolin were applied as primary and secondary dressings, and the patient returned to clinics the day after for final medication and discharge, showing a reduction of the wound area of 15% (Table 2).

This patient had starting levels of proteins in the exudate at Visit 1 comparable to the previous cases, but they increased to values higher than Cases 1 to 3 at Visit 2 with a significant protein concentration being found in the Melolin (Figure 2, Case 4). After surgery, the levels of protein concentrations appeared to be relatively low in the exudate, but higher in both the primary and secondary dressing. The TNFα concentration remained at similar values in the exudates and dressings at all visits (Figure 3A, Patient 4). Conversely, IL-6 showed a high exudate concentration value at Visit 1 to then be significantly reduced at Visits 2 and 3 in both exudates and primary dressing, but increased in Melolin at Visit 3 as observed in Cases 1 and 2 (Figure 3B, Patient 4).

In this patient, the concentration of PDGF-BB in the Visit 1 exudate was relatively higher than the other previous cases at Visit 1, but dropped at constantly lower levels in the exudates of Visits 2 and 3 (Figure 3C, Case 4). Noticeably, Melolin absorbed relatively high levels of this growth factor, similar to the previous cases at Visit 2, but it also showed relatively high levels in Atrauman (Figure 3C, Case 4).

The number of cells in the exudate of this patient was also relatively high since Visit 1 (210,370), peaking at Visit 2 (374,375) and registering a significant decrease at Visit 3 (137,666) (Table 3). The characterisation of the subpopulations in the exudate of Visit 3 showed a relatively high density of MPO^+ neutrophils and $iNOS^+$ M1 macrophages, with a scarce density of $CD206^+$ M2 macrophages and a significant presence of CD105+ progenitor cells in the form of single cells and aggregates (Figure 4, Case 4). A similar pattern appeared in the dressings where neutrophils and M1 macrophages were mainly observed to establish contacts with Melolin and M2 and progenitor cells with Atrauman (Figure 5, Case 4).

2.5. Case 5

A 36-year-old female, with a BMI of 24.2 without a history of diabetes and smoking presented an IGTN of the proximal nail fold (retronychia) on the left hallux unstageable (Table 1), showing inflammation and low levels of drainage.

At Visit 1, Melolin was applied as wound dressing and the patient returned to the clinic for Visit 2 after 4 weeks to undergo a total nail avulsion of the nail with phenolisation of the nail matrix (Figure 1, Case 5). Atrauman and Melolin were applied as primary and secondary dressings, and the patient returned to clinics the day after for final medication and discharge showing an increase in the wound area of 38.9% (Table 2).

Noticeably, the exudates showed non-detectable levels of proteins and relatively low levels absorbed into Melolin at Visit 2 and into both Atrauman and Melolin at Visit 3 post-surgery (Figure 2, Case 5). The levels of TNFα in the exudate were also non-detectable at Visit 1, but they increased pre-surgery at Visits 2 and 3 and were absorbed at similar levels (ca. 100 pg/mL) in Melolin at Visit 2. At Visit 3 both Atrauman and Melolin absorbed similarly higher amounts (Figure 3A, Case 5). Wound exudates and dressings at all stages showed constant levels of IL-6 and PDGF-BB (ranges: 70 to 150 pg/mL, Figure 3B,C, Case 5), with Atrauman retaining levels of PDGF-BB significantly higher than Melolin at Visit 3, post-surgery (Figure 3C, Case 5).

This patient showed the highest exudate cell number at Visit 1, which underwent a decline at Visit 2 to return to levels similar to Visit 1 after surgery at Visit 3 (Table 3, Case 6). These exudates showed relatively low densities of all the cell phenotypes investigated (Figure 4, Case 5), but the analysis of the same subpopulations adhering to the primary and secondary dressings at Visit 3 showed a tendency of MPO+ neutrophils, CD206+ M2 macrophages and CD105+ progenitor cells to be adhering more on Melolin than Atrauman (Figure 5, Case 5).

2.6. Case 6

A 17-year-old female with a BMI of 18.8 without a history of diabetes or smoking presented an IGTN of the fibular sulcus of the left hallux stage IIB (Table 1).

On visit 1, Melolin was applied as wound dressing and the patient returned to the clinic for Visit 2 after 20 days to undergo a bilateral partial nail avulsion of the nail with phenolisation of the nail matrix. After the surgery, Atrauman and Melolin were applied as primary and secondary. The participant returned to the clinic 24 h after the surgery for a follow-up appointment showing a wound reduction of 5.4% (Table 2, Case 6). The wound bed was entirely granulating and serosanguineous exudate was observed. Erythema and swollen tissues were localised distally to the interphalangeal joint and no signs of infection were observed. The wound was redressed with Melolin and the participant discharged.

As per Case 5, the total protein concentration levels were also undetectable in all the exudates and dressing collected with the exception of the Melolin retrieved at Visit 3 (Figure 2, Case 6). This patient showed relatively high levels of TNFα, IL-6 and PDGF-BB concentrations in all samples with the exception of the Atrauman at Visit 3, where no detectable values were obtained (Figure 3A–C, Case 6).

The exudate cell numbers were reduced from Visit 1 to Visit 2, but sharply increased post-surgery at Visit 3 (Table 3, Case 6). In this exudate, the various subpopulations under investigation had a relatively low density (Figure 4, Case 6), but relatively higher levels of adhering MPO^+ neutrophils and $CD105^+$ progenitor cells were observed in Melolin (MPO^+ and $CD105^+$ cells) and Atrauman ($CD105^+$ cells) (Figure 5, Case 6).

2.7. Protein Adsorption

The gel electrophoresis of the eluted proteins clearly showed different patterns of adsorption for the two types of dressings. Atrauman led to the adsorption of only one main protein band that was putatively identified as a 68 kDa albumin (Figure 6, Lanes 2 to 5, black arrow) [32]. The peak of elution of this protein occurred upon incubation in 30% *v*/*v* and 50% *v*/*v* isopropanol/water media. In the case of Melolin, more protein species were eluted (Figure 6, Lanes 6 to 9, black arrow and bracket). Proteins in the molecular weight range of 250 kDa to 75 kDa are likely to include, among others, immunoglobulin, cold fibronectin and fibrinogen (Figure 6, Lanes 6 to 9, bracket) [32]. These were mainly released upon incubation with 10% *v*/*v* and 30% *v*/*v* isopropanol/water media, indicating that proteins were either loosely bound to the Melolin fibres or likely to be still in a soluble state entrapped within its mesh.

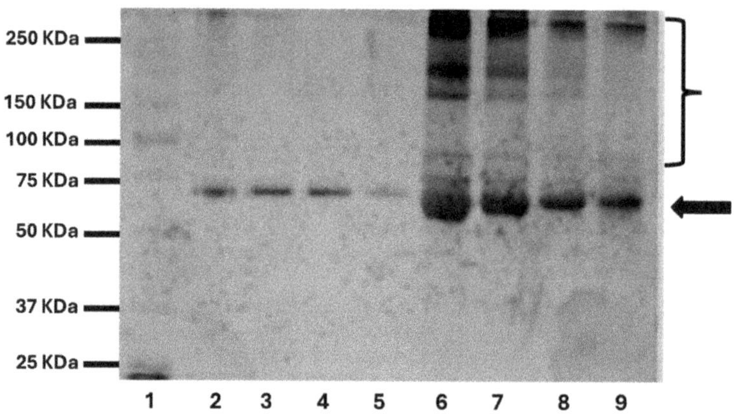

Figure 6. Protein elution profiles from different types of wound dressing. Lane 1: Molecular weight standards, Lanes 2 to 5: proteins eluted from Atrauman, Lanes 6 to 9: proteins eluted from Melolin. Lanes 2 and 6: proteins eluted by a 10% *v*/*v* isopropanol/water washing, Lanes 3 and 7: proteins eluted by a 30% *v*/*v* isopropanol/water washing, Lanes 4 and 8: proteins eluted by a 50% *v*/*v* isopropanol/water washing, Lanes 5 and 9: proteins eluted by a 70% *v*/*v* isopropanol/water washing. Arrow indicates a 68 kDa protein putatively identified as human serum albumin [32]. Bracket indicates a range of high-molecular-weight proteins putatively including cold fibronectin and immunoglobulins. Experiments were performed on the dressing of each patient providing reproducible results.

3. Discussion

While many studies have highlighted the role of specific cytokines, growth factors and cell phenotypes in acute and chronic wounds, no clear biochemical and cellular pathway of healing or non-healing has been unequivocally identified [25–28]. The main obstacles found by these investigations are likely to be related to the different types of wounds, patients' health conditions and comorbidities, treatment protocols and analytical methods adopted.

At the same time, the effect of the wound dressings' physicochemical properties and biocompatibility has been neglected despite many studies have demonstrated that the interactions occurring between proteins and cells with the surface of medical implants are inevitably altered, leading to the formation of a film of adsorbed proteins and to phenotypical changes in adhering inflammatory and tissue cells [16,32].

The present work was designed to study the interactions that the wound dressing biomaterials have with proteins and with cells present in the exudate. The aim was to find out whether these interactions could affect the healing process and be harnessed to establish and monitor potential biomarkers of healing or non-healing. It was hypothesised that the identification of any specific biochemical or cellular pattern either in the wound exudate or at the surface of the retrieved dressings would not only shed light on the therapeutic role or adverse effect of specific wound dressings on tissue repair, but it would also turn the retrieved dressing into a prognostic device.

To this end, the study was designed to analyse the effect that two types of dressings with different physicochemical compositions could have on acute wounds as those generated by a relatively limited surgery, ingrown toenail avulsions, on six patients with no relevant comorbidities.

To highlight the advantage of focussing on the wound dressing/protein/cell interactions rather than the wound bed, biochemical and phenotypical markers found in contact with the dressings were compared with those of the wound exudate. In addition, the clinical cases were selected on the basis of the combined use of the primary dressing, Atrauman and the secondary dressing Melolin when in contact with the wound exudate for a relatively short period of time, 24 h. Such a short implantation time enables the analysis of the early interactions between biochemical and cellular species with the dressing, thus emphasising any effect caused by the biomaterial surface physicochemical properties.

As expected, a glance at the clinical assessment did not show any clear link between the patients' reported general clinical history and the 24 h healing response to the surgery. However, it was clear that according to the Martinez-Nova classification [33], Case 3 presented a less invasive nail fold/nail plate ratio (IIA) compared to Cases 1, 2 and 6 whose conditions were classified as IIB, to Case 4 who was classified as III and to Case 5 who was unstageable. Indeed, in Case 3, the surgical procedure caused a wound of a size (Visit 2, 29.6 mm^2) comparable to that of Case 1 and significantly smaller than all the other cases, but the wound size in this patient was significantly reduced after only 24 h of treatment with Atrauman and Melolin. All the cases showing a reduction of the wound size were reported to have a reduction of the cell numbers in the exudate at Visit 3. The cases where wound healing did not appear to progress (Cases 1 and 6) or to regress (Case 5) showed increased cell numbers in the exudate. This clinical observation corresponded also to the ability of this patient's wound to show low levels of cell numbers before and after surgery in the exudate with a population of $CD105^+$ cells adhering in clusters, particularly at the surface of the Atrauman knitted fibres (Figure 5, Case 3, Atrauman, CD105) 24 h after surgery. In this case, there was no detectable $CD105^+$-cell in the superimposed Melolin secondary dressing, indicating that these progenitor cells had not been subtracted from the wound bed [34,35]. This seemed to distinguish Case 3 from all the other cases. In particular, the cases with less wound reduction, while showing adhesion of $CD105^+$ cells on Atrauman fibres, they revealed cell penetration across Atrauman into Melolin where they adhered on its fibres (Figure 5, Cases 1, 2 and 4, CD105). More noticeably, the worsening wound size conditions of Case 5 corresponded to a high level of penetration of $CD105^+$-cells within the secondary Melolin dressing with no traces in the primary Atrauman dressing and in the exudate (Figures 4 and 5, Case 5, CD105). These results seem to indicate that any absorption of exudate from the wound by the more hydrophilic Melolin secondary dressing has subtracted from the exudate cells playing an important role in the healing process, while the more hydrophobic Atrauman, as primary dressing in direct contact with the wound, has made the same cells available to the healing process at the interface with the wound bed. Likewise, Case 6 showed less penetration in the Melolin dressing and some levels of $CD105^+$ cells on the Atrauman fibres (Figure 5, Case 6, CD105), but to a lesser extent than all the other cases except Case 5.

CD105 is a marker of endoglin, a transmembrane protein relevant to angiogenesis and wound healing, mostly expressed by endothelial cell progenitors [34], mesenchymal stem cells and fibroblasts. Its presence in wounds has been observed as early as two days after injury [35]. The present work demonstrates that, while only weak positive staining was observed in exudates 24 h after surgery, cells expressing this marker can be detected more reliably by analysing the retrieved wound dressings.

Case 3 clearly also showed a distinct profile of inflammatory cell interaction with the dressings when neutrophils (MPO^+ cells) [36], M1 macrophages ($iNOS^+$ cells) [37,38] and M2 macrophages ($CD206^+$ cells) [39] were investigated (Figure 6, Case 3). In this case, no neutrophils or M1 macrophages were observed, but the regenerative M2 phenotype population appeared to be enriched at the wound bed/Atrauman interface.

Among all the other cases showing a relatively smaller wound reduction in 24 h, neutrophils (and to a lesser extent M1 macrophages) were observed and appeared in both the primary and secondary dressings, while in the case of the deteriorating Case 5 and not progressing Case 6, neutrophils were mainly absorbed by Melolin (Figure 5, MPO). These data, together with the absence of any significant $CD206^+$ cell in the Atrauman dressing of Cases 5 and 6, seem to indicate a wound environment in a pro-inflammatory status rather than the activation of a regenerative pathway.

Alongside its different engineer of the fibres in a tulle rather than hydrogel structure, Atrauman appears to minimise protein adsorption limiting it to the adsorption of albumin (Figure 6, Lanes 2 to 5), a relatively hydrophobic protein known to 'passivate' biomaterials surface in terms of cell adhesion [16,32]. This can be explained by the presence of the impregnation of this type of dressing with relatively hydrophobic triglycerides [6]. Although this type of coating has been introduced by the manufacturer to reduce adherence of the dressings to the wound [6], the results of this study demonstrate that the coating also contributes to the albumin-driven passivation of the biomaterial surface thus explaining the relatively limited adhesion of cells on its fibres. On the contrary, Melolin was shown to absorb and adsorb more protein species among which the presumptive identification made in this study indicates the possible presence of 'cold fibronectin', IgG and fibrinogen (Figure 6, Lanes 6 to 9); proteins known to promote the adhesion and activation of platelets, inflammatory and tissue cells [32].

The insights provided by the present investigation are likely to be relevant also to the use of other types of wound dressings. Indeed, previous papers have compared the swelling properties of Melolin to other absorbent dressings including the carboxymethylcellulose-based devices Aquacel and Kerracel and the alginate-based Kaltostat [40,41]. In particular, Uzun et al. have reported a swelling of approximately 20% wt/wt in Kaltostat and 19% wt/wt in Aquacel [40], while 25% wt/wt in Kaltostat and 15% wt/wt in Aquacel were observed by Minsart et al. [41]. The percentage of Melolin swelling has been reported to be 18% wt/wt thus making its exudate absorbing potential similar to Kaltostat and Aquacel [40]. Therefore, although not used in the present study, it can be speculated that the effect of both Kaltostat and Aquacell when adopted as secondary dressings would lead to results similar to that observed with Melolin raising questions about the use of highly absorbent dressings in cases where a healing pathway is, as in the case of acute wounds, in progress. To fulfil the need to remove excessive exudate volumes while preserving a favourable cell population in the wound bed, absorbent dressings such as the carboxymethyl cellulose-based Kerracel should rather be used. In fact, while absorbing a relatively high volume of exudates, Kerracel is known to undergo a high swelling of its fibres capable of obstructing the penetration of the cells throughout its mesh [42].

When compared to the exudates where no clear links could be found between the total cell number (Table 3), cell subpopulations (Figures 4 and 5) and wound healing, the profiles of these cell biomarkers in the wound dressings show the potential advantage that wound dressings can offer as tools to monitor healing processes. This was not necessarily the case for the studied biochemical markers where the only trend seems to be that the concentrations of the total protein content and of TNFα, IL-6 and PDGF-BB were higher in Melolin than Atrauman, post-surgery.

4. Materials and Methods

Clinical treatments. The study of 6 clinical cases of onychocryptosis, commonly referred to as an ingrown toenail (IGTN), treated with surgical excision and redressed with a combination of Melolin (Smith and Nephew, Watford, UK) and Atrauman (Hartmann Buckingham, UK) wound dressings was performed at the Leaf Hospital (University of Brighton, Eastbourne, UK). The experimental protocol was ethically approved by the University of Brighton Ethics Committee (Brighton Research Ethics Application Manager, Ref: 2023-11385-Forss) and the Health Research Authority Ethics Committee (Integrated Research Application System, Project ID: 318917). The ethics panels' approval included the recruitment of patients from the age of 16 years. Patient Number 6 (17 years old) was recruited following the signing of the consent form by both the patient and parents. In addition, all researchers involved in the collection, storage, use and disposal of human samples received formal training to comply with the UK Human Tissue Act regulations. Eligibility criteria include subjects with an active IGTN with moderate levels of exudate and without clinical signs of infection. Participants for this study were recruited between April and July 2023. During the nail surgery assessment appointment (Visit 1) eligible subjects were approached by a dedicated research podiatrist. The participant information sheet was provided to eligible subjects. Following the appropriate time for consideration of the participant information sheet and discussion with the research podiatrist, consent to participate was gained through the completion of the consent form. Subjects who were unable to provide informed consent were excluded from the evaluation. Surgical treatments were individually agreed with participants and followed the best practice principles. Procedures taken at each visit are summarised in Table 4.

Table 4. Study protocol followed at each visit.

Visit 1 Nail Surgery Assessment Appointment	Visit 2 Surgery Day	Visit 3 24 h Post-Surgery Follow Up
- Recruitment and consent. - Collection of demographic and clinical data. - Collection of Exudate.	- Collection of last Melolin applied 24 h before surgery. - Collection of Exudate (after nail removal, before phenol application).	- Collection of Atrauman and Melolin applied after surgery. - Collection of exudates.
- Application of Melolin. - Subject advised to redress daily with Melolin.	- Application of Atrauman and Melolin. - Subject advised to keep the dressings in place until Visit 3.	- Application of Mepore. - Subject discharged.

On Visit 1, participants' demographic and baseline clinical data were collected alongside exudate sampling (Table 4). Participants were tested for peripheral arterial disease (PAD) and peripheral neuropathy (PN). PAD was assessed by analysing the posterior tibial (PT) and the dorsalis pedis (DP) artery of the left foot (LF) and the right foot (RF) with an 8MHz Doppler ultrasound. PN was assessed by analysing 10 areas of LF and RF with a 10-g Semmes-Weinstein monofilament. In addition, IGTNs were staged according to the onychocryptosis classification outlined by Martinez-Nova et al. [34] (Table 5).

Table 5. Onychocryptosis classification adopted to stage participants' IGTN at Visit 1.

Stage	Description
I	Erythema, slight oedema, and pain. Nail fold does not exceed the limits of the nail plate.
II	A. Increased pain, oedema, erythema, hyperesthesia, serum drainage, and/or infection. Nail fold exceeds the nail plate < 3 mm. B. Increased pain, oedema, erythema, hyperesthesia, serum drainage, and/or infection. Nail fold exceeds the nail plate > 3 mm.
III	Granulation tissue and chronic hypertrophy of the nail fold. Granulomatous or hypertrophic tissue widely covers the lateral nail plate.
IV	Serious chronic deformity of the toenail, both nail folds and distal fold. Hypertrophic tissue completely covers lateral, medial and distal nail plates.

On Visit 1, the IGTN exudate was collected using a swab (FLOQSwabs 520CS01, COPAN Diagnostics, Murrieta, CA, USA) and diluted in 0.5 mL of sterile phosphate buffer saline (PBS) pH 7.4. Melolin dressing was applied to the wound according to the wound management guidelines. Participants were advised to change the dressing regularly and to apply Melolin dressing 24 h before the surgery appointment (Visit 2).

On Visit 2, the Melolin wound dressing was removed, and two sections (1.5 cm × 1.5 cm) were cut where the exudate was absorbed. Each section was collected either in 5 mL of sterile PBS for cell studies or in sterile deionised water for protein adsorption studies.

At this stage, surgery was performed by experienced podiatrists following the latest Royal College of Podiatry nail surgery guidelines. Participants underwent either partial or total nail avulsion under local anaesthetic with phenolisation of the nail matrix of the hallux. The procedure involved the following stages: after peri-surgical skin disinfection, a digital nerve block of the hallux was performed by injecting 3% *w*/*v* plain mepivacaine hydrochloride (Scandonest, Septodon, Maidstone, UK). A tourniquet was then applied to the base of the hallux and kept in place for the entire procedure (for a maximum of 20 min). After the partial or total removal of the toenail, 80% *v*/*v* liquified phenol (Phenol Swab-it, PodoPro, Huddersfield, UK) was applied twice for one minute to ablate the nail matrix and the tourniquet removed. Depending on the clinical needs, the surgery resulted in wounds of different sizes, as shown in Table 2, Column Visit 2.

The exudate sample was collected as described for Visit 1, after the removal of the nail, but prior to the phenol application.

Following surgery, Atrauman was applied to the wound as the primary dressing, while Melolin was added as the secondary dressing. Participants were booked for a 24 h post-surgical follow up (Visit 3), as per clinical guidelines.

On Visit 3, both the primary and secondary dressings were removed, cut into two sections (1.5 cm × 1.5 cm), and collected in sterile PBS and deionised water as described for Visit 2. Subsequently, the exudate sample was collected as for Visits 1 and 2. Participants were finally medicated by applying a Mepore (Molnlycke Health Care, Oldham, UK) on the wound bed and discharged.

The maximum length and width of the wounds were measured by a research podiatrist by using a sterile paper ruler and photos were taken at every visit. The wound area was then calculated using ImageJ software, as elucidated in Figure 7A,B.

Biochemical and cellular studies. For biochemical and cellular experiments, the collected samples were transferred to the laboratories of the School of Applied Sciences and Centre for Regenerative Medicine and Devices, University of Brighton, within 2 h from collection.

Protein concentrations in both exudates and eluates of the dressings were measured by using Bradford's assay (BioRad, Watford, UK), while TNFα, IL-6 and PDGF-BB concentrations were measured by using ELISA (Abcam, Cambridge, UK). The choice of these three factors was made on the basis of their widely accepted role in the healing process, whereby TNFα is involved in the early acute phase of inflammation, IL-6 contributes to the acute inflammatory process while playing a role in its transition to healing steps, and

PDGF-BB is released by both activated platelets and macrophages considered the most potent inducer of fibroblast proliferation.

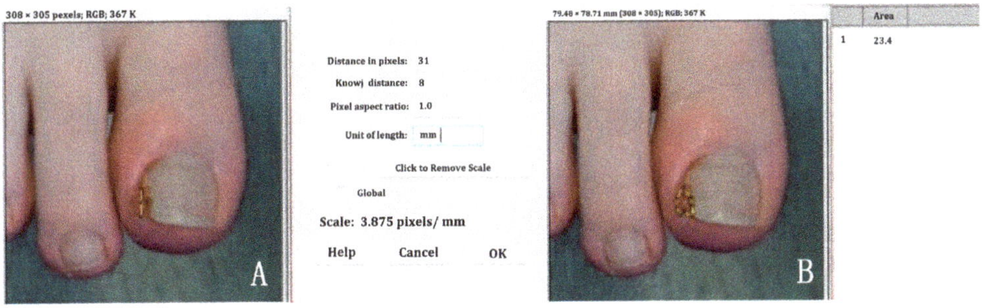

Figure 7. Wound images analysed by ImageJ software. (**A**) Software calibration was obtained using the function 'straight line' and inserting the known distance (i.e., wound length) manually measured during the visit. (**B**) Subsequently, the wound area was calculated after drawing the wound edges with the function 'polygon sections'.

Cells were separated from the exudates by centrifugation at 1000× g and counted by haemocytometer after resuspension in 100 µL of PBS and finally processed as smears for immunostaining by applying 10 µL on microscope glass slides. Three markers of inflammatory cells were studied: (i) myeloperoxidase (MPO) for neutrophils [35], (ii) CD68 for the monocytes/macrophages overall population [36], (iii) induced nitric oxide synthase (iNOS) for pro-inflammatory macrophage (M1) phenotype [37], (iv) CD206 for post-inflammatory macrophage M2 phenotype [38], and (v) CD105 for haemoprogenitor cells [34] by confocal microscopy. Immediately after smearing on the glass slides, cells were fixed in formalin for 10 min, washed three times with PBS and then treated for 1h with 3% w/v bovine serum albumin solution as blocking agent to eliminate any subsequent non-specific binding of the antibodies. After further washes in PBS, the samples were incubated in antibody (rabbit anti-human MPO, CD68, iNOS, CD206 and CD105 Abcam, Cambridge, UK) solution diluted 1:100 in the same blocking solution for 1 h, room temperature. Following the same washing procedures, a secondary FITC-conjugated goat anti-rabbit IgG antibody solution diluted 1:100 in the same blocking solution was added for 1 h at room temperature and in dark conditions. Confocal microscopy was performed on all smears and dressing samples at ×20 magnification.

The biochemical and cellular data were related to the adsorption of proteins on the dressing fibres where the binding strength was analysed by a previously published method [30]. Briefly, after 2 h of transportation, the incubation in sterile deionised water was established to be sufficient to remove the excess proteins entrapped in the dressing mesh, but not tightly bound to their fibres. At arrival, the excess water was removed from the dressings by contact with tissue paper. Dressings from each patient were then sequentially immersed in increasing concentrations of isopropanol/water solutions (IsoPOH/Water, 10%, 30%, 50%, 70% v/v) to detach proteins from the fibre surface according to their binding strength. The eluted proteins were freeze-dried overnight and then resuspended in 10 µL of electrophoresis sample buffer (BioRad, Watford, UK). Electrophoresis was performed according to a standard sodium dodecyl sulphate poly(acrylamide) gel electrophoresis (SDS-PAGE) method using a Mini Protean electrophoresis kit (BioRad). The electrophoresis was performed at 100 mV for 2 h. To enhance the detection of protein species bound to the fibres in low amounts, a sensitive silver staining (BioRad, Watford, UK) of the gels was adopted. Protein electrophoretic profiles were documented by image analyser by visible light (BioRad, Watford, UK).

Statistical analysis. Biochemical and cell data were analysed by ANOVA two-way test from n = 3 using GraphPad Prism version 8 software. Data were considered significantly different at $p \leq 0.05$.

5. Conclusions

The current study provides evidence of the different interactions that biochemical and cellular components establish with Atrauman (a dressing manufactured in the form of woven knitted fibres made of a synthetic polymer) and Melolin (a hydrocolloid engineered as different layers of polyester and cellulose non-woven fibres). When the two dressings are combined as primary and secondary dressings, it appears that any condition (e.g., excessive exudate absorption by the hydrogel-based absorbent layer) leading to the removal of endoglin-expressing cells ($CD105^+$) and/or M2 macrophages by absorption into the secondary dressing can impair healing. This appears to be the case when the hydrogel-based Melolin absorbs relatively high levels of these two types of cells in its mesh. At the same time, the predominance of adhesion of M2 macrophages and $CD105^+$ cells with the knitted fibres of the primary dressing Atrauman was linked to a healing pathway. These findings also suggest that the rapid detection or absence of these two types of cells on the Atrauman fibres can be harnessed as a prognostic tool in healing/non-healing. However, to be adopted in clinics as prognostic tools, the tests of the interactions between cells and dressing will require further efforts to develop methods of detection of these cell phenotypes that are rapid, cost-effective and easy to interpret.

Author Contributions: Conceptualization, M.S.; methodology, S.S., G.M., J.R.F., L.R. and N.T.; investigation, S.S., G.M. and J.R.F.; data curation, M.S., S.S., G.M. and J.R.F.; writing—M.S.; writing—review and editing, M.S., G.M., J.R.F., N.T. and L.R.; supervision, M.S., J.R.F. and L.R.; project administration, M.S.; funding acquisition, M.S. All authors have read and agreed to the published version of the manuscript.

Funding: This research was funded by the UKRI Engineering and Physical Sciences Research Council, grant number EP/W023164/1 and The APC was funded by the UKRI.

Institutional Review Board Statement: The study was conducted in accordance with the Declaration of Helsinki, and approved by the Institutional Review Board (or Ethics Committee) of the University of Brighton (Brighton Research Ethics Application Manager, Ref: 2023-11385-Forss, 25 January 2023).

Informed Consent Statement: Informed consent was obtained from all subjects involved in the study.

Data Availability Statement: Raw data are available in the University of Brighton Open Repository.

Conflicts of Interest: The authors declare no conflicts of interest.

References

1. Olsson, M.; Järbrink, K.; Divakar, U.; Bajpai, R.; Upton, Z.; Schmidtchen, A.; Car, J. The humanistic and economic burden of chronic wounds: A systematic review. *Wound Repair Regen.* **2019**, *27*, 114–125. [CrossRef] [PubMed]
2. Raziyeva, K.; Kim, Y.; Zharkinbekov, Z.; Kassymbek, K.; Jimi, S.; Saparov, A. Immunology of Acute and Chronic Wound Healing. *Biomolecules* **2021**, *11*, 700. [CrossRef] [PubMed]
3. Shi, C.; Wang, C.; Liu, H.; Li, Q.; Li, R.; Zhang, Y.; Liu, Y.; Shao, Y.; Wang, J. Selection of Appropriate Wound Dressing for Various Wounds. *Front. Bioeng. Biotechnol.* **2020**, *8*, 182. [CrossRef] [PubMed]
4. Weller, C.D.; Team, V.; Sussman, G. First-line interactive wound dressing update: A comprehensive review of the evidence. *Front. Pharmacol.* **2020**, *11*, 155. [CrossRef]
5. Punjataewakupt, A.; Aramwit, P. Wound dressing adherence: A review. *J. Wound Care* **2022**, *31*, 406–423. [CrossRef]
6. Barrett, S.; Rippon, M.G.; Rogers, A.A. Effectiveness of wound contact layers in enabling undisturbed wound management: A case series. *J. Wound Care* **2023**, *32*, 134–144. [CrossRef]
7. Pawar, M.; Tripathi, N.; Patwa, P.; Mistry, P.; Hosamani, A. A prospective, comparative study of outcomes with Melolin, collagen sheet and traditional vaseline gauze dressing for healing of skin graft donor site in burns cases. *Int. J. Surg. Sci.* **2021**, *5*, 239–241. [CrossRef]
8. Feng, F.; Zhao, Z.; Li, J.; Huang, Y.; Chen, W. Multifunctional dressings for wound exudate management. *Prog. Mater. Sci.* **2024**, *146*, 101328. [CrossRef]

9. Sood, A.; Granick, M.S.; Tomaselli, N.L. Wound Dressings and Comparative Effectiveness Data. *Adv. Wound Care* **2014**, *3*, 511–529. [CrossRef]
10. Harding, K. *World Union of Wound Healing Societies (WUWHS) Consensus Document*; Wound exudate: Effective assessment and management; Wounds International: London, UK, 2019.
11. Blazeby, J. Bluebelle pilot randomised controlled trial of three wound dressing strategies to reduce surgical site infection in primary surgical wounds. *BMJ Open* **2020**, *10*, e030615. [CrossRef]
12. Harle, S.; Korhonen, A.; Kettunen, J.A.; Seitsalo, S. A randomised clinical trial of two different wound dressing materials for hip replacement patients. *J. Orthop. Nurs.* **2005**, *9*, 205–210. [CrossRef]
13. O'Donnell, T.F.; Lau, J. A systematic review of randomized controlled trials of wound dressing for chronic venous ulcers. *J. Vasc. Surg.* **2006**, *44*, 1118–1125. [CrossRef] [PubMed]
14. Cullen, B.; Gefen, A. The biological and physiological impact of the performance of wound dressings. *Int. Wound J.* **2023**, *20*, 1292–1303. [CrossRef] [PubMed]
15. Diegelmann, R.F.; Evans, M.C. Wound healing: An overview of acute, fibrotic and delayed healing. *Front. Biosci.* **2004**, *9*, 283–289. [CrossRef]
16. Kondyurina, I.; Kondyurin, A. Foreign Body Reaction (Immune Response) for Artificial Implants Can Be Avoided: An Example of Polyurethane in Mice for 1 Week. *J. Funct. Biomater.* **2023**, *14*, 432. [CrossRef]
17. Raffetto, J.D.; Ligi, D.; Maniscalco, R.; Khalil, R.A.; Mannello, F. Why Venous Leg Ulcers Have Difficulty Healing: Overview on Pathophysiology, Clinical Consequences, and Treatment. *J. Clin. Med.* **2021**, *10*, 29. [CrossRef]
18. Goto, T.; Saligan, L.N. Wound Pain and Wound Healing Biomarkers From Wound Exudate: A Scoping Review. *J. Wound Ostomy Cont. Nurs.* **2020**, *47*, 559–568. [CrossRef]
19. Patel, S.; Maheshwari, A.; Chandra, A. Biomarkers for wound healing and their evaluation. *J. Wound Care* **2016**, *25*, 46–55. [CrossRef]
20. Agyare, C.; Osafo, N.; Boakye, Y.D. Biomarkers of wound healing. In *Wound Healing-Current Perspectives*; Intech Open: London, UK, 2018; pp. 24–30. [CrossRef]
21. Heil, F.; Babitzki, G.; Laferriere, A.J.; Ooi, C.H.; Hidalgo, M.; Massard, C.; Martinez-Garcia, M.; Le Tourneau, C.; Kockx, M.; Gerber, P.; et al. Vanucizumab mode of action: Serial biomarkers in plasma, tumor, and skin-wound-healing biopsies. *Transl. Oncol.* **2021**, *14*, 100984. [CrossRef]
22. Birincioğlu, İ.; Akbaba, M.; Alver, A.; Kul, S.; Özer, E.; Turan, N.; Şentürk, A.; İnce, İ. Determination of skin wound age by using cytokines as potential markers. *J. Forensic Leg. Med.* **2016**, *44*, 14–19. [CrossRef]
23. Nirenjen, S.; Narayanan, J.; Tamilanban, T.; Subramaniyan, V.; Chitra, V.; Fuloria, N.K.; Wong, L.S.; Ramachawolran, G.; Sekar, M.; Gupta, G.; et al. Exploring the contribution of proinflammatory cytokines to impaired wound healing in diabetes. *Front. Immunol.* **2023**, *14*, 1216321. [CrossRef] [PubMed]
24. Burian, E.A.; Sabah, L.; Karlsmark, T.; Kirketerp-Møller, K.; Moffatt, C.J.; Thyssen, J.P.; Ågren, M.S. Cytokines and Venous Leg Ulcer Healing—A Systematic Review. *Int. J. Mol. Sci.* **2022**, *23*, 6526. [CrossRef]
25. Ashcroft, G.S.; Jeong, M.J.; Ashworth, J.J.; Hardman, M.; Jin, W.; Moutsopoulos, N.; Wild, T.; McCartney-Francis, N.; Sim, D.; McGrady, G.; et al. Tumor necrosis factor-alpha (TNF-α) is a therapeutic target for impaired cutaneous wound healing. *Wound Repair Regen.* **2012**, *20*, 38–49. [CrossRef] [PubMed]
26. Johnson, B.Z.; Stevenson, A.W.; Prêle, C.M.; Fear, M.W.; Wood, F.M. The Role of IL-6 in Skin Fibrosis and Cutaneous Wound Healing. *Biomedicines* **2020**, *8*, 101. [CrossRef] [PubMed]
27. White, M.J.V.; Briquez, P.S.; White, D.A.V.; Hubbell, J.A. VEGF-A, PDGF-BB and HB-EGF engineered for promiscuous super affinity to the extracellular matrix improve wound healing in a model of type 1 diabetes. *NPJ Regen. Med.* **2021**, *6*, 76. [CrossRef] [PubMed]
28. Zgheib, C.; Xu, J.; Liechty, K.W. Targeting inflammatory cytokines and extracellular matrix composition to promote wound regeneration. *Adv. Wound Care* **2014**, *3*, 344–355. [CrossRef]
29. Li, D.; Niu, G.; Landén, N.X. Beyond the Code: Noncoding RNAs in Skin Wound Healing. *Cold Spring Harb. Perspect. Biol.* **2022**, *14*, a041230. [CrossRef]
30. Varela, P.; Sartori, S.; Viebahn, R.; Salber, J.; Ciardelli, G. Macrophage immunomodulation: An indispensable tool to evaluate the performance of wound dressing biomaterials. *J. Appl. Biomater. Funct. Mater.* **2019**, *17*, 2280800019830355. [CrossRef]
31. Krzyszczyk, P.; Schloss, R.; Palmer, A.; Berthiaume, F. The role of macrophages in acute and chronic wound healing and interventions to promote pro-wound healing phenotypes. *Front. Physiol.* **2018**, *9*, 419. [CrossRef]
32. Motta, A.; Migliaresi, C.; Lloyd, A.W.; Denyer, S.P.; Santin, M. Serum protein absorption on silk fibroin fibers and films: Surface opsonization and binding strength. *J. Bioact. Compat. Polym.* **2002**, *17*, 23–35. [CrossRef]
33. Martínez-Nova, A.; Sánchez-Rodríguez, R.; Alonso-Peña, D. A new onychocryptosis classification and treatment plan. *J. Am. Podiatr. Med. Assoc.* **2007**, *97*, 389–393. [CrossRef] [PubMed]
34. Schoonderwoerd, M.J.A.; Goumans, M.J.T.H.; Hawinkels, L.J.A.C. Endoglin: Beyond the Endothelium. *Biomolecules* **2020**, *10*, 289. [CrossRef] [PubMed]
35. González Muñoz, T.; Amaral, A.T.; Puerto-Camacho, P.; Peinado, H.; de Álava, E. Endoglin in the Spotlight to Treat Cancer. *Int. J. Mol. Sci.* **2021**, *22*, 3186. [CrossRef] [PubMed]

36. Kolarova, H.; Klinke, A.; Kremserova, S.; Adam, M.; Pekarova, M.; Baldus, S.; Eiserich, J.P.; Kubala, L. Myeloperoxidase induces the priming of platelets. *Free. Radic. Biol. Med.* **2013**, *61*, 357–369. [CrossRef]
37. Chistiakov, D.; Killingsworth, M.; Myasoedova, V.; Orekhov, A.N.; Bobryshev, Y.V. CD68/macrosialin: Not just a histochemical marker. *Lab. Investig.* **2017**, *97*, 4–13. [CrossRef]
38. Wilmes, V.; Kur, I.M.; Weigert, A.; Verhoff, M.A.; Gradhand, E.; Kauferstein, S. iNOS expressing macrophages co-localize with nitrotyrosine staining after myocardial infarction in humans. *Front. Cardiovasc. Med.* **2023**, *10*, 1104019. [CrossRef]
39. Wollenberg, A.; Mommaas, M.; Oppel, T.; Schottdorf, E.M.; Günther, S.; Moderer, M. Expression and function of the mannose receptor CD206 on epidermal dendritic cells in inflammatory skin diseases. *J. Investig. Dermatol.* **2002**, *118*, 327–334. [CrossRef]
40. Uzun, M.; Anand, S.C.; Shah, T. In vitro characterisation and evaluation of different types of wound dressing materials. *J. Biomed. Eng. Technol.* **2013**, *1*, 1–7.
41. Minsart, M.; VanVlierberghe, S.; Dubruel, P.; Mignon, A. Commercial wound dressings for the treatment of exuding wounds: An in-depth physico-chemical comparative study. *Burn. Trauma* **2022**, *10*, tkac024. [CrossRef]
42. Bishop, A. Factors influencing dressing choice in wound care: A discussion. *Br. J. Nurs.* **2023**, *32*, S12–S20.

MDPI AG
Grosspeteranlage 5
4052 Basel
Switzerland
Tel.: +41 61 683 77 34

Pharmaceuticals Editorial Office
E-mail: pharmaceuticals@mdpi.com
www.mdpi.com/journal/pharmaceuticals

www.ingramcontent.com/pod-product-compliance
Lightning Source LLC
Chambersburg PA
CBHW040840250926
51850CB00007BA/1365
9783725866601